LEARNING FROM THE PATIENT

Learning
from the Patient

❖ ❖

PATRICK J. CASEMENT

Foreword by Robert S. Wallerstein, M.D.

THE GUILFORD PRESS
New York   London

Published by The Guilford Press
A Division of Guilford Publications, Inc.
72 Spring Street, New York, N. Y. 10012

Printed in the United States of America

This book is printed on acid-free paper

Last digit is print number: 9 8 7

Library of Congress Cataloging-in-Publication Data

Casement, Patrick.
  [On learning from the patient]
  Learning from the patient / Patrick J. Casement.
    p.   cm.
  Reprint (1st work). Originally published: On learning from
the patient. London; New York: Tavistock Publications, 1985
  Reprint (2nd work). Originally published: Further learning
from the patient. London; New York: Routledge, 1990.
  Includes bibliographic references.
  Includes index.
  ISBN 0-89862-559-9   —ISBN 0-89862-157-7 (pbk.)
  1. Psychotherapist and patient.   2. Psychoanalysis.
3. Psychotherapy.   I. Casement, Patrick.   Further learning
from the patient.   II. Title.
  [DNLM: 1. Physician–Patient Relations.
2. Psychotherapy.   WM 420 C3375o]
RC480.8.C38 1991
616.89'14—dc20
DNLM/DLC
for Library of Congress   90-14210
                                                        CIP

*To the many
who have helped me to learn*

❖ ❖

Acknowledgments

I am indebted to Arthur Hyatt Williams, whose enthusiasm first prompted me to start writing this book; to many colleagues and friends, who provided me with the stimulus to persevere and gave me valuable criticism throughout the writing of it; to David Tuckett for his advice on the revision of Part One; Jim Gomersall for his help in revising Part Two; also Harry (H. A. Williams) for his inspiration and encouragement to look beyond dogma; Fran Acheson, Dilys Daws, Martin James, Michael Parsons, and Eric Rayner for their help with particular chapters; and Josephine Klein for her painstaking work of editing each chapter, and the book as a whole, before it was presented for publication. Most particularly, I wish to thank "Joy" (Chapter 13) for being herself, her parents for their permission to publish my work with her, and all my patients and students for their contributions to my understanding of the analytic process, without which I could not have written this book, and my family for their forbearance throughout. And finally I wish to acknowledge my gratitude to Robert Wallerstein for his generosity in agreeing to write the Foreword to this volume.

The author and publishers wish also to thank the editors of various journals for their invitations to contribute those papers that formed the nucleus for Part Two, and to acknowledge permissions received to use material that has been published before, the details of which are given in relation to the chapters in question. We would also like to thank Faber and Faber Ltd. for permission to reproduce material from *Four Quartets* by T. S. Eliot in Chapters 10 and 12, and from *Collected Poems* by Edwin Muir in Chapter 20.

Contents

Preface

This volume combines my two books on the theme of its title, *On Learning from the Patient* (Tavistock 1985) (Part One) and *Further Learning from the Patient* (Routledge 1990) (Part Two).

In Part One I examine the first principles of psychoanalytic practice as I see it, in terms of learning from the patient in the course of the analytic session. Indispensable to this is the technique of *internal supervision* by means of which analysts can monitor the interaction between themselves and their patients, and their impact upon the analytic process. In Part Two I go further in exploring the nature of the analytic process, and I illustrate the kind of results that can emerge when we follow it. I also suggest ways in which we can help to preserve the analytic space from influences that can interfere with that process.

Following the patient's lead has always been an important principle of psychoanalysis and analytic psychotherapy. But, in practice, there has been a tendency for some analysts to become inappropriately controlling through being dogmatic, which interferes with the analytic process. Learning to learn from the patient provides a balance against this, helping to preserve the analytic space more clearly for the processes within it.

I have come to regard the nature of the repressed unconscious as sometimes surprisingly positive and creative; even pathology may be seen as an indication of *unconscious hope*. What has been repressed is not necessarily dangerous, except in so far as it is thought to be so. There may be some inherent destructiveness in the primary unconscious, but I believe that we should not overlook our patients' positive search for what they need, so often indicated by the unconscious prompts and cues they give to the analyst.

I have become increasingly aware of the ways in which patients unwittingly seek out the help and experience they need for recovery and health. The manner of this unconscious search defies common sense but it can involve analysts in a process which represents what the patient is just becoming capable of facing in the analysis. The past, as it was, is reexperienced in the present but with a difference: the analyst neither collapsing nor retaliating, as past objects often had. For the analyst to be guided by the patient's unconscious search, in this process, is not to be unjustifiably controlled by the patient: it is to be aided by the unconscious processes that interact within the analytic relationship.

August 1990   PATRICK CASEMENT
                                                      London

❖ ❖

Foreword

There is by now a very respectable body of literature about both psychoanalysis and the varieties of psychoanalytic psychotherapies as treatment modalities, that is, as techniques for ameliorating mental and emotional disorders—enough so that one needs to look at new offerings in this category from the viewpoint of how they relate to the existing corpus and what novel or altered perspectives they bring to the subject. It is also true, however, that by and large the books in this area are theory driven; that is, they elaborate a theory of technique from within the larger framework of an overall *general* psychoanalytic theory of the mind, of its development, and of its normal and abnormal functioning. The theory of technique is then the derivative conceptual structure that guides the effort to restore mental functioning in desired directions in accord with the requirements for mental balance determined by that theory.

Given this approach to the organization of most of our literature on psychoanalysis as therapy, it should be no surprise that this literature is almost entirely framed within the traditional kinds of one-body psychology to which, in erecting their understandings of the human mind, our various theoretical perspectives in psychoanalysis are naturally disposed to a considerable extent (though some will feel this to be an arguable assumption). This is true even when those theoretical perspectives are avowedly object-relational or interpersonal in their conceptions of the driving motivational forces in human personal and interpersonal functioning. It is just this fact that has always underpinned the uneasy dialectical tension between theory (theory in general, and its derivative theory of technique in particular) and actual technique, that is the actual clinical operations in the consulting rooms with their "natural" two-body interactional language. Patrick Casement is not the first to call attention to this dialectic with his observation that, to the practicing clinician absorbed in the transference and countertransference interactions in the consulting room, the existence—in the background—of an explanatory theoretical structure serves often primarily as a shield against bewilderment and anxiety, rather than as a true guide to and determinant of our actual clinical operations. The link between theory *qua* theory and technique *qua* technique is just too elastic and loose-jointed.

Perhaps out of fear of falling into the opposite difficulty in writing books on treatment, the risk of producing a reductive caricature of the complex psychoanalytic treatment process—a stereotyped "cookbook" akin to the listing of typical dream symbols in pop psychology dream interpretation books—most psychoanalytic authors have avoided writing about the nature of treatment and the treatment process from the clinical phenomenal base of therapeutic interactions, building up to clinical theory, and even to overarching general theory, within which these phenomena can be convincingly enough and comprehensively enough ordered. Freud, who through his long and prolific career wrote so little about actual issues of clinical technique and treatment, had in fact warned against the difficulties of this task in 1913: "Anyone who hopes to learn the noble game of chess from books will soon discover that only the openings and end-games of an exhaustive systematic presentation and that the infinite variety of moves which develop after opening defy any such description. This gap in instructions can only be filled by a diligent study of games fought out by masters. The rules which can be laid down for the practice of psycho-analytic treatment are subject to similar limitations."

It is this daunting challenge which Casement has so successfully taken up, without making any claim to being a "master," since it is central to his approach that psychoanalytic therapy is a process of "interactive communication" to which analyst and patient *both* bring their characters propensities, forged within the crucibles of their own personal histories, which *both* experience in ways that seem plausible and persuasive in the light of their own characteristic expectations and apprehensions (with those of the analyst hopefully more governed by the present and less by the past than in the case of the patient), and in which *both* (but again, hopefully, more the patient) pull for a "role responsiveness" that actualizes wished for and/or feared role relationship patterns. Given all of this, no one's perceptions can always be veridical, analysts do—being human—make mistakes of both understanding and of intervention, and no analyst need claim to be a "master," only an open and forthright enough searcher who is willing to, in accord with the book's title, "learn from the patient."

The concepts that Casement either borrows and utilizes—and he has acknowledged major indebtedness to Winicott, Bion, and Langs and has (I think) a far less acknowledged debt to Gill—or devises include trial identification, communication by impact (a graphic description of projective identifications), "holding" and "containment" (as the demonstration that the analyst can tolerate the patient's most extreme affective discomforts and pressures "without collapse or retaliation"), unconscious corrective cues and prompts from the patient (as pointers to the analyst's failures of empathic understanding), the patient's "unconscious hope," to be responded to as a form of striving for what is *needed* in terms of growth and phase-specific developmental needs and to be distinguished from what is sexually and aggressively *wanted*, and the application of (Winnicott's) "period of hesitation" in order to provide the patient the "analytic space" to search out his own destiny in the fullest possible freedom and autonomy. Uniting all of these is the central notion of "internal supervision," a learned but ultimately semi-automatic preconscious process by which the analyst constantly scans behaviors and verbalizations from the point of view of how these might be experienced by the patient, in light of the patient's history and character, and quite apart from how they were formulated and consciously intended by the analyst.

And corollary to all this are many clinical examples, both good and bad from the author's perspective, that illustrate Casement's various operative maxims; to listen unflaggingly for the unconscious cues from the patient pointing to the analyst's (usually unintended) contributions to the patient's transference perceptions; to keep from intrusive or preemptive or overly general interpretations, by way of what he calls "half-interpretations" that give the patient room for his unique and specific transference particularization; to refrain from deflecting the transference intensity by premature genetic recourse to the absent figures from the distant past, and so forth.

Casement carries this off elegantly, eloquently, and informatively enough so that this book can be wholeheartedly recommended as useful and thought-provoking (perhaps in different ways) to the broad range of practitioners from clinical novice to seasoned analyst. There is, however, another intent to my Foreword as well. This volume is actually two books by Casement, the first, *On Learning from the Patient*, published in Great Britain in

1985, together with the second, *Further Learning from the Patient*, being published there now, in 1990. It is a mark of the parochialism of our psychoanalytic enterprise worldwide that the first book, which made a very impressive splash in the psychoanalytic world in Britain (and to a considerable extent on the Continent as well), has been almost unremarked and unread in America, despite very favorable reviews. The occasion of the publication here of its successor is now a happy opportunity to bring both books together into one volume for American publication and, hopefully, for a significant and well-deserved American impact.

I will close with a caveat. I started with the observation that most of our literature about treatment and setting is about the theory of technique, beginning with one's overall theoretical perspective, and then within that framework deriving and trying to apply a theory of technique to the understanding of the treatment and change process. This book is a happy effort to correct that imbalance, to start with the phenomena of the consulting room, the clinical interplay of transferences and countertransferences, and to build from that to useful and unifying clinical theorizing, trusting thereby to arrive at what Casement calls "theory rediscovered," that is theory emerging ultimately from the consideration of the clinical interactions. But building back to a consistent theoretical clarity and comprehensiveness that make coherent explanatory sense out of the total clinical enterprise laid out before us is really beyond the scope of this volume and is perhaps, anyway, not the author's special forte. But no one volume can do all things in so complex an enterprise as the interplay of psychoanalytic theory and psychoanalytic technique. Those integrative efforts will have to be for readers on their own, which in the spirit of Casement's book, is the way I think he would want it to be.

August 1990　　　　　　　　　　ROBERT S. WALLERSTEIN, M.D.
　　　　　　　　　　　　　　　　San Francisco, California

❖ PART ONE ❖

First Principles

❖ ❖

Introduction

... the psycho-analyst needs to be able to
question himself as often as, and as long as,
he is unsatisfied, but should not spend too
much time looking for the answer in books. The
time we have is limited, so we must read people.

(BION 1975: 17)

A number of observations have prompted me to write this book.
For example, there is a common myth that the experienced analyst
or therapist understands the patient swiftly and unerringly. Although some patients try to oppose this, risking the retort that they
are "resisting," other patients do expect it. Perhaps it satisfies a
wish to find certainty. Some therapists also appear to expect it of
themselves; perhaps to gratify an unacknowledged wish to be
knowledgeable or powerful. It is not surprising, therefore, how
often student therapists imagine that immediate understanding is
required of them by patients and supervisors. This creates a pressure to know in order to appear competent. Interpretations offered
to patients may then be taken "off the peg," culled from the
writings or teaching of others—who in turn have accepted such
formulations as time-honored, even though overuse rapidly
degrades these insights into analytical clichés. I have therefore
tried to suggest ways in which psychoanalytic insight can be rescued
from this self-perpetuating cycle and discovered afresh with each
patient.

Our creative learning from patients can be inhibited by the
impression that everyone else seems to understand their patients
so much better than we do, or is apparently less prone to being
muddled, confused or caught up in making mistakes. It is my

conviction that we can learn as much from our mistakes as from the times when we more readily get it right. And when we follow the patient most closely, and the interaction between the analyst and the patient, we learn from the patient. And what we learn, or re-learn, are the first principles of psychoanalytic theory and technique. This is the focus of Part One.

There have been some genius analysts, such as Freud and Winnicott, who learned naturally how to learn from their patients. It would, however, be inhibiting and misleading if others were to emulate either that genius or the brilliance of well-known writers on psychoanalysis. I believe that the majority of analysts and therapists are more ordinary, sincere hard workers—not necessarily brilliant—who seek the truth with such care as they are able. I count myself amongst those who strive to become better therapists with time and more experience, and I address myself especially to my fellow travelers in this quest.

The world of unconscious communication between people is strange and often awesome. It can also be complicated and confusing. This has led to a regrettable divide between specialists in the unconscious who have developed an esoteric language, with which they speak to each other more precisely, and the majority of nonspecialists who feel excluded by this. I therefore wish to illustrate some of the dynamics of the unconscious mind, and of the helping relationship, in ways that I hope will be understandable to anyone in the related helping professions and to the interested lay reader.

There are some unquestioning believers in psychoanalytic circles; there are also skeptics in the real world outside. Amongst these, I think, are many who might have more respect for psychoanalytic ways of working if they could have a clearer sense of what it involves. These may be glad of an opportunity to follow some of what goes on in the mind of a therapist, as he struggles to get to know and to understand the complex mysteries of another person's mind and ways of being.

Opportunities for learning from the patient are there in all caring professions. It is mainly because the analytic consulting room offers a "research space," within which we can best study the dynamics of this intimate interaction of the therapeutic relationship, that I address myself more directly to analysts and therapists. I hope, nevertheless, that those in allied caring professions will be able to play with the ideas I explore here and relate them to their own spheres of work.

I have tried to share, as openly as feels tolerable, some of the difficulties which are commonly encountered in the extraordinary but challenging process of becoming a therapist and an analyst. It is my hope that others may learn from this too, and be encouraged.

I cite authors whenever I quote from them, but I know that I am not able to designate all influences upon me: the thinking of others has often been a part of my own for so long that I cannot always recall what I have learned from whom. Sometimes, however, there may be parallels of which I could have no knowledge because I have not yet read what many others have written. My apologies, therefore, to those authors who may feel that their works should have been cited. But I believe that parallel "discovery" has its own value; and I think that clinical work feels specially validated when a path that others have travelled before is happened upon independently. The difference is that the analyst (or therapist) has sometimes been led to this by unconscious processes in the patient—not by dogma. Of course, we might arrive at the same point more directly by following "maps" that others could have provided, but insight that is applied too readily from established understanding is seldom as effective as that which is arrived at from working with the patient.

Note: Some of the ethical issues arising from the use of clinical material from patients' therapy, and from students in supervision, are discussed in Appendix II.

❖ 1 ❖

Preliminary Thoughts on Learning from the Patient

> However experienced we are we still know very
> little indeed about how to bring up children, of
> whatever age. We are beginning to know that we
> do not know—that is something.
>
> (BION 1975: 147)

THE HELPING RELATIONSHIP REEXAMINED

There are many different caring professions, but the psychodynamics of any helping relationship may be universal. It is important, therefore, to become familiar with the ways in which "helper" and "client" interact and communicate to each other.

For this study I use the analytic consulting room as a setting in which we can examine the therapeutic relationship, looking in particular at the patient's perception and unconscious monitoring of the therapist.

Many of the examples I give are from sessions with people who were seen once or twice a week in analytic psychotherapy. Most of these people (had they been differently referred) could have found themselves with a social worker or counselor, a doctor or priest, or intermittently in a mental hospital. Some of the work discussed was with patients who were seen more than twice weekly; a few were seen five times a week. In Chapter 2, Example 2.4, I give a clinical illustration from my own earlier experience as a social worker.

My focus throughout is more on technique than on theory. But I do not wish to define or to prescribe ways of working which others should follow. Instead, I raise issues and questions, the answers to which will often lie in the work experience of the individual practitioner. From this, I hope others will also learn to learn from their patients, and to tune more finely their own technique to the changing needs of the individual patient.

For the ease of writing I shall not always refer to the therapist as "him or her." Instead, I will often use "him" as a short-hand and other variants will be treated similarly. Likewise, I frequently use "therapist" to stand for any professional helper who works psycho-dynamically. The exceptions are when I am referring specifically to a psychoanalyst seeing a patient in five-times-a-week analysis, or a social worker seeing a client.

PSYCHOTHERAPY: A WORLD OF PARADOX

There are many paradoxes in psychotherapy. I will mention just a few.

For each person there are always two realities—external and internal. External reality is experienced in terms of the individual's internal reality, which in turn is shaped by past experience and a continuing tendency to see the present in terms of that past. Therapists, therefore, have to find ways of acknowledging both realities and the constant interplay between them.

There are many different ways of remembering. In everyday life, memory is usually thought of as conscious recall. When uncon-scious memory is operating another kind of remembering is some-times encountered—vivid details of past experience being relived in the present. This repetition of the past is by no means confined to good times remembered, as in nostalgia. More often it is what has been fearful in the past that is reexperienced in the course of analysis or therapy. This is believed to be because of an uncon-scious search for mastery over those anxieties which had earlier been unmanageable.

Nobody can know his or her own unconscious without help from some other person. Repression maintains a resistance to what has been warded off from conscious awareness; and yet, clues to unconscious conflict still emerge in derivative forms which another person may be able to recognize. If this unconscious communica-tion can be interpreted in a meaningful and tolerable way to a patient, what previously had been "dealt with" solely by repression can begin to enter conscious awareness and become subject to conscious control or adaptation: "Where id was, there ego shall be" (Freud 1933: 80).

It is usual for therapists to see themselves as trying to understand the unconscious of the patient. What is not always acknowledged is that patients also read the unconscious of the therapist, knowingly or unknowingly. Therapists can no longer claim to be the blank screen or unblemished mirror, first advocated by Freud, because they too are people and no person can be blank or unblemished. Every analyst and therapist communicates far more to the patient about himself than is usually realized. It is important to take this clinical fact into account.

Therapists try not to make mistakes, or to get caught up in defensive behavior of their own. There will, nevertheless, be occasions when this happens. Frequently, patients make unconscious use of these mistakes in ways that throw new light on the therapeutic process. The ensuing work with a patient is often enriched by the experience of the therapist being able to learn from the patient. In this way the therapy is restored from what might otherwise have become seriously disruptive.

In the course of this book I intend to show how I have come to deal with some of these issues in my everyday work, by formally developing a process of internal supervision, analyzing from the patient's perspective what I think is happening. It is this process of internal supervision, and learning to listen, that I wish to share with the reader. I believe that this offers ways out of the many dilemmas that are inherent in psychotherapy.

Knowing and the Use of Not-Knowing

Therapists sometimes have to tolerate extended periods during which they may feel ignorant and helpless. In this sense students are privileged: they have license not to know, though many still succumb to pressures that prompt them to strive to appear certain, as if this were a mark of competence. The experienced therapist or analyst, by contrast, has to make an effort to preserve an adequate state of not-knowing if he is to remain open to fresh understanding.

Bion, perhaps more than anyone, was explicit about the need for openness to the unknown in every individual. He did not advocate any comfort in knowing. Instead, he was clear about the anxiety with which analysts can react when they are genuinely faced by the unknown. He said: "In every consulting room there ought to be two rather frightened people; the patient and the psycho-analyst. If they are not, one wonders why they are bothering to find out what everyone knows" (Bion 1974: 13).

Analytic theories are built up to define more clearly the framework in which analysts and therapists work. These are necessary, if analytic interpretation is not to become a matter of inspired guesswork. Theory also helps to moderate the helplessness of not-knowing. But it remains important that this should be servant to the work of therapy and not its master.

Freud described the tendency towards dogma in his paper "The Future of an Illusion": "And thus a store of ideas is created, born from man's need to make his helplessness tolerable" (Freud 1927: 18).

It is all too easy to equate not-knowing with ignorance. This can lead therapists to seek refuge in an illusion that they understand. But if they can bear the strain of not-knowing, they can learn that their competence as therapists includes a capacity to tolerate feeling ignorant or incompetent, and a willingness to wait (and to carry on waiting) until something genuinely relevant and meaningful begins to emerge. Only in this way is it possible to avoid the risk of imposing upon the patient the self-deception of premature understanding, which achieves nothing except to defend the therapist from the discomfort of knowing that he does not know.

By listening too readily to accepted theories, and to what they lead the practitioner to expect, it is easy to become deaf to the unexpected. When a therapist thinks that he can see signs of what is familiar to him, he can become blind to what is different and strange.

Similarity and Sameness

It is a fact of the unconscious that, in any unfamiliar situation, elements that can be regarded as familiar are responded to as signs. They can be seen as warning signals, that a bad experience could be about to be repeated. They may also be seen as signs of security. Either way, the unknown is treated as if it were already known.

It is possible to see these responses in the phenomenon of transference. A patient is confronted by the unknown in the therapist, whom he seeks to know in order to lessen the anxiety of being in the presence of someone who remains unknown. The therapist will also sometimes react to the unfamiliarity of the patient in terms of what is already familiar. Everyone finds it easier to respond in this way—thinking that the unknown is already known and therefore can be understood—rather than to remain in a more prolonged state of not-knowing.

Bion encouraged analysts to hold together their knowing and not-knowing in what he called "binocular vision" (Bion 1975: 63–4). The analyst can learn to follow with one eye those aspects of a patient about which he knows he does not know, while keeping the other eye on whatever he feels he does know. There is a creative tension between this knowing and not knowing.

Sets, Subsets, and Symmetry

When a therapist is confronted by unconscious communication from a patient, he will often encounter elements of primary-process thinking. It is necessary, therefore, to have ways of listening to this that will allow for the paradoxical logic of the unconscious.

In his book *The Unconscious as Infinite Sets* (1975), Matte Blanco[1] uses two concepts from the mathematics of set theory which elucidate in an interesting way these issues of similarity and sameness.

One concept is that of "set," defined as a collection of all things that have a common element. So we can construe, for instance, a set of all cats. There can be a subset to this of all black cats. We can also, if we like, construe a set of all black things, with a subset of all black cats.

Another concept that Matte Blanco uses is that of "unconscious symmetry." This postulates a kind of logic which is basic to primary-process thinking. Unconsciously, we assume all relationships to be symmetrical. For instance, if John is angry with Mary, Mary is unconsciously experienced as also angry with John: they are linked by the relationship of anger. If John is to the left of Mary, in primary-process thinking Mary can equally be to the left of John: they are linked by the relationship of side-by-sideness. Similarly, if Mary is the mother of John, in this "logic" of symmetry John can also be the mother of Mary: they are joined by the relationship of mother/child. The baby thus creates the mother who creates the baby, and vice versa. Likewise, the baby feeds the breast that feeds the baby.

There can be innumerable applications of symmetry in psychoanalytic listening, and in clinical experience. "Self" and "other" may be interchangeable, and this is true of patient and therapist. The part is often equated with the whole, the part-object with the whole-object. Similarly, "inside" and "outside" are frequently treated as the same. As Freud pointed out, in the unconscious there is neither negation nor contradiction. There is also no concept of time (Freud 1915: 187).

Sets, Transference, and Countertransference

If transference is considered in terms of unconscious sets, one can often identify what triggers this process. There is then an expectation that the present will be like a similar situation belonging to a previously formed unconscious set.

The sense of similarity, between past and present, can be initiated by either patient or therapist. Most often it has been thought of as the patient attributing elements of past experience to the therapist, or the therapeutic situation, and then responding to this as if the past had spilled into the present. It is, however, evident that the trigger for transference can also be unwittingly created by the therapist behaving in a way that echoes some aspect of the patient's past.

We could illustrate these phenomena diagrammatically by two circles *(Figure 1)*. If one circle is used to represent a set of "present experience," and the other a set of "past experience," anything in the area of overlap can be regarded as belonging to either set. (This overlap may represent a similarity between the past and present of the patient, or of the therapist.)

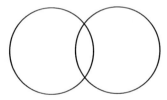

Figure 1

From a conscious viewpoint, whatever the similarity may be, past and present can still be distinguished as different. However, because there is no sense of time in the unconscious, anything in the area of overlap can be seen unconsciously as belonging equally to the past or to the present. It is this misperception of similarity as sameness that brings about the phenomenon of transference, whereby previous experience and related feelings are transferred from the past and are experienced *as if* they were actually in the present. This is why the phenomenon of transference can have such a sense of reality and immediacy.

There may be a similar unconscious overlap between the experience of "self" and "other." What comes from whom, in any two-person relationship, is not always clear. This is because the processes of communication can be either projective (one person putting into the other) or introjective (one person taking in from the other).

As well as responding to objective elements of similarity, patients also respond to their perception of external reality in terms of their changing inner states of feeling. For example, a patient may become aware of a growing dependence upon the therapist. This can evoke an unconscious set to which other experiences of dependence belong. The patient's internal reality (particularly in the clinical setting) may be seen to include additional elements being currently linked, such as feelings of dependence being associated with an actual separation pending. This can result in a more specific subset around that conjunction, evoking responses in the patient which duplicate earlier experiences of separation-at-times-of dependence. These specific elements coming together in the present sometimes give an important indication of the particular time in a patient's life which is being relived in a transference experience.

This helps to explain why even a short break in the therapy, during a regression to more infantile dependence, is often more traumatic to a patient than a long holiday had been earlier in the therapy. Some people expect patients to be able to draw upon the fact of having coped during an earlier absence of the therapist. Clinical experience illustrates that patients are affected more by the current state of their inner reality than by their adult experiences, however recent.

This reexperiencing of the past is not necessarily confined to the analytic relationship. I shall first give an example of it occurring in a patient's home.

Example 1.1

A patient (Mrs. P.) found herself crying in a distraught way after her four-year-old son had gone to bed. She could not think what had come over her. Her associations to this incident included the fact that her son had been very difficult earlier in the day. He would not do what she asked him. She had told him to go to his room, and when he refused she had screamed at him. He had then obeyed her and was no further trouble.

Mrs. P. thought that her crying had had something to do with this incident, but she wondered why it had upset her so much. It was particularly strange as her son had been quite all right later on. She wondered if it had to do with the fact that he had not been able to settle for the night until she suggested that he get into his father's bed, after which he had gone straight to sleep. It was only then, when she was on her own, that she had become so extremely upset.

Discussion: If we abstract the themes in this sequence we can see the triggers to the distraught crying more clearly. There was a mother/child relationship, with a child being difficult to handle and a mother screaming. Later, there were two people together in bed with the patient outside and crying. These particular elements could be regarded as belonging to familiar subsets, each related to unmanageable childhood experiences.

Mrs. P.'s mother used to scream at her when she was difficult to deal with, after her brother had been born. Eventually, the patient had refused to eat—to the point where (at the age of four) her mother had sent her to a home until she recovered her "correct weight." The memories evoked by the coming together of these specific elements in the present included that of her brother being allowed to stay with her mother, here represented by the son allowed to be alone with his father.

The concepts of sets and symmetry can help us to see that the patient, as a screaming mother, evoked in herself an identification with her son as the child being screamed at. Secondly, the excluding relationship (which in childhood had been that of mother with brother) was being unconsciously experienced here as equivalent to the present relationship of husband with son. Each relationship combined the elements of parent/child and an experience of someone being excluded.

(This patient is referred to again in Chapter 6, Example 6.4.)

Countertransference Responses to the Familiar

Therapists are trained to monitor their countertransference responses to a patient so that they do not respond inappropriately to a patient as to a "transferential object." (I discuss other aspects of countertransference in Chapter 4.)

I wish to suggest that, in one important respect, patients continue to be exposed to unacknowledged countertransference activity by the therapist. This is because therapists tend to develop an attitude (not unlike a transferential relationship) to their own theoretical orientation or clinical experience. As with transference, there is a tendency to experience a feeling of *déjà vu* when there are elements of similarity between a current clinical situation and others before it. This can prompt a therapist to respond to new clinical phenomena with a false sense of recognition, drawing upon established formulations for interpretation. The unconscious dynamics that contribute to this "countertransference response to the familiar" include the therapist's anxiety, and a need to feel more secure, particularly when under stress with a patient. There is also a natural investment in one's own way of interpreting.

Example 1.2
In a series of clinical seminars, in which we were looking at "failed cases," the following interchange between a therapist and patient was reported. A female patient had been in twice-a-week therapy for three months with a male student therapist. Clinical material was presented from the penultimate session before the therapist was due to go away for his Easter holiday.

> PATIENT: You will have to listen to me with extra care to-day because I have just been to the dentist. His drill slipped and he has hurt my tongue. It is difficult to talk.

> THERAPIST: (*relating this immediately to the pending break*): I think you are afraid I will be careless with you; that I may not exercise enough care with you with regard to my Easter holiday, so that my words could bore holes in you and leave you feeling hurt when I have gone.

> PATIENT: No, not at all. (*Silence.*)

> THERAPIST: I think you are using the silence as a way of leaving me before I leave you.

> PATIENT: No. In fact I was thinking of leaving therapy anyway. I think things are better. My outside relationships are better.

> THERAPIST: (*prompted by a recent seminar on ending therapy*): Do you feel this improvement is due to work we have done together, or do you see this as your own achievement?

> PATIENT: I see it as my own achievement.

The therapist was able to persuade the patient to allow some time to think over this sudden decision to leave therapy. In the next session the patient told her therapist she had decided that she could not afford her therapy any more. She could spend the money she would save on a course for learning to teach English to foreigners.

Discussion: The patient began by telling the therapist there had been some kind of injury, which now made it difficult for her to speak to him or to make herself understood. The therapist did not appear to recognize any derivative communication in what the patient was saying to him. ("Derivative communication" is used to mean the indirect communication of thoughts or feelings unconsciously associated to, or derived from, whatever has primarily provoked them.)

The therapist listened mainly in terms of theory, and a premature assumption that this patient was referring to the pending holiday break. Even if this interpretation could have been correct in content, it was wrong in timing. By butting in here, the therapist leaves no space for the patient to experience what is described. By preempting the patient's possible anxiety about the therapist becoming careless, the therapist ironically then *becomes* careless.

Let us again abstract the themes. The therapist accepted the reference to a current carelessness as referring to the dentist. But, if we again think in terms of sets, the careless dentist belongs to a set of "careless professionals" to which the therapist could also belong if he had been experienced recently as careless in the therapy.

By intervening too quickly, the therapist missed a chance of listening for further leads about an injury, to see whether this referred to him or not. There may be an allusion here to some recent interaction with the therapist in which the patient has felt hurt. If so, this could be making her experience the current difficulty in communicating with him. If he were to recognize the less obvious communication to him it would need special care in listening. The patient tells him so.

The therapist proceeds to relate the patient's opening statements to the holiday break. There is a clinical tradition for thinking of material before a holiday in terms of the break, but here it sounds rather bookish. The patient replies by disagreeing with the interpretation. The therapist responds to the ensuing silence with a further interpretation to do with the holiday break. The communication gap widens.

When the therapist does not understand the patient's allusion to something getting in the way of her communicating to him, even when she has pointed out that he will need to listen with special care, the patient considers terminating work with this therapist. She rubs his nose in this by saying her outside relationships are going better. A nuance here could suggest that these other relationships are going better than the present relationship inside the consulting room.

The therapist aims to assess the reality of this readiness for leaving. He thus moves into a new gear, which makes it obvious to the patient that he accepts her thought of leaving as virtually decided. The patient presses home her dissatisfaction. The improvement referred to feels like her own achievement, not a shared thing, nor thanks to the therapy. When the patient's decision to end is made final, she offers her therapist a parting comment which may contain the key to her feeling of injury. She is going to teach others to learn her own language (English). There is a sense in this sequence of the therapist having failed to learn her language.

Instead he had imposed his therapy-language upon her, feeling prompted to do so by what seemed to be a familiar clinical situation. The traditional responses here, to do with holiday breaks or silences, are therefore not related to the more specific communications from this patient.

It is very easy to make this kind of mistake: and it is not only students who rely upon the understanding of others, and the knowledge of theory, to bolster a feeling of competence. Using a familiar element for orientation amongst the unfamiliar can be misleading, although it may bring some relief. In *Three Men in a Boat* (Jerome K. Jerome 1889), when the three companions were lost in Hampton Court maze one of them noticed that they had passed the same half-eaten bun before. This did not mean they knew where they were; it only demonstrated that they were going in some kind of a circle.

AN EXERCISE IN INTERPRETIVE REORIENTATION

As an analogy, the process of analytic listening and interpretive linking could be loosely compared with that of looking for a sequence in mathematics. The difference, of course, is that with patients we are dealing with human processes that are not susceptible to any such proof or disproof of accuracy.

Let us consider the following sequence:

$$- - 2\ 2\ 4\ 4\ - -$$

One response could be to interpret this as two pairs: 22 44. We then have two numerical entities which can be linked by the multiple 2. Equally, however, they could be linked by the addition of 22. We do not yet have enough to go on, to know which sequence this belongs to. If it is the former we would expect to find the sequence to be extended, either before or after, as 11 22 44 88. If it belongs to the latter we would expect it to be extended as 00 22 44 66.

If these sequences were to represent clinical material, it would be a grossly premature interpretation to assume the relationship between 22 and 44 to be simply that of one number being twice the other. We need to be aware of the other possibility, so that we will wait for more of the sequence before trying to interpret. After waiting we can more confidently see which of these sequences is more probably being represented.

Let us add to the sequence:

1 22 44 8

We can now eliminate one of the possibilities that had been previously considered; i.e. the sequence is not going to evolve as 00 22 44 66. Instead, it looks as if it could be (1)1 22 44 8(8); but it might still be premature to think we understand the sequence. For instance, the missing numbers in the sequence could turn out to be as follows:

61 22 44 89

We would then have to abandon all assumptions we have made so far, being back in the area of not-knowing; and the sequence has to be returned to a state of apparent non-sense, as 6 1 2 2 4 4 8 9.

If this were clinical material, once again we would have to listen to more of the sequence. We would also need to allow passive recall of prior details which might contain elements of the same sequence. If we add to this now, before and after, we could have the following:

3 6 1 2 2 4 4 8 9 6

At first sight this might look like a meaningless sequence of random numbers. However, if we look at it from a different viewpoint, we can discover that it makes sense if we rearrange it around a new axis. What had seemed to be non-sense will become meaningful if we break it up thus:

3 6 12 24 48 96

The above illustration, like any analogy, has its shortcomings. Of course no psychoanalytic listening can be so mechanical, nor should it be regarded as absolutely right or wrong. Nevertheless, the illustration does represent the clinical experience of discovery that follows when we realize that we have missed something essential, when our initial assumptions are not borne out by what follows later in the sequence—or what may have gone before (perhaps unnoticed).

Reorientation in a Session

When in a session with a patient it can be important to sustain a sense of not-knowing, beyond the initial impression of having understood. Often the patient will provide the missing factor(s) that can point to the unconscious meaning which hitherto had remained elusive. I will illustrate this from the work of a female therapist.

Example 1.3

A patient of twenty-five was in her second year of three-times-a-week therapy when she became pregnant. As the elder of two sisters she had longed for this, her younger sister already being married with a child.

During the first months of the pregnancy the patient had treasured the privacy of her personal secret. No-one knew about this except her husband, her GP, and her therapist. Her secrecy was important to her because she had suffered all her life from her mother's intrusive attempts to control every aspect of her existence. Her marriage had helped to establish a much needed separateness from this widowed mother; and the patient had chosen to live at a sufficient distance from her to limit the mother's tendency to interfere.

The patient had been carefully preserving this period of privacy concerning her pregnancy, for as long as this could be prevented from becoming public knowledge. She then came to a session in great distress. Her sister had just been to see her and had guessed she was pregnant. She had directly challenged the patient, who felt obliged to tell her. She was now so upset because her mother would have to be told too, and the timing of this had been forced upon her by circumstance.

Since the moment when her sister had asked about the pregnancy the patient had had a splitting headache. Her therapist interpreted this in terms of the patient's familiar anxiety that once again her mother could become an intrusive influence in her life. The patient agreed. She had hoped to have had at least another month before having to resume dealings with her mother. The pregnancy had been her first experience of real privacy from her mother's compulsive interference. Even her marriage had not been immune from that. Her headache continued to be very painful.

Silent reflection: The therapist was reminded, by the patient's allusion to the marriage, that there had been similar anxieties then. The patient had experienced her future husband as threatening to invade her. Having only just begun to win some mental and emotional space from her mother, the patient had become afraid she might be about to lose this to her husband; and her marriage could become just another version of being owned by someone else, unconsciously representing her mother.

When the therapist thought about this reference to the patient's marriage she felt prompted to reorientate her listening around the issue of pregnancy. Until then, she had been regarding the headache as a symptomatic expression of the patient's fear of being taken over again more directly by her mother. She had not perceived this as an allusion to her unborn baby. This was already inside the patient's body. Could it be that the patient was unconsciously experiencing the baby as representing her mother taking her over from inside?

The therapist offered a tentative interpretation. Could the patient be experiencing her baby as a threat, perhaps as an embodiment of her mother's invasiveness which previously she had been trying to combat externally?

The patient was able to think around this for herself. Yes, she believed this could be true. She had been afraid of being invaded physically, and of being taken over emotionally, when she got married. The baby could be an even greater threat to her, on the same two counts. It was as if she could never get away from her mother, and she could not get away from her own pregnancy. She was afraid of damaging her baby by hating it as a representation of her mother.

After a silence, the patient elaborated further. she said it felt like an unthinkable thought that she could hate her own baby. She added that perhaps her headache had been an expression of the conflict between her protective love for the baby and her life-long impulse to get away from anything threatening to invade her privacy. She continued to think aloud around this. For her, it was an entirely new discovery that she could have hostile feelings towards the baby she so much wanted.

Later in the session she realized her headache had lifted for the first time in several days. She felt convinced that this conflict in her feelings about the baby had been the key to her headache, which both the therapist and she had been missing until then.

Discussion: As a result of following the patient's cues, it became possible for the therapist to recognize that the current conflict might have to do with the baby. It was as if her baby might represent a "Trojan horse," by which all she had most feared from her mother could take her over—literally from within. The patient's subsequent realization that she could hate her baby, as well as love it, carried the conviction of discovery. It was after all her own; the thought had not been put into her by the therapist.

The patient would have been let down if her therapist had continued to work over the patient's more direct and conscious fears concerning her mother. Equally, if the therapist had interpreted earlier the likelihood of the patient having ambivalent feelings towards her baby, that insight (though true) would have been premature and persecutory to the patient. In this case the therapist's slowness allowed time and space for the patient to arrive at this realization for herself, in a way she could tolerate and make her own.

Insight Offered or Imposed?

When patients feel they are not being understood, it is not always easy for them to communicate this to someone whose professional claim is to know about these things. The patient may also encounter the ultimate and irrefutable reply, that if the patient does not know something consciously it is because the patient is unconscious of the alleged truth being offered by the analyst. But it is not always just offered. It is sometimes dogmatically stated; and even a patient's rejection of an interpretation can be invoked as proof of its truth, and as evidence of the patient's defensiveness in response to it.

The analyst or therapist, as an implicit prophet of the unconscious, has a position of power in these matters which he must handle with great caution. Some patients do not find it easy to stand up to a therapist. Nevertheless, because they cannot always be right, therapists need help from the patient's cues towards better understanding. These cues are most often oblique rather than direct, unconscious rather than conscious.

In trying to understand the patient, a therapist waits until he feels that he can recognize a thread of meaning that can be identified and interpreted. But, in this work of interpreting, how can therapists avoid imposing their own theoretical bias upon their patients? Bion advocated that an analyst should approach each session without desire, memory or understanding (Bion 1967a; also 1967b: 143-45). The desire (for instance) to cure or to influence, the active remembering of the previous session, and the illusion of understanding in terms of what is theoretically familiar, all contend against the kind of openness to the patient's individuality that is the hallmark of psychoanalysis at its best.

Whose Resistance?

When a patient fails to acknowledge some truth about himself, as presented by the therapist, or agrees verbally without any significant shift in his life or in the therapeutic relationship, it is common to regard this as due to unconscious resistance within the patient. It may be so; but sometimes it can be an indication that there is, in this lack of change, an unconscious cue to the therapist to reassess his assumptions about the patient, his theory or his technique. There may be something the therapist has not yet recognized, or acknowledged, and the therapist can be resistant too. Listening for unconscious symmetry in the patient's communications can often help to indicate what it is that has been overlooked. Potential stalemate in a session may then lead on to renewed movement.

Example 1.4
At a clinical seminar a female therapist discussed some work involving a male patient who continually shouted. In presenting a session, the therapist demonstrated this shouting to the seminar group. We were told by the therapist that she had tried many times, and in many ways, to understand this behavior in the therapy. So far, nothing had helped it to alter.

When one member of the seminar group asked the therapist how she felt about being shouted at in this violent-sounding way, she replied: "Well, one thing I know about myself is that I don't have difficulties with aggression or violence."

Discussion: By listening to the interaction here in terms of symmetry, we could formulate that *someone* was failing to get through to *someone*. What we had been assuming, previously, was that the therapist had been failing to get through to the patient—hence no change. But the interaction took on a fresh perspective once we realized the patient could be failing to get through to the therapist. Perhaps the shouting was an attempt at achieving this.

We could also wonder whether the therapist was only able to cope with being with an aggressive (even violent) patient by shutting off a part of her own responsiveness. The group had felt far less comfortable about the shouting than the therapist. So, if the patient were trying to get through to the therapist (but was failing to do so) perhaps he was demonstrating exasperation, or despair of being heard, by shouting louder.

Having considered that the resistance producing the stalemate might partly be coming from herself, the therapist reflected upon this and became more able to hear what previously she had been missing in her patient's communication. She later reported to the seminar group that the patient had quietened down. The patient was now feeling heard.

The Issue of Control

It is easy to rationalize that patients should not be allowed to control their own therapy, as if this might "render the therapist impotent"—to use a familiar phrase. But if the therapist insists on controlling the entire therapy, might that not equally render the *patient* impotent? Sometimes, of course, a therapist has to stand firm with a patient. There are also times when a patient has to stand firm with the therapist, in the name of his or her own truth. Such occasions can be misunderstood if a therapist is anxious about being manipulated or controlled by the patient. This often indicates that a therapist is feeling under stress; in which case it is usually more fruitful to listen to the sense of pressure, as an unconscious communication from the patient, rather than to react to it prematurely around an issue of control.

THE THERAPIST'S RESPONSIVENESS TO CUES FROM THE PATIENT

Several patients have pointed out how they first became able to trust me through discovering that I was willing to learn from them. For some this may be how they first come to find a basic trust. Unless this is rooted in experience it can remain an insubstantial hope.

Example 1.5
Early in her analysis Mrs. B. (who had been severely burned when she was eleven months old) was telling me that the continuing pain from this experience and the attendant memories were making her hair go gray. I began looking more closely at her hair (over the back of the couch) to see if I could see signs of this graying. When I could not see any trace of this, I wondered whether it was an invitation for me to be closer to the patient. Perhaps if I were *very* close to her I would be able to see *some* gray hairs. I began to explore this as an appeal for me to be closer, thinking (to myself) that the patient was trying some hysterical manipulation on me.

Mrs. B. became very distressed. When I listened to her distress, which was a crying from deep inside, I realized I had completely missed the point. I had been looking for outward signs of going gray. When I listened more closely I was able to interpret quite differently. The patient had been trying to tell me about her *inside* world, in which the scars from her childhood experiences made her feel that she was growing prematurely old. Part of the problem was that her emotional scars were not visible. She and I were having to deal with those other scars which had not yet healed.

Discussion: Although I had hurt this patient by my misunderstanding, by my focusing on the outside (where others too had found their reassurance that she had recovered from the accident), I was given an opportunity to be guided by the patient to recover from my mistake. She gave me another chance. This time I was able to recognize what she had been trying to tell me, in her enigmatic reference to her graying hair, and it turned out to be an important moment in her analysis. Mrs. B. frequently referred back to this occasion. She told me that this was when she had begun to believe she could risk some dependence upon me. I had let myself be guided by her, which meant I could learn from her.

After her accident, Mrs. B. had felt that her mother no longer seemed able to respond to her cues, or to her needs, in the same way as before. It was therefore crucial to her that I was learning to follow the cues she gave to me; and this became the basis for much of what later emerged in her analysis.

(This patient is referred to again in Chapters 5 and 7.)

I have noticed that as I have learned more about psychoanalysis, and about being a therapist, I have also become able to learn more from my patients. This has made me wonder about the different quality of relating that has resulted from this.

With some patients I have had to rely much more upon what I already know from the theory of psychoanalysis, and what I have learned about analytic technique, for that is often how I find (or maintain) my role. With them I have gone more by the book than by intuition, and I have remained more classically the same. With other patients, particularly with those from whom I feel I have learned most, I have found myself becoming responsively different to each of them. What does this imply? Which group of patients might be said to have had the better analytic experience: those with whom I preserved myself more firmly the same, or those in response to whom I allowed myself to be molded into a more individual analyst?[2]

I have no easy answers to these questions. I can only eliminate the obvious extremes. If firmness becomes rigidity, it offers a false security to analyst and patient alike. On the other hand, the opposite extreme of an unreflecting flexibility amounts to "wild analysis" with serious risks of unresolved countertransference difficulties being acted out within what is meant to be a therapeutic relationship (see Chapter 3 for an example of this).

There remains a type of analytic interrelatedness, that can be seen more clearly in some analyses than in others, but which may be a factor in all. I am thinking here of certain parallels with the parent–child relationship, that is so often presented for sorting out in the course of an analysis. To illustrate this I shall briefly digress.

ANALYSIS AND THE NURSING TRIAD

Growing children need their parents to be able to respond differently according to different developmental stages. For example, a mother has to learn her infant's language if she is to respond according to the varying needs of her baby. Some mothers develop more skill in this than others. This difference has many determinants. There is the mother's own experience of being mothered; this will have left a set of images of mothering in her mind. A mother-to-be also has her own innate potential for being a mother to her baby; this potential can either be realized, or it can be interfered with.

From reading Winnicott I have come to think in terms of a "nursing triad," whereby the mother is emotionally held while she holds the baby. The biological father may be absent, but there needs to be someone in the new mother's life whose chief function is to be there to support the mother-and-baby as they begin to get to know each other. In particular the new mother needs to be believed in as capable of being a "good enough mother" to her own baby (Winnicott 1958: 245).

Where this holding of the mother (as mother to her baby) is absent, there can be serious disruptions of the subsequent mothering. If the mother feels undermined as mother she may begin to resent her baby, which can come to represent her sense of failure as a mother. (Society sometimes reinforces a mother's insecurities here, when attention is more often focused on the mother than upon those who have failed to give her the support she has needed.). This lack of confidence in herself can be aggravated by other people's readiness to tell her what to do, and by others taking over and seeming to be better mothers to her baby. There may also be an internal erosion of confidence from bad childhood experiences of being mothered, or (in the present) of not being believed in or supported as a mother. Added to that there is sometimes a persecutory awareness of the baby's failure to thrive or to feel secure in the mother's handling. All these factors can contribute to a tendency to neglect the baby, even to give in to impulses to attack a baby who represents an attack upon herself as a mother.

If, on the other hand, a mother feels adequately held (as mother to her baby) she is more able to learn from her baby how best to be the mother which, at that moment, her baby most needs her to be. To begin with, this means learning her baby's language and individual rhythms; and these will not be the same as in the books, or the same as the baby next door, or the average baby that some child experts seem to speak of (with their "milestones" and so on). These will also not be the same as in the case of any other baby that the mother previously may have had. Each baby is different.

A mother who thus allows herself to respond to the individuality of each of her babies will, in some measure, find herself being a different mother to each. She will also find herself changing with time, through her continuing to learn from her baby/child in response to changing developmental needs (Winnicott 1965b: Chapter 7).

The father (or father substitute) comes into this too. From the beginning that holding presence is of crucial importance to the mother, and the child benefits or suffers according to the quality of that support. The "father" later comes into a different role, as the child moves into discovering about triangular relationships. Still later the adolescent presents different needs again, requiring a firmness which "belongs to containment that is non-retaliatory, without vindictiveness, but having its own strength" (Winnicott 1971: Chapter 11).

The Patient, the Analyst, and the Internal Supervisor

I have covered the above, familiar, ground in some detail as I believe that similar dynamics apply in the analytic relationship. We can see this most clearly in relation to students.

Student analysts and therapists have a particular need to be professionally held while they learn about the analytic holding that a patient needs in therapy. They should be able to draw upon the experience of their own analysis; they can also be held by their knowledge of theory and of technique, to have the security to continue to function analytically even under pressure. But, in addition, there needs to be a supervisory holding by an experienced person who believes in the student's potential to be in tune with the patient and to comment helpfully.

However, students need to be able to develop a style of working which is compatible with their own personality; so there will be something essential missing if he or she becomes too much of a *pastiche* of the training analyst, or the supervisor, however unconscious that may be.

Amongst the pitfalls of a supervisor (and here I draw upon what I have learned from those I have supervised) is the danger of offering too strong a model of how to treat the patient. This can mislead students into learning by a false process, borrowing too directly from a supervisor's way of working rather than developing their own. Some students can be seriously undermined in this way, feeling as if the treatment (or even the patient) has been taken over by the supervisor.

Here there are echoes of the mother who feels she is being told how to be a mother, and the results can be similarly disturbing to the student's analytic attitude towards the patient. For, if a patient comes to represent the student's difficulties in believing in himself as a therapist, he will have problems in working with that patient.

Winnicott was careful always to respect a mother's understanding of her own child. He therefore used to emphasize that he was only an expert on mothers and babies in general. Although he might be useful to a particular mother, it was she who continued to be acknowledged as the person who knew her own baby better than anyone else (Winnicott 1965a: Chapter 1).

As with the mother, this holding of the student therapist is first experienced as coming from outside. Transitionally the experience of supervision is usually internalized. Ultimately this needs to develop into an internal support that is autonomous and separate from the internalized supervisor. So, in order to emphasize this further development, I have come to think in terms of an internal supervisor (see Chapter 2).

When the internal supervisor remains poorly individuated there is a tendency for therapists to rely too much upon the thinking of others. But, any strong adherence to a particular school of theory, or position on technique, can itself become intrusive. The analytic process can easily become tilted in a predetermined direction, which means it then ceases to be truly exploratory or psychoanalytic. It is not surprising that the critics of psychoanalysis can point out how Freudian patients seem to have Freudian dreams, whereas Jungian or Kleinian patients are said to have dreams that fit in with the different theoretical position of *their* analysts. Here, I think, we have evidence of patients being taught to speak the language of the analyst; and not only language. Parallels may be found, among analysts and therapists, with mothers who assume they know best what their baby needs. We also hear of mothers who did not trust their own judgment sufficiently, having been misguided by authorities on childrearing (Truby King among others) into believing they could bring up their babies by the book rather than "by the baby."

If "the book" is given too much importance, then the choice of book becomes a crucial issue. Many bitter controversies might have been avoided if more analysts had questioned their belief in the overriding importance of a fully integrated theory.[3] When analysts and therapists go rather more "by the patient," and less by the particular theoretical orientation by which they feel supported, it becomes easier to notice when a patient feels out of tune with what is being said or with how the analysis is being conducted. Some patients may need a different style of analysis. It is important that therapists leave themselves room in their technique to allow for this. The analytic process becomes seriously restricted if therapists define themselves out of this possibility in the name of their own chosen orthodoxy.

In order to guard against the distorting influence of theoretical bias I find it useful to keep asking myself two questions, before and after interpreting or when supervising: (1) "Is the patient's individuality being respected and preserved, or overlooked and intruded upon?"; (2) "Who is putting what into the analytic space, at this moment, and why?"

Psychoanalysis has the potential for enabling a rebirth of the individual personality. It is a tragedy if this comes to be limited to a process nearer to that of "cloning," whereby the patient comes to be "formed in the image" of the analyst and his theoretical orientation.

Learning from the Patient

In his book *Orthodoxy* (1908), G.K. Chesterton imagines:

> an English yachtsman who slightly miscalculated his course and discovered England under the impression that it was a new island in the South Seas... who landed (armed to the teeth and talking by signs) to plant the English flag on that barbaric temple which turned out to be the Pavilion at Brighton. (Edition 1961: 9)

If a therapist trusts in the analytic process he will often find himself led by the patient to where others have been before. The importance for the patient is that any theoretical similarity to what previously has been conceptualized in relation to others shall be arrived at through fresh discovery, not preconception.

The therapist's openness to the unknown in the patient leaves more room for the patient to contribute to any subsequent knowing; and what is thus jointly discovered has a freshness which belongs to both. More than this, it may be that a significant part of the process of therapeutic gain is achieved through the patient coming to recognize that the therapist can learn from him or her. The patient is thus given a real part to play in helping the therapist to help the patient and, to that end, to discover what is needed in that patient's therapy.

Patients benefit from a therapist's willingness to find out, even that which is already "known," through working clinically with them. This feels better by far than using short-cuts to understanding, based on what is borrowed from others—and which patients also borrow. Fresh insight emerges more convincingly when a therapist is prepared to struggle to express himself within a patient's language, rather than falling back upon old thinking.

When I let patients play a part in how their therapy evolves I do not find myself being made helpless because of this. At times I may even have to become drawn into a "harmonious mix-up" within the analytic relationship (Balint 1968). There are, of course, other times when I have to maintain an adequate firmness, without which a patient could feel insecure and deprived of the opportunity to experience confrontation with someone clearly separate and different from himself. For instance, when a patient is ready to find a therapist's otherness (or what Winnicott calls "externality") the therapist has to be able to respond to the patient's attacks, upon him and the therapy, without collapse or retaliation (Winnicott 1971: Chapter 6).

Therapists need confidence in the analytic process if they are to be able to tolerate the vicissitudes of being used by their patients in these different ways. They need to be able to follow the patient, without feeling too much at sea to function analytically. For this they will need an adequate orientation to hold them near enough on course, or to help them back on course when they become lost.

In the treatment setting, it is a function of the internal supervisor to hold the analyst (or therapist) who is learning to hold the patient. This provides the structure of an internal "nursing triad," which can help the therapist to find an inner play-space where the clinical options can be explored (silently or with the patient) rather than remaining blinkered by past thinking that often functions too much like a set of rules.

In the rest of this book I intend to examine various aspects of the interaction between a patient and the analyst or therapist. It is my belief that therapists could risk being less tenacious in their adherence to particular theoretical positions if they allowed themselves to be more receptively open to what their patients communicate to them at so many diverse levels.

When a therapist learns to follow the patient's cues, and listens to the resulting dialogue between the two viewpoints of "binocular vision" (Bion 1975), of knowing and not-knowing, he will frequently find himself led towards the understanding which is needed.

❖2❖

The Internal Supervisor

INTERNAL SUPERVISION: A QUEST FOR BALANCE

Therapists are often related to by the patient as a transferential object, representing aspects of earlier relationships, and yet also as a real object. This means that they have to be able to remain well disposed towards a patient even when they are being treated as someone with attitudes that may be quite alien.

In order that a patient can relate to the therapist, as freely as possible in terms of the patient's inner reality, it has long been accepted that the analytic process should be protected from needless interference from the therapist's own personality. However, in order to avoid becoming intrusive in the therapy, some therapists become defensive in trying to be as little in evidence as possible. Unfortunately, falling over backwards (in trying to achieve this) can become just as intrusive as falling forwards into the center vision of the patient's awareness. As far as possible, the therapist's presence therefore has to remain a transitional or potential presence (like that of a mother who is nonintrusively present with her playing child). The therapist can then be invoked by the patient as a presence, or can be used by the patient as representing an absence.

This is the world of potential space (Winnicott 1971: Chapter 3) which is part real and part illusory, and here I use the notion of illusion as belonging to the experience of playing (ludo = to play). In this space the patient needs to be allowed opportunities for optimum experience, without interference from the therapist.

In order to preserve for the patient the creative potential of this space, therapists have to learn how to remain close enough to what the patient is experiencing for this to have a feeling impact upon himself while preserving a sufficient distance still to function as therapist. But that professional distance should not leave him beyond the reach of what the patient may need him to feel. A therapist has to discover how to be psychologically intimate with a patient and yet separate, separate and still intimate.

In their day-to-day functioning, therapists have to feel their way amidst many paradoxical pulls and pushes; and they have to acquire a sense of balance if they are to feel at ease in this therapeutic *pas de deux*. What is needed, therefore, is more than just those external aspects of the nursing triad referred to in the previous chapter.

Support from a supervisor or analyst can offer *hindsight* on what has been missed in an earlier session; it can also offer *foresight* in relation to what may be yet encountered. Therapists still need to develop a capacity to function with more immediate (but not instant) *insight* within the momentum of the analytic process. Not even that which is sometimes called the "internalized supervisor" meets all that is required here.

As a counterbalance to the many pressures upon a therapist in a session, I have found it useful to think in terms of an internal supervisor (Casement 1973).[1] I first began to articulate the need for this in supervising others. I noticed that trainees in supervision often lean too heavily upon the advice or comments of a supervisor, which creates a barrier between the social worker or therapist and the client or patient. The effect of this becomes evident in the trainee's subsequent clinical work. I therefore came to see that formal supervision alone does not adequately prepare a student to deal with the immediacy of the therapeutic present.

THE DEVELOPMENT OF AN INTERNAL SUPERVISOR[2]

What I am calling the internal supervisor has origins that derive from before the experience of supervision and its development continues far beyond it. I shall trace this here with particular reference to therapists, as they are specifically required to have personal analysis as a part of their training. In other helping professions, all the other stages described here are similar.

During Personal Analysis

Writing from the point of view of an analyst seeing a patient, Sterba (1934) stresses that it is important to enable a "therapeutic ego-dissociation" within the ego of the patient. This, he points out, is achieved by interpreting the transference. One result of this is that the patient is encouraged to observe with the analyst what he (the patient) is experiencing. The two aspects of this split have sometimes been referred to as the "observing ego" and the "experiencing ego." In this paper, Sterba also introduces the notion of "an island of intellectual contemplation." So, when therapists have become genuinely involved in their own analysis, they too will have experienced this need to find within themselves (as patient) that island of contemplation—from which they could observe with their analyst what they were experiencing in the transference.

It is here, in their own experience of being a patient, that therapists establish the first roots of what later becomes the internal supervisor. Something is added to this in each phase of training and subsequent clinical work. As our experience grows, so we build on what has gone before.

Being Supervised

This may be considered in three separate phases, as the function of supervision during the early stages of training is different from what is needed later.

1. When therapists first begin to treat a patient they have limited resources to draw upon. They have what they know of theory. They have what so far has been experienced in their own analysis. They may also have some knowledge of the work of other people, as this has been written about or has been presented in clinical seminars.

However, the only direct experience of being in a therapeutic role that student therapists have had before is often in some other discipline, as a doctor or psychiatrist, as teacher or as social worker. At times, particularly when being stressed by a patient, there can be a strong pull to revert to type—calling upon earlier modes of functioning that are familiar. This can hinder a fuller learning of the new mode of functioning that is required of a student in becoming a therapist or an analyst.

Therefore, when a student therapist begins to work with training cases under supervision, the supervisor has a crucially important function in holding the student during this opening phase of clinical work—while he or she is learning to hold the patient analytically. The supervisor provides a form of control, making it safe for the therapist and patient to become analytically engaged, and helping a student to understand and to contain what is being presented by the patient. The foundations are laid down here for working independently later on.

At the outset, students naturally rely a good deal upon the advice and comments offered by the supervisor. With time, these supervisory insights should become more integrated into the ongoing work with a patient. Sometimes, however, they continue to impinge upon this as elements of borrowed thinking.

2. During the course of being supervised, therapists need to acquire their own capacity for spontaneous reflection within the session, alongside the internalized supervisor. They can thus learn to watch themselves as well as the patient, now using this island of intellectual contemplation as the mental space within which the internal supervisor can begin to operate.

3. Towards the end of training, I believe that the process of supervision should develop into a dialogue between the external supervisor and the internal supervisor. It is through this that therapists develop the more autonomous functioning that is expected of them upon qualification.

Working without Formal Supervision

After therapists first qualify there is an important period of consolidation. In his teaching and supervising, John Klauber used to emphasize that it takes at least ten years to become an analyst after being qualified. Bion stressed that "becoming" is a process which begins, continues, and is never completed. We should always be in a state of becoming (Bion 1975: 26). At the time of qualifying, a more autonomous internal supervisor may be forming in the therapist; but I hope there will never be a time when therapists cease from this "becoming" or imagine that they have "arrived."

Supervising Others

When therapists have an opportunity to supervise others, they can enter into a further phase of growth that recapitulates much of what has gone before. The sequence is like a spiral in which they can find themselves back at a beginning, the beginning of training or the beginning of a treatment. They are back where they have been before, but also where they have never been before.

Just as we can see our own errors more clearly in others, so too in supervising others. Here there are endless opportunities for therapists to reexamine their own work, when looking closely at the work of the person being supervised. Not infrequently; supervisors will be seeing reflections of their own difficulties with technique. We do not always do as we teach others to do, but we can learn a lot by trying to do so.

When I have followed the work of my supervisees from an interactional point of view[3] it has brought home to me how closely patients follow the work of their therapists, monitoring their moods, noticing their timing, wondering about the unconscious implications of their comments (what clues these may give the patient beyond the attempted inscrutability of the therapist). I had not realized before how much I too must give away of myself in the manner of my own interventions, or the mode of my responses to a patient.

Renewed Reflection

Once I had come to recognize this unintentional maneuvering of the patient by those I supervise, it became imperative for me to monitor my own work more closely. Some therapists might be surprised by how often they could be falling into modes of intervention that they have questioned when supervising someone else. This realization can stir into life a renewed cycle of learning about technique, and about our own contribution to the responses that we see in our patients.

TRIAL IDENTIFICATION

As a part of the internal supervision that I am suggesting, I often find it helpful to use trial identification (Fliess 1942). This can also be thought of as related to empathy in seeking to understand a patient. Reik (1937) pointed out that we develop empathy as a capacity to share in the experience of others, not just *like* our own but *as* our own.

Money-Kyrle linked this to the analyst's familiarity with his own unconscious:

> It is just because the analyst can recognize his early self which has already been analyzed, in the patient, that he can analyze the patient. His empathy and insight, as distinct from his theoretical knowledge, depend on this kind of partial identification. Identification can take two forms—introjective and projective. We may therefore expect to find both forms in the analyst's partial identification with his patient. As the patient speaks, the analyst will as it were become introjectively identified with him, and having understood him inside, will reproject him and interpret. What I think the analyst is most aware of is the projective phase—that is to say, the phase in which the patient is the representative of a former immature or ill part of himself, including

his damaged objects, which he can now understand and therefore treat by
interpretation, in the external world. (Money-Kyrle 1956: 360–61)

It is therefore not just the patient who needs to develop the
capacity for a therapeutic dissociation within his ego, such as Sterba
describes. The therapist also has to be able to maintain this benign
split within himself, whereby his experiencing ego is free to move
between himself and the patient, between thinking and feeling.
Kris refers to this as "regression in the service of the ego" (Kris
1950). The analyst uses a controlled regression within himself in
order to cross the boundary between his conscious (rational)
thinking and his unconscious (primary-process/irrational) thinking. Allowing himself this freedom to enter a state of listening
reverie, alongside the patient, he can monitor what it may feel like
to be the patient (in whichever context).

Now, when I use trial identification I do so in a number of
different ways. I may, for example, think or feel myself into
whatever experience is being described by a patient. I may also put
myself into the shoes of the other person being referred to. From
each of these viewpoints it is possible to pick up elements of the
patient's object-relating that might otherwise be missed.

In addition to these more usual ways of monitoring a patient
through trial identification, I also try to put myself into the
patient's shoes in his or her relationship to me. I try to listen (as
the patient might) to what it crosses my mind to say, silently trying
out a possible comment or interpretation. This helps me to recognize when a patient could mishear what I wish to say, because of
its ambiguity or due to an unfortunate choice of words. Or, I put
myself into the patient's position and reflect upon my own last
comment. Frequently this will alert me to the unintentional, and
unconscious communications that a patient could read into what I
have just said. Then, when I listen to the patient's subsequent
response, it becomes easier to see when this has been actually
provoked by me by my timing or manner of interpreting.

I first learned to monitor the therapeutic interaction in this way
by trial-identifying with the patient when following the clinical
presentations of people whom I supervised. With practice it becomes possible to use these two viewpoints simultaneously, the
patient's and one's own, rather like following the different voices
in polyphonic music.

This capacity to be in two places at once—in the patient's shoes
and in one's own simultaneously—can only be encompassed if
therapists can develop a capacity to synthesize these apparently
paradoxical ego states. It is here, I believe, that the processing

function of the internal supervisor comes to the fore. It is more than self-analysis and it is more than self-supervision.

THE INTERNAL SUPERVISOR AND PLAY

Winnicott pointed out that:

> *psychotherapy is done in the overlap of the two play areas, that of the patient and that of the therapist.* If the therapist cannot play, then he is not suitable for the work. If the patient cannot play, then something needs to be done to enable the patient to become able to play, after which psychotherapy may begin. The reason why playing is essential is that it is in playing that the patient is being creative. (Winnicott 1971: 54)

I regard playing as one of the functions of the internal supervisor, and it is through this that the therapist can share in the patient's creativity. It is also here that he can discover a balance between what he knows of the nature of the unconscious and the pitfalls of premature assumption.

RESISTING PRECONCEPTIONS: AN ANALOGY FROM GEOMETRY

I wish to give an example of imaginative play in relation to psychotherapy. I also want to illustrate how there can be several different versions of "original" image (or meaning) referred to, when we recognize that unconscious derivative communication frequently employs defensive forms of reference such as splitting and projection, displacement and reversal, etc. Here, I wish to illustrate some of these processes by using an imaginary shape from geometry.

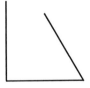

Figure 2

Suppose, for instance, that we are trying to make sense of a shape suggested by three lines of equal length (Figure 2). Let us also suppose that the three lines are joined, with two forming an angle of 60 degrees and the other line forming a right angle. If we are predisposed to find a triangle, we might regard the key to this shape as conveyed by the two lines at 60 degrees. The line at 90 degrees could then be regarded as out of place. If we play with this, as we might with a dream image (Figure 3), we could think of the 90 degrees angle as displaced—perhaps suggesting a defensive need not to represent the shape of a triangle in its undisguised form. Prompted by that explanation, we could begin to think that we are "really" being presented with a derivative representation of an equilateral triangle.

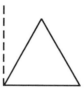

Figure 3

With the analytical predisposition to look for Oedipal material, it would be easy to formulate some triangular interpretation, regarding the "discovered" triangle as having been defensively represented. We could think of the original shape as derived from a hidden triangle, being indirectly rather than directly alluded to.

If however we take another look at our imaginary shape we could orientate ourselves instead around the right-angle, and see the 60 degrees angle as a displacement—perhaps from another right angle (Figure 4). We might be looking at a derivative from a square, with one side unstated. Or we could be looking at a square-shaped "U" or a "container"; or (upside down) it could be a "cover," that is if we do not confine ourselves only to the world of geometry.

Figure 4

It is this capacity for playing with a patient's images that Bion encouraged when he spoke of the analyst's use of "reverie" (Bion 1967b: Chapter 9). He also gave a graphic illustration of this in his last paper to the British Psycho-Analytical Society (1979, unpublished). He showed us how he arrived at a patient's particular question "Why?" in the context of a patient's dream, in which the dreamer was being looked down upon by a crowd of people who were on a staircase that divided into the shape of a "Y."

UNFOCUSED LISTENING

Before giving an example of using internal supervision I wish to introduce the notion of "unfocused listening." I regard this as a first step beyond that of the familiar "evenly suspended attention," with which analysts are encouraged to listen to the overall drift of a patient's communications.

When I think that I am beginning to understand what is being communicated in a session, I find that it helps me to avoid preconceived ideas about this if I first abstract the recognizable themes from what a patient is saying, and hold these provisionally away from the overt context. Also, if I sometimes listen to the identified themes with unconscious symmetry in mind, it helps to show up the different possible meanings that can then emerge.

For instance, if a patient were to say "My boss is angry with me," this can be silently abstracted as "someone is angry with someone." *Whose anger with whom* then remains unclear, and this can be considered with a more open mind than otherwise would be possible. It could be a statement of fact, objectively reported; it could be a reference to the patient's anger, projected onto the boss; it could be a displaced reference to the transference, the therapist seen as angry; or it could be an oblique reference to the patient being angry with the therapist. In practice, this balancing of different potential meanings needs to be integrated into the normal process of internal supervision.

THE INTERNAL SUPERVISOR AT WORK: AN EXERCISE IN APPLICATION

I shall now use a clinical vignette as an "exercise," because we can more readily learn to recognize the various clinical options when we are not subjected to the pressures that exist in an actual therapy session. However, this is not intended as a model for conscious and active monitoring, or for choosing an interpretation in the session; nor should it be allowed to interfere with the therapist's "free floating attention" during the session.

In order that we can develop a more subliminal use of the internal supervisor when we are with a patient, it is valuable to use (or, in a Winnicott sense, to "play" with) clinical material outside of the session. A musician plays scales, or technical studies, in order that these can become a natural part of his technique. So too in psychotherapy: when a therapist is "making music" with a patient he should not be preoccupied with issues of technique. That technique can be developed by taking time, away from the consulting room, for practicing with clinical material. Then, when in the presence of a patient, the process of internal supervision is more readily available when it is most needed.

> *Example 2.1*
> A widow (Mrs. J.) in her early forties comes to a session with these opening statements to her male therapist:
>
>> PATIENT: I have been wondering whether to go to a clairvoyant. (*Pause.*) I found a book of John's on his bookshelf, called *Father and Son*. I remember him talking about it as having been important to him, but I don't recall now what he said. I once started it, but I never really got into it. I suppose one day I ought to finish it. (*Pause.*) I like reading, particularly Proust. It was John who first put me in touch with that. I'm glad he did. I began reading it again recently. That should fill a good many hours anyway. (*Pause.*)
>>
>> I had a dream: *I saw a girl who was in difficulty in a fast running river. I thought she might be drowning, and wondered whether I should dive in to help her to get to safety.* I woke up before I did anything about it. (*Pause.*) I wonder whether it is true that you see all of your life again when you are about to drown. I wouldn't have thought that there would be time. But the mind is very strange. Perhaps we will never know whether we can see our lives that clearly unless we are actually drowning.

Passive Recall

I have deliberately not given any background to this session as I want to illustrate the usefulness of allowing the material of a session to evoke particular memories from earlier work with the patient. This helps a therapist not to enter a session laden with preconceived ideas, gained from earlier sessions. The paradox, of course, is that we do need to have an overview of the progression of any psychotherapy, while at the same time being able to leave that on one side to be recalled as needed.

We are here reminded that Mrs. J.'s husband (John) died less than a year ago; and we need to know (from an earlier session) that Mrs. J. had recently decided to buy a house away from London. She had given as her reasons for this that she wanted to get away from the constant reminders of John, in the house in which they had lived since they married; and she wanted her son (her only child) to go to the secondary school near where she had chosen to live. He was to start there after the summer holiday.

Mrs. J.'s decision to move away from London had arisen suddenly, after only six months therapy. We could therefore wonder whether she was afraid of getting into her deeper feelings, and whether this move might include an element of flight into health. (Her stated reasons were clearly important to her, so the therapist had resisted interpreting her move in case she took it as an attempt to control her decision about this.)

At this point in the therapy there were only five weeks until the therapist's summer holiday, and Mrs. J. was planning to stop her sessions then. This ending felt abrupt and premature, but it was not until after this session that there was any open thinking about her other options.

Abstracting the Themes

As we "play" with this clinical material, using unfocused listening, we can note that there are several themes that are recurring. The clairvoyant suggests a wish to know about the future. If, however, we apply the concept of unconscious symmetry here we may be alerted to a possible primary-process equivalence of past and future. The unconscious theme therefore could be to do with a wish to make contact with *someone who is difficult to reach*, or *someone unreachable* (in the past or the future). We do not know whether this primarily refers to the husband, to the therapist representing the husband, or to the therapy. The clairvoyant could also be an unconscious metaphor for the patient's wish to have an alternative therapist, either because of the imminent end of therapy or because the patient may have experienced the therapist as not foreseeing enough.

There are several details around the theme of *something unfinished*. For instance, there is the book that has been only partly read. This could refer equally to the unfinished relationship to the husband, or to the therapy that Mrs. J. has only partly got into, or both. We can note too that, in the dream, Mrs. J. begins to feel that she should dive in to rescue the drowning girl; but she wakes before

she acts upon this. The death of her husband leaves much else that
is unfinished, the marriage relationship and John's relationship
with their son; and there is the title of the book which may be a
further unconscious clue.

There is also a clear implication of *lost time*, in Mrs. J's reference
to Proust's *A la recherche du temps perdu*. The time lost most
obviously refers to the cut-short marriage, but it could again
prompt us to think of the therapy which is about to be cut short.
Perhaps she has not had enough time to deal with the painful
experiences that she has been through. Mrs. J. points out she has
a kind of self-therapy in mind; reading Proust will fill many hours.
There is a wish to recover time lost, to go over the past again,
perhaps to keep memories alive. Mrs. J. may be thinking about how
else one can recall one's life. Does she have to be near to drowning
to find out? This could be another reference to her wondering
whether there would be time enough for that, perhaps also alluding
to the planned ending of her therapy.

We might think of the father/son relationship. If we apply
symmetry to this too, we are hearing about a *parent/child relationship*. Does this only refer to her son and his dead father? Could it
also refer to herself as a child, and her father? (Her own father had
died of a heart attack when she was twelve.) She may well be
identifying with her son and his experience. They had both lost a
father, at a similar age and in a similar way. We can wonder about
the transference. Is the therapist representing her father here, who
is about to be lost to Mrs. J. before she is ready? The pattern of loss
is apparent in all three sectors of her life, as if there were some
unstoppable repetition operating. We can see this in her
childhood, in her marriage, and now in her therapy—as it might
seem to her.

Is this premature ending of therapy really so unstoppable? Has
the therapist been going along with this as inevitable? Mrs. J. could
in fact get to London quite easily. It is only an hour away from her
new home. Perhaps the therapist is referred to in the dream, as the
person hesitating to rescue someone who is drowning.

Choice of Interpretation: Some Examples

There are of course many possible responses to this material. Part
of the work of internal supervision is to assess which could best
serve the interests of the patient and of the therapeutic process. I
shall give different possibilities, enlarging upon the options that

might flash through my mind if I were to allow myself a "period of hesitation" (Winnicott 1958: Chapter 4) before intervening.

Therapists need time to reflect, but the human mind can also work very quickly (like that of a drowning person) as long as the therapist is not himself feeling drowned by the quantity (or impact) of what a patient is saying. If he is feeling overwhelmed, it is often more useful to listen first to the form of the communication (its sheer weight or volume) before he risks getting lost in the detailed *content.*

Relating Details to the Therapy

A fairly common kind of interpretation here would be to play back the detail of the patient's communication, relating this to the therapy. But, when this is too all-embracing, it becomes like a lecture not an interpretation. For instance I have heard some responses to a patient that went something like:

> "I think you would like me to be a clairvoyant, so that I could lessen your anxiety by knowing how things will be for you in the future. Also, as with the book that you have only begun to read, you may be wondering what is being left 'unread' by leaving your therapy early. We now do not have time to look more thoroughly at your past life, or your future; so it may be that in your dream you could be the drowning person, which suggests that I am represented as the person who is hesitating to dive in to rescue you. Instead of having further therapy you plan to read Proust to yourself, which could be your attempt to be a therapist to yourself, recovering what you can of your past life and doing this on your own."

This covers most of what the patient has said, and brings it quite neatly together around the therapy. It may even be that it is all correct. Internal supervision, however, would help us to recognize that it lacks focus. This becomes even clearer if we use trial identification. What could a patient's response be to this? Suppose she were to say "Yes" to this long interpretation, what would she be saying "Yes" to?

We might also pick up a sense of the patient being bombarded by such an all-embracing interpretation. The patient could either be impressed by the skill of the therapist, in being able to fit everything together like this (if it did fit), or she could feel irritated by the basic assumption that everything is being related to the therapist as if it were bound to be so.

This style of interpretation is unlikely to enhance the therapeutic process. It leaves no room for the patient to offer leads of her own, towards distinguishing which part of what she has communicated is most urgent to her at this point in the session.

A Full Transference Interpretation

What I am here calling a *full* transference interpretation is that in which it is possible to bring together the three elements that are usually linked in a dynamically complete interpretation of transference: (a) the patient's present life; (b) the therapeutic relationship; (c) the patient's past. (NB: It is often forgotten that it may take several sessions, or even weeks, before a full transference interpretation can be convincingly offered to a patient, whether based on a dream or other communications.) A transference interpretation here could be formed by linking together the following elements in the patient's current experience: in her present life (the ongoing impact of her husband's death); in her childhood (the death of her father); and in the therapeutic relationship (the impending end). We could therefore interpret:

> "You are concerned with a repeating pattern of premature endings: the death of your husband, and in your childhood of your father, and now I may have come to represent husband *and* father as we approach the ending of your therapy."

Many therapists would accept this kind of interpretation as applicable, and perhaps as necessary, here. It is more focused than the previous example, because it draws upon a fuller abstracting of the themes, and it offers a single integration of these around the focus upon premature endings.

Our internal supervision, however, should point out the predictability of such an interpretation. It is almost a standard comment, and patients who have had regular interpretations of this kind expect the therapist to do exactly this again, with almost whatever they say. Trial-identifying with the patient can prompt us to recognize when a patient could reply: "I thought you might say that." This is not proof of the accuracy of an interpretation so much as of the expectability of it. And therapists do not need to tell patients what they already know.

In this session, it is possible that the patient might be able to use this particular transference interpretation because it has impact. The fact that the therapy does not have to end could emerge out of this. Equally, the patient might recognize, perhaps for the first time, the extent to which the death of her husband has come to be reenacted within the therapy even to the extent of the patient setting up a premature ending of the treatment.

My main reservation, in this instance, would be to do with the timing. It would carry more conviction, if the therapist were to wait until it becomes clearer that the patient is needing this kind of interpretation. Here it could appear to be arrived at more by rule of thumb.

The Deepest Anxiety

Another possible interpretation, aimed at the patient's deepest anxiety in this sequence, could be to pick out the unconscious implications of the dream. (We need to know that Mrs. J. had repeatedly been angry with the hospital and the doctors, that they had not done more to save her husband's life.)

It is possible to see a reference in the dream to some life-saving action that is withheld. We could wonder about Mrs. J.'s earlier signs of projected guilt, in blaming others. (The therapist had previously heard her pleading that she had not realized that a mild heart attack could be so quickly and fatally repeated. She had thought that her husband had recovered more than he had. She had been relieved when they had been able to resume a normal life, after he had recovered from his first heart attack.)

We could wonder about Mrs. J.'s unconscious guilt, and her possible collusion with her husband's resumed level of normal activity. Had she been blaming herself for not having taken the risk to his life more seriously? Does the drowning girl (in the dream) represent her husband whose life had been at risk? Does the dream represent her husband as a girl because the undisguised truth here could have been too painful to the patient? If we think this to be so, and if we believe that the patient needs to face this pain along with her unconscious guilt, we could say:

> "I think that you are blaming yourself for what you see as your part in your husband's death, as if you feel there might have been something you could have done to have saved him from this. So, in the dream, there is a person that you recognize as drowning but you wake up to reality before you have acted upon this."

Here there is a technical problem. If a therapist prematurely interprets some assumed unconscious guilt, he can be experienced by the patient as suggesting that she should feel guilty. If he claims to see evidence of unconscious guilt, or the assumed cause of such guilt, before the patient begins to be aware of this, that assumption of the therapist can no longer be regarded merely as the patient's projection or transference.

By using trial identification, we can assess more sensitively whether this patient is actually indicating a readiness for an exploration of possible unconscious guilt; or might this focus for interpretation merely induce guilt without leaving time, in this session or even in the remaining therapy, for it to be worked through? Our listening to that possible intervention, from the position of the patient, might prompt us to remain cautious and not yet to offer any interpretation aimed at her supposed unconscious guilt.

Finding a Bridge to an Interpretation

It is important that therapists should find ways to interpret to patients, which do not interfere with the drift of their own emerging thoughts. It is also important that they do not preempt a patient's experience, by interrupting what he or she is beginning to feel, or by anticipating what is not yet being felt by the patient. It will often be the case, therefore, that therapists do not have sufficient evidence for any interpretation as such. This does not mean that they ask questions to elicit the evidence they lack. Equally it does not always mean that they just remain in silence until further information emerges. Sometimes a patient is better able to continue if a therapist simply indicates that he has been following.

So, instead of interpreting, there are occasions when a therapist has to look for an intermediate step that brings to a manageable focus what has been said so far. This should maintain as fully as possible the patient's freedom to continue in any direction, rather than in a direction indicated by comments from the therapist.

Here, for instance, we cannot assume that the reference to drowning necessarily relates to the therapy more than to anything else. If the therapist had forgotten, or did not know, that this patient was currently approaching the anniversary of her husband's death, it would be a hurtful assumption to presume that her distress was to do mainly with her therapist. It might therefore be preferable, at this point in the session, not to assume any reference to the therapist even if it might be around. Instead we could look for a more neutral way of playing back the themes to her.

We can note the theme of things that are unfinished. We can also recognize a sense of urgency in the dream. We could therefore show that we are aware of this by saying something like:

"Running through what you have told me, I notice that there are several references to things left unfinished; and there is also a sense of urgency in the dream about a person who might be drowning."

From a neutral playback such as this, the patient could lead on to the issue of whether or not to end her therapy; or she could surprise us by leading straight into the anniversary mourning. This may, or may not, subsequently come to be linked to the proposed ending of her therapy. If it is not, we might again feel it to be important that we offer a way of leaving the patient to find this for herself, preferably without her being directed to it. A further bridge comment, which might serve that purpose, could be:

"One question, that you may be asking yourself in your dream, is whether all endings have to be unstoppable and final. There is a fast-flowing river which cannot be stopped, but it may be possible to rescue the girl from drowning. "

The Most Urgent Anxiety

One way of focusing an interpretation here would be around the sense of urgency, which is clearly indicated in the dream. Some action is called for, to save someone from drowning. The most immediate context for this dream is likely to be the fact that the time for therapy is running out.

If we feel that the patient is needing to recognize the self-destructiveness in her premature ending of therapy, and there is not much time left to deal with this, we might say to the patient:

"I think you are anxious about the approaching end of your therapy. Time is running out, as things stand, and you may be wondering whether I will do anything to prevent what (in your dream) is represented as a drowning."

Our trial identification here might still prompt us to pause before offering this interpretation. The patient may be waiting for the therapist to stop her leaving. If he were to act upon this wish she could experience this as manipulative—even as a seductive move by him. She might get to this on her own, from a half-interpretation as described in the preceding section (pp. 44–5).

The therapist would have to balance the possible gains or losses for this patient. If he does not preempt her recognition of the need for her therapy to continue, she might arrive at this for herself and could accept any decision to continue therapy more clearly as her own. On the other hand, if the patient's self-destructiveness is being denied, it would amount to a collusion if the therapist were to sit back passively without challenging her. He would have to assess the patient's readiness to recognize the self-destructiveness for herself, or her degree of unconscious resistance to seeing this, before deciding upon whether to confront her. Depending upon the particular patient, quite different courses here might be preferred.

I have offered five contrasting ways of responding to this material, and of course there are others. No therapist could consciously explore so many options (even silently) within an ongoing session unless a patient happens to allow time for this. Nevertheless, some of this reflection might be fleetingly noted, even if only at a preconscious level. It is always important that therapists learn to recognize alternative ways in which they might respond.

I have given a sample of what I am calling "playing scales" with clinical material, in order to illustrate some of the technical issues. If a therapist does not rush in to interpret, internal supervision can more easily process the options that are available and the implications of each.

FROM SUPERVISOR TO INTERNAL SUPERVISION

The shift from an initial dependence upon the external supervisor, via the internalized supervisor, to a more autonomous internal supervision is a slow process—and at times it will not be steady. To illustrate some stages in this development I will give a brief clinical example of each.

Internal Supervision Being Absent

Example 2.2
A patient was being seen in therapy three times a week with a male therapist. She spent the first half of a session swamping her therapist with details of depression, promiscuous sexuality, scenes of violence, etc. There was a general feeling of no containment or control anywhere.

The therapist stayed silent, unable to find any meaningful way into the session. The patient then left the session to go to the toilet, which she always did at least once in every session. Upon returning, she closed the consulting room door and appeared to change the subject.

Comment: The therapist might have been able to find release from his sense of paralysis if he had commented on the form of this patient's communication, her pouring out of details and her need to relieve herself of anxiety (in the toilet), as indicating her fear that her therapist could not offer the relief or the containment she was so urgently in search of.

The session continued as follows:

> PATIENT: I cannot sleep unless I have the windows and doors all tight shut.
>
> THERAPIST: Was your mother like that?
>
> PATIENT: Yes... (*Lots of details followed.*)

Comment: Important opportunities for following the patient can be lost when a therapist diverts the session by introducing a new focus of attention. So, when a therapist points the patient to the past (as in a transference interpretation), it is as well to check whether he or she could be taking refuge from stress in the session by a defensive maneuver of flight to the past.

Discussion: Upon presenting this material in supervision, the therapist had initially been pleased with the wealth of new detail from his patient's childhood, which followed from this single question. After all, therapists are told that one indication of an effective interpretation is that new material emerges from the patient. If, however, we follow this sequence from an interactional viewpoint, suspending our trial identification equally between therapist and patient, we arrive at a quite different formulation of this exchange.

Before the therapist's first intervention we can see that the patient's behavior in the session was similar to her life outside. She was pouring out detail, as discharge rather than as a communication, and the themes were of noncontainment, both sexual and aggressive. My trial identification with the therapist here highlights the pressure he is under from the patient. The patient then leaves the session, to get rid of her discomfort into the toilet. This is further discharge of unease through action. There is no containment.

Upon resuming her session, the patient's first communication (nonverbal and verbal) had to do with doors and windows. These could be symbols for the containment she is needing. She points out that, for her, they have to be firmly closed if she is to feel secure. However, the therapist thinks that he is being given a cue to explore this "symptomatic behavior" in terms of the patient's childhood so he asks about the patient's mother.

If we again listen to this interactionally, we can sense the therapist's unconscious communication to the patient. There are a number of qualities to this particular question. It puts a pressure on the patient to answer it. (Is the therapist feeling under pressure; and he is reversing this onto the patient, i.e. unconsciously retaliating?) It deflects the patient from the present to the past. (Is the therapist needing a breather from what had been around in the session up until then?) It deflects the patient away from the therapist onto the patient's mother. (Is there something that is uncomfortable for the therapist to stay with, in the therapeutic relationship?) These are all possible reasons for him resorting here to a deflection of the focus in the session.

When the patient follows the unconscious lead given to her by the therapist, she may be joining him in a shared search for relief from something that *both* could have been finding difficult to cope with in the present. If the therapist were using his own trial identification he might have been prompted to reassess this sequence. The patient is responding to a deflective lead provided by the therapist.

The willing production of new detail here therefore does not indicate an intuitively apt question. It could instead be evidence of a shared defense, the therapist and patient together moving off to past history where feelings are more distant and where the details discussed do not refer specifically *either* to the patient *or* to the therapist. Talking about the mother's pathology can become a collusive avoidance of the present, and of the relationship between the patient and therapist—not all of which is transference. It will also be noticed by the patient that this avoidance of the present has been instigated by the therapist, with the result that what had been difficult for the patient to contain could be seen as uncontainable by therapist and patient alike.

Using the Internalized Supervisor

Example 2.3

A therapist seeing a male patient early in therapy found herself being overactive in several sessions. This seemed to be in response to a characteristic passivity with which this patient had approached life, including the question of referral for therapy.

In the session immediately prior to the therapist coming for supervision, the following interchange took place:

PATIENT: I can't remember where we left off at the end of the last session.

THERAPIST: Perhaps if you let your mind wander you will be able to remember.

During the supervision I had said that this reply could confirm the patient's impression that he should try to link one session with the other. The notion of staying with the present, whatever that may lead to, is not yet clear to this patient.

The next session began as follows:

PATIENT: I am trying to let my mind wander, to see if that helps me to remember the last session. I'm not sure that it's going to work for me.

THERAPIST: I may have given you a misleading impression in what I said last time. What I meant to say was that it doesn't matter in therapy whether one session clearly links up with the previous one, or not. You can start anywhere, and we can see where it goes.

PATIENT: Well, I am now thinking about learning to swim with my older sister helping me. She knew just when to hold me and when to let go, so that I could begin to swim on my own. The same happened when I was learning to ride a bicycle. She started by holding the steering wheel for me, and the saddle. She later just held the saddle while I steered; and then she began to let go until I was riding on my own.

Discussion: This patient responded immediately with memories that related to the need to shift from someone steering or holding him (both being forms of controlling) to letting go—so that he could be free to use the psychotherapeutic process more autonomously and actively than had been happening hitherto.

This example illustrates a therapist drawing upon her previous supervision (using the "internalized supervisor"). In recognizing and responding to the patient's cue, in this next session, she also shows that she is beginning to develop and to use her own internal supervision.

Using Internal Supervision

In order to point to the use of internal supervision in settings other than just therapy and analysis, I include here a vignette from my own earlier experience as a social worker.

Example 2.4
Teddy, as his mother called him, was twenty-four when I first met him. For two years he had been treated at home, on stelazine, as a catatonic

schizophrenic. He had formerly been treated in a mental hospital until his mother insisted on having him back home.

Teddy's mother asked me to see him because she felt it might be possible to begin getting through to him; he had started to give single-word answers to questions. I agreed to see him once a week. His mother began to bring him to my office, leading him by the hand, and she would then wait downstairs until he was ready to go home. It was as if he were a toddler being taken to playschool.

During the first few weeks I was able to get three different one-word responses from Teddy: "Yes," "No" and "Not really." From these answers, and by asking specific leading questions, I was able to gather from him that he had a brother four years younger than himself. I was also able to get some details about his home and school, and the fact that he had had a job for two years after leaving school. For some reason that was unclear he had been dismissed from that job, since when he had remained permanently not speaking.

Internal supervision: Although it could be thought that I was making progress with Teddy, by getting these details out of him, I became very uneasy about the nature of the interaction between myself and him. Nothing seemed to be achieved during my attempts at using silence with him: nothing other than factual information was being gained through this active questioning.

I imagined myself in his place, wondering what it might be like having a social worker intermittently firing questions at me like that. It soon struck me how persecutory that could be. It was as if I were trying to force myself through Teddy's near total exclusion of the outside world: and his mode of answering seemed to be a compromise between his need to defend himself from intrusion and the pressures (from me) for him to speak. I resolved to try a different approach.

When Teddy next came to my office I had moved our chairs from their previous position (almost face to face) to being more nearly parallel. When we were seated I began to speak—half to Teddy and half to myself.

SOCIAL WORKER: I have arranged the chairs differently today for a reason that I will try to explain. I have been thinking how it might feel being you here, with a social worker who has been firing all these questions at you. I have also wondered if it might be easier for us both if I didn't sit so directly opposite you—looking as if I am expecting you to look back at me. (*Silence.*)

When I imagine being in your place, with all those questions coming at me, I feel as if someone were trying to get inside me—forcing me to give away bits of myself that I might not want to give away. (*Silence.*) I have an image of being surrounded by people trying to force me to talk, and wanting to hide from them. I can also imagine myself not talking to anyone, as a way of trying to build a wall around me to keep people out. (*Pause.*)

Unfortunately, until today, I have been failing to recognize that you might be needing to keep up a wall of silence as a way of keeping me out and at a safe distance. (*Teddy turned his head towards me with a look of interest.*)

TEDDY: It's funny you put it like that. I have often thought of myself as hiding under a manhole cover, in a drain, with people trying to find me—and sewage down below. I'm not afraid of drains. It's people that smell. They make it difficult for me to breathe. My mother suffocates me. She treats me like a little boy. I am really a man inside, you know. She doesn't realize that.

I was astonished. Teddy had been almost entirely silent for over two years. The only exceptions had been his single-word answers, with which he had parried questions from those around him. Now, quite unexpectedly, he was beginning to express his own thoughts and feelings.

Discussion: By putting myself in his place, I had come to recognize Teddy's need for his defensive withdrawal. Only when I stopped being an "impinging object" could he begin to feel free to reach out to me—as someone he could begin to relate to. In particular, I had to be aware of his need for space and separateness in a world that had become persistently intrusive. Like other people, I had originally responded to his silence by also becoming intrusive. It was only by using trial identification, to monitor his experience of me, that I became aware of the nature of this interaction.

We still had far to go beyond this beginning, but it was a start that Teddy was able to build upon. After six months he persuaded his mother to desist from bringing him. Thereafter he always came on his own, and he began to use his sessions spontaneously without any leading from me. In the second year he found himself a job in a toy shop. There he could relate to parents and children on his own terms.

In the rest of this book I shall give other illustrations of internal supervision being used clinically, or missing. I hope also to show how this process needs to settle into a background level of functioning. Too active a preoccupation of self-monitoring can disturb the free-floating attention (see Chapter 5). But, there are many times too when the analytic work can be rescued from foundering by learning to sense how a patient could be experiencing the therapist, in the kind of ways that I have been describing.

❖ 3 ❖

Internal Supervision: A Lapse and Recovery

In this chapter I wish to show how patients respond to a therapist's errors. The example I shall give is of a time when I failed to remain in a professional role. We will see how the patient gives unconscious prompts towards a recovery of the therapy when this is in danger of collapse.

I shall also use this clinical sequence to demonstrate the different clinical perspectives that are opened up when one examines the therapeutic relationship from a viewpoint that takes into account the unconscious interaction between patient and therapist, in which each is responding to cues from the other.

AN INTERACTIONAL VIEWPOINT OUTLINED

Since the papers on countertransference by Heimann (1950) and Little (1951), it has been increasingly recognized that the analytic relationship is one in which there are two people interacting. Each is seeking to get to know the other. Consciously or unconsciously each is affecting the other. This dimension to the analytic relationship is implicit (and sometimes explicit) throughout the writings of such authors as Balint, Winnicott, Bion, Sandler and Searles, to name just a few. Langs, on the other hand, has made an extensive study of these phenomena.[1]

It is no longer adequate to think of the analyst as the one who observes and interprets, and the patient as the only person in this relationship who presents evidence of unconscious communications and pathology. Patients do not see the analyst as a blank screen. They scrutinize the analyst, who aims to remain inscrutable, and they find many clues to the nature of this person they are dealing with. They sense the state of mind of the analyst and respond accordingly.

Analysts and therapists often give away more about themselves than they realize. They might not speak openly about themselves, and they can be careful about personal questions, but they do not remain a closed book to the patient. Like a child who watches the mother's face for signs of pleasure or indications of mood, patients listen for similar signs from the therapist and there are many available.

Patients monitor changes in the manner of the therapist's presence, for instance his state of relaxation or his fidgeting in sessions. They also note the unconscious implications indicated by the nature of his comments. These interventions are not always interpretive—making conscious what is emerging from the patient's unconscious. They may be directive, suggesting what the patient should do or feel; or intrusive, as with questions; or they may be deflective, inviting a change of focus, which can suggest that the therapist is avoiding something difficult in the session.

Patients notice the selection and timing of the therapist's interventions. They ask themselves why this is commented on and not that, and why the therapist intervenes when he does, rather than sooner or later (or not at all). Patients also pick up the therapist's anxiety when he is overactive or interruptive in a session. Likewise they wonder about prolonged silences, particularly when a flood of the patient's strong feelings has been expressed. Has the therapist been overwhelmed by the patient?

At least unconsciously, and sometimes consciously, patients will be interpreting the therapist to themselves. They even offer unconscious interpretations to the therapist (Little 1951: 381). When the therapist is seen as defensive he is also seen as feeling threatened. This raises anxiety about his capacity to contain the patient. One response is for the patient to behave protectively towards the therapist, by displacing more difficult feelings onto others, or introjectively against themselves. A patient's more hopeful response challenges the therapist's defensiveness, drawing his attention to whatever appears to be amiss. Patients always note the degree to which a therapist is ready to stay in touch with what is being communicated. So, it is important that therapists recognize elements of objective reality in the consulting room to which a patient could be responding. It is here in particular that trial identification offers valuable insight to the therapist.

Whenever I say something in therapy, or continue to say nothing, I am having an effect upon the patient. I therefore need to listen for the patient's responses to my input, some of which initially may be beyond my immediate consciousness. Listening to myself in the place of the patient can help to bring the dynamics of this interaction more into the field of my awareness.

Frequently, patients show a double response to a therapist's contribution to a session. At one level they respond to the external reality; at another they elaborate on it in terms of past experience and their inner reality. So, even when a patient's responses can be considered as transference, these are often initiated by external triggers in the session from the therapist (see Chapter 5).

It follows that I often cannot understand what a patient is trying to communicate to me until I can identify the nature of my own contributions in a session to which a patient may be responding. When I can identify the trigger(s) to a patient's responses I am able to understand the patient differently and (I believe) more pertinently. Therefore, like a blind man, I try to listen for the different kinds of echo that are reflected back to me from each step that I take in a session. This is how I think of an interactional viewpoint to listening. It helps me to be in touch with my own effects upon a patient as distinct from what arises more autonomously from within the patient. I also try to monitor the patient's effects upon me. The use of an interactional viewpoint is implicit throughout this book. I outline it here because I give specific examples in this chapter, and in Chapter 5, of my own early attempts at using this way of listening to patients. I shall look more extensively at the nature of patients' unconscious cues and prompts in Chapter 8.

INTRODUCTION TO THE CLINICAL PRESENTATION

The clinical work I use to illustrate the theme of this chapter was undertaken at a time when I had not yet worked out my thoughts as in Chapter 2; so I had not established internal supervision as a regular process in my listening. Previously, I had used this mainly when I knew that I was under stress, or when the patient was in crisis; I still had to learn that there is an additional need for self-monitoring at times when the therapy seems to be going well. What follows, therefore, are two occasions of countertransference folly.

Whenever a therapist acts upon his countertransference, there is a need for self-analysis to understand what has been happening and why. There is also a need to attend to the disruptive effects of this upon the therapy. Here an interactional view to listening turns out to be particularly helpful, the more so as I was not being supervised on this case at the time reported. We will see how the patient indicates the various levels at which she was responding to my stepping out of role. She also demonstrates how perceptively she had been following my part in her sessions.

Had I remained unaware of acting out my countertransference, my intrusive behavior could have brought this therapy to an abrupt and destructive close. Fortunately, I was able to recover from this lapse through recognizing the patient's unconscious prompts. I could easily have missed the significance of these cues, if I had not already become aware of the ways in which patients can reflect their valid perceptions of the therapist's unconscious (Langs 1978).

BACKGROUND TO SESSION[2]

Mrs. A. was in her sixties when she entered once-a-week therapy. She was referred for severe anxiety attacks with a history of manic-depressive mood swings. Initially, therapy had failed to contain the patient, and she was hospitalized. Lithium carbonate therapy was begun by the psychiatrist, who took over the treatment. Later, at the request of Mrs. A., I was asked to resume her psychotherapy while she was still in hospital. This began to be more meaningful to her and she was discharged from the hospital. Not long afterwards, her wish for the medication to be discontinued was also agreed to.

Mrs. A. began to make significant progress in many areas of her life. The anxiety attacks ceased over a period of two years, and there was no reoccurrence of the earlier uncontrollable mood swings. The patient was pleased with her progress and so was I. This situation, however, led to a more relaxed relationship, with me "soft-pedalling" during a period that seemed to be a prelude to ending therapy. At the time, I rationalized this shift towards a more realistic and mutual relationship in terms of my residual belief that it might enable the transference relationship to be worked through and relinquished more easily. I no longer believe that. It was a left-over from my earlier work, as social worker and as inexperienced therapist.

What I did not know at this time was that the patient was

approaching a crisis in her marriage. Stresses had been developing at home because her husband had relied upon his wife's readiness to avoid conflict by her dutiful compliance to his wishes and demands. During therapy Mrs. A. had discovered that she could stand up for herself with her husband, even if doing so led to conflict, but this growth in her was creating pressures for change in the marriage. There had been hints of this problem in the past, but a more direct presentation of these marital difficulties was postponed until I had attended to the period of professional laxity here described.

RECENT BREAKS IN THE THERAPEUTIC FRAME[3]

About two months prior to the session to be quoted, Mrs. A. had been praising her dentist (Dr. X.). Even though it meant traveling a long distance to see him, she had been treated by this same man for years, as he had always been careful and thorough in his work. Recently she had been able to combine her weekly visits for therapy with going to this dentist, whose surgery was just down the road from my consulting rooms.

Here I fell into a countertransference gratification as a result of my own need for a good dentist. I felt tantalized by the patient's unsolicited testimonial of her dentist, and asked her if she would mind giving me his name as I was looking for a reliable dentist for myself. Mrs. A. readily gave this and said she was glad to be of help. She hoped that I would find Dr. X. as good as she always had.

Comment: We will see later a typical split between the patient's conscious pleasure at being able to be of help and her unconscious resentment at the implications of this request for *her* attention to *my* needs. We will also see how one exception often leads to another.

Two sessions before the one to be presented, I asked the patient for another favor. Mrs. A. had been speaking of her occasional difficulty in getting to sleep, and of how useful she had found a relaxation tape to be. This tape was so effective for her that she had never yet heard it to the end it as she was always asleep by then. I said I would be interested in hearing this tape. Mrs. A. replied by saying that she could tell me where I could get it. She then correctly assessed that I was hinting at borrowing *her* tape. She said that perhaps I would prefer to hear it before making the commitment of buying a copy for myself. She offered to bring it with her the next week to lend to me. Her husband could make her a copy in case she needed to use it while I had the original.

Comment: My listening has veered completely away from the patient. As with the earlier reference to her good dentist, I am responding like an envious child. Each time Mrs. A. indicates that she has something good, I have wanted some of it for myself and I have asked the patient to provide it for me. The patient is unlikely to miss the unconscious implications here concerning difficulties I might be having in managing something in myself. She may be wondering whether I am telling her that I too am having sleeping problems, as I seem to be asking her obliquely to help me with this. My countertransference gratification is clearly evident.

I thanked Mrs. A. and accepted her offer. She brought the tape to her next session; and her last words in that session were: "I don't know why, but to-day doesn't seem to have been as helpful as I had hoped."

Comment: I have not yet responded to the patient's unconscious efforts to alert me to this role-reversal; and my accepting the loan of the tape, even after having had a week to reflect on the implications of this action, could confirm the patient's fear that I have not yet recognized my need to attend to something wrong in the therapy. It also demonstrates a continuing lack of alertness in my self-supervision. Her closing words express a sense of disappointment about the session. This time, however, I notice her unconscious prompt and I am able to make use of it in the following session.

THE SESSION

Mrs. A. came in and sat down. I handed back the tape and thanked her for letting me listen to it. I made no further reference to this, not wanting to lead into a discussion about it, and neither did she. She put the tape on the table between us and left it there throughout the session.

Internal supervision: By leaving the tape on the table the patient could be indicating that this remains an issue to be attended to.

Mrs. A. proceeded to show me a new Bible, which her husband had just given to her for a wedding anniversary present. Her husband knew that it was just what she wanted. I looked at it briefly and handed it back to her, saying that it was certainly a very beautiful Bible.

Internal supervision: I am still caught into the quasi-social relationship, which I had initiated earlier. The patient demonstrates a split response. She uses the same kind of break in the frame, handing something else to me for my approval. We may also speculate that Mrs. A. has become concerned about my seductiveness, in my neglect of the usual professional boundaries, and this could be why she is symbolically bringing her husband in here. She may be reminding me that she is a married woman.

> Mrs. A. said she had had a terrible week and could not think why. Nevertheless, she had been able to sleep every night except the last. She had been using her copy of the relaxation tape, made for her by her husband, but the previous night she had not used it because she was afraid she might not wake up in time and could miss her session.

Internal supervision: The patient may be rebuking me for having caused her to sleep badly. There could also be some wish to miss the session expressed in her anxiety about oversleeping.

> Mrs. A. said she could not remember what had happened during the last session. She went on to say that she had had a fall during the week. She had thought for a moment that there might have been something wrong with *her,* that she could have had a blackout; but she came to realize that this was not what had happened. She had tripped over a badly laid paving-stone: "It was very uneven and dangerous. It really isn't safe leaving pavements in that condition. So many people fall over them, and some get seriously hurt, but the authorities always find ways to shelve the blame. They still don't do anything to put it right."

Internal supervision: The patient may be commenting on my recent behavior. Has she introjected my own tripping up? And has this come to be enacted in her falling, she wondering at first whether it might have been *her* fault? She later realized that it was not something wrong with herself, but was due to the unevenness of what she had been walking on. This feels like an unconscious reference to the unevenness of my work with her, and my failure to maintain a sufficiently secure basis for the therapy. The patient points out that this unevenness could be dangerous. The themes continue around blame being shelved and nothing being done about it. If this does refer unconsciously to the unevenness of my recent work, the patient may be expressing her fear that nothing will be done about putting things right.

> Mrs. A. continued by saying that over the weekend she had suddenly developed a terrible abscess under the root of a front tooth, that resulted

in the worst pain she had ever experienced. She had phoned Dr. X. (the dentist), and he had told her to come right over. She went to see him that Monday. He had examined her carefully and said that she certainly had an abscess; but there was nothing wrong with her tooth, so she must be run down or something. She could not think why this should be so. True, she said, she had gone away to St. Mary's Rest Home recently, hoping to come away feeling much better, but she had left there feeling just the same.

(Note: As I recognized that it was an important session in this therapy, I made notes on the clinical sequence immediately afterwards. At this point they continue verbatim—as far as I could recall what was actually said. I quote direct from those notes.)

> PATIENT: I'll say this for Dr. X., he did something they don't often seem to do nowadays. When there's poison there underneath I think it is better to lance it, or in some other way to help the poison to come out, and that is exactly what he did. He removed a filling, which allowed the abscess to drain out, and it feels much better now. He gave me penicillin too, which probably helps, but it always makes me feel terribly exhausted. Doctors often just give you a pill, or whatever, and expect that to deal with the problem without doing anything more about it.

Internal supervision: The patient now speaks of work done thoroughly, where the root-cause of something wrong is radically and carefully dealt with. She compares this with other more casual ways of dealing with patients. Mrs. A. reports having fallen, and then developing this abscess, but she continues to look for proper treatment. It is also worth noting that an earlier break in the frame, concerning the dentist, had been left unattended to and may be alluded to here.

Comment: If this contrast is thought of as referring to the therapy, it is not surprising that therapists are not always willing to recognize their work reflected by patients in ways like this.

> THERAPIST: I believe you are pointing out to me some of what has been wrong with your recent sessions. Last week you had come expecting that something troubling you would be properly attended to. You left feeling that the session had not been helpful.
>
> PATIENT: I didn't think I was criticizing you in what I was saying, but I suppose it is possible that I was. I don't claim to be much good at understanding these things.

Internal supervision: The patient is prepared to consider that she could be expressing criticism of me. She speaks of herself as not claiming to be much good at understanding these things. This may be a further introjective reference to me as a therapist who does claim to understand these things, but lately has been failing to do so.

> PATIENT: I've got some good news to tell you. Although John [her husband] and Anne [her daughter] are both being rather difficult still, James [her son] has been a great help. An old lady's electric kettle had not been working. She had taken it to the Electricity Board repair-desk, where she was told it needed a new heating element and this would cost £4 if someone else could fit it for her, or £10 if she left it at the desk.

(Note: It so happened that the patient's fee was also £10 per session.)

The patient continued:

> The old lady could not afford to pay that, so she had offered it to Anne for her annual charity bring-and-buy sale. James offered to look at the kettle, and shortly afterwards came back with it mended. He'd seen that the flex was all rotten, and needed renewing, and the plug was also cracked in two places. He'd replaced the flex and the plug, and the kettle was working perfectly. James now plans to see what other electrical things this old lady has that might have dangerous flexes or plugs, and he will be checking everything over for her. It could have been lethal. Fancy someone at the Electricity Board not seeing that this was wrong, and handing it back in that condition! They of all people should have known better. I suppose nowadays there are lots of people who don't do a proper job. They just sit back and take the money, and don't bother about the consequences.

Internal supervision: The themes remain the same—jobs not done properly; faults are left that could be lethal—and there are references to more than a single fault being revealed upon proper inspection; and we hear of people (who should know better) failing to recognize what is wrong. It happens that there is more than one break in the usual boundaries to therapy, which were still needing to be dealt with. I also note this reference to money being taken for poor work. As this session is the last of the month, and the patient would be expecting to receive the monthly account, it is difficult not to feel that she is making some reference to me here—seeing me as recently having been sitting back in the therapy.

> THERAPIST: You are giving me more examples of jobs not being done properly, because people do not bother to see what is wrong, compared with James taking the trouble to look into what was wrong and putting right those faults that could have been seriously dangerous or even lethal. I think you are still wondering whether I am bothering to do a

proper job here, or am I just sitting back and taking the money without adequately dealing with what is wrong.

PATIENT: Well, now that you come to point this out, I have been wondering about the way in which you work. For instance, it is like a machine; let's say a tape recorder (and she looks at the tape on the side-table), where something is wrong so that only some of what is being said is recorded. When you play it back, there are bits that are so faint you cannot hear it properly. Now, take something like my visits to St. Mary's. I know you know, at least I assume you know, that that is something important to me and yet you don't ask me about it. I might go on for a whole session to see if you will, but you don't. So when you don't, I'm not sure if you really care. On the other hand, I have assumed it must be because you want to leave me room to say what else may be on my mind. But you do sometimes ask. For instance, you always asked about my leg after my accident, and would offer me the footstool when I was having to keep my leg up as much as possible.

Internal supervision: The patient has been following my way of working very closely, and has been trying to understand why I work in this way. In particular, she is trying to understand why I have been inconsistent. She indicates the tape as a part of what is wrong. She goes on from there to give an example of a listening machine that is not functioning properly. There is a strong impression that these may be derivative references to my lapses in attention, my recent failures to listen adequately. The patient goes on to wonder whether I care. In her example, she refers to a time when I had been functioning more appropriately, leaving her space to say what was on her mind; but she concludes with a further reference to my inconsistency. The offering of the footstool is also a move away from the formal therapeutic relationship, and is referred to along with the other exceptions.

THERAPIST: I think that the key to this is that you have experienced a confusing degree of unevenness in the way I have been working with you. Part of you would like me to offer a more social kind of relationship; and when I do you may be consciously glad of that, as with the footstool. But you actually need me to remain a therapist in this relationship. (*Pause.*) When I have been more clearly a therapist you have been able to make sense of what I do, so long as I have been consistent. What has been confusing to you has been when I have shifted between being therapist at one moment and being more social with you at another, thereby entering into superficial exchanges with you that result in my not listening or attending adequately to the underlying problems. My borrowing of the tape is an example of this, and it has become a further source of confusion to you.

PATIENT: I must admit I was very surprised when you said you would be interested in hearing that tape, but I thought it was nice to see you being human and to be of use to you. After all, you have been a great help to me in the past.

Internal supervision: The patient feels free to acknowledge her surprise at my behavior, now that I indicate I am prepared to look at this myself. She softens this, nevertheless, perhaps in order not to hurt me as she may not now be sure how much criticism I can take.

THERAPIST: I was not helpful to you on this occasion, as you pointed out to me at the end of the last session. You had, after all, told me where I could obtain a copy of this tape without involving you; but instead I took the short-cut of borrowing it from you. That was a break in the usual relationship here, and it has been threatening to be harmful to your therapy unless this is recognized and properly dealt with. Otherwise, as with the tooth abscess, it could fester.

PATIENT: That was another occasion when you surprised me: you said Dr. X. must be a very good dentist for me to travel all this way to see him, and you then asked me for his name. It was so unlike you to ask, but again I felt it was good to be able to be helpful to you.

Internal supervision: The patient points to each time she has felt that I have stepped out of role. She expresses a rationalized pleasure along with her surprise. The way in which she explains her pleasure includes an unconscious recognition of my having turned her into my helper, my unacknowledged therapist.

THERAPIST: So we have more than just one occasion when I can be seen as reversing roles with you, where you found yourself put into the position of having your own needs overlooked while you were being asked to attend to requests of mine. It may seem reassuring to find that I am human, and that you can be of help to me, but as far as your therapy is concerned this has led to a diversion from your reasons for coming to see me. I believe this is why you have been pointing out to me the contrast between people who do their jobs thoroughly and those who do not. When you pay me it is for me to do my job as therapist, and to do that carefully and attentively; not to have me sitting back and being social with you.

I handed her the account, which she accepted with a knowing smile showing that she understood what I had just been saying to her. This was the end of the session.

The patient returned the following week feeling reassured by the work done in the session just quoted. She began to talk about the state of her marriage, and stresses in the family, that had been alluded to briefly before but she had felt unsure about discussing these in depth. Mrs. A. confessed that she had begun to wonder whether there was any point in continuing with her therapy, but she was now relieved to find that it felt all right to go on. She was beginning to feel positive about her therapy again.

Discussion: Mrs. A. demonstrates a degree of awareness of her therapist's state of mind that can be most disconcerting. Some people might wish to regard this as unusual, but it is probably typical. A patient will monitor the therapist either quite consciously (as some patients will point out) or unconsciously. Mrs. A. has an intuitive grasp of what constitutes a secure framework for therapy. She notes every occasion when I crossed the boundaries necessary for insight-promoting psychotherapy. She unconsciously recognizes the countertransference implications of these transgressions, and in the interests of her own therapy she contributes persistent unconscious supervisory efforts (Langs 1978) towards having these dealt with.

At the point in this clinical sequence when I was sliding into a state of "countertransference neurosis" (Racker 1968) the patient shifted into the role of unconscious therapist to me (Searles 1975). Only when I began to recognize the outstanding breaks in the therapeutic boundaries did I start to listen around these as a primary issue to be attended to. It is this awareness that prompts me to focus my listening on the derivative rather than the manifest levels of the patient's communications, and that leads me eventually towards the necessary work of putting things right. As I begin to recover my role as therapist, the patient feels safe enough to point out other departures from the more usual therapeutic framework. When these are attended to, she is able to resume meaningful therapy.

❖4❖

Forms of Interactive Communication

> It is a very remarkable thing that the *Ucs.* of one
> human being can react upon that of another,
> without passing through the *Cs.*
>
> (FREUD 1915: 194)[1]

There are times when the most important communication from a
patient is unspoken. The process of a therapist's internal supervision can often help to identify this interactive dimension, so that
it begins to make sense. Patients clearly demonstrate that the
dynamics involved are by no means just theoretical, nor are they
confined to analytic therapy. The forms of communication illustrated here are universal. Too often they are not recognized or
they are seen as bewildering: the communication then remains
unacknowledged or not understood.

COMMUNICATION BY IMPACT

Patients often behave in such a way that they stir up feelings in the
therapist which could not be communicated in words. I have found
it useful to consider this form of interaction under a general
heading of *communication by impact*.

As a basic example of this, let us consider an infant's cry and the
mother's response to its impact upon her. This is one of the most
primitive ways by which one human being acts upon another, and
is reacted to. A mother's response to her crying infant is usually to
draw upon her maternal intuition, to sense the specific meaning of

this particular cry. To that end she will often put herself empathically in the infant's position, or in her own mother's position when she herself was crying in a similar way, in order to distinguish between one kind of crying and another.

In psychotherapy, therapists are often subjected to the unspoken cries of those who come to consult them. As with the mother and her infant, therapists have to be able to listen within themselves to draw upon their own experience of distress (whether that had been contained or not). If therapists persevere in their wish to understand, even when they are experiencing the confusion or pain which some patients induce in them, times will occur when the unconscious purpose of these pressures becomes apparent.

Some patients need to be able to have this kind of effect on the therapist, as an essential way of communicating what otherwise may remain unspeakable. When a therapist is able to understand the unconscious purpose of communication by impact, and can find ways of interpreting this, which help to make sense of it, then the patient can begin to feel that someone is really in touch with them—even with their own most difficult feelings.

EXPERIENCES RELATING TO ROLE-RESPONSIVENESS

I shall not attempt to define this concept prior to giving an example.

Unconscious Communication Evoked through the Therapist's Response to the Patient

Example 4.1
My first experience of being in any kind of supervisory role to another therapist was when I had just qualified as a psychotherapist. A colleague would sometimes let off steam to me by complaining about a particular patient of hers. This patient was described as coming from a good family, with parents who had maintained a good marriage, who had provided her with all that she could have needed in her childhood and in her education. The patient, however, was always complaining about her parents. She was described to me as "so persistently ungrateful" that the therapist felt exasperated, and she wondered whether she could continue to work with her. The therapist could not see that there was anything to complain about.

Discussion: I was aware of the possibility that I was hearing a straightforward example of countertransference, such as my training had taught me to beware of. It could have been that the patient had become a transferential object to the therapist, representing some unresolved conflict of her own. What I knew of the therapist made me feel that this was not unlikely: I had gathered, from what she said about her family, that she sometimes thought of her own daughters as ungrateful.

Superficially, therefore, it looked as if there could hardly be a clearer example of countertransference, as it was first described (Freud 1910: 144-45). I sensed that my colleague also thought of her response to this complaining patient as a countertransference problem, to be dealt with outside the patient's sessions. This may have been why she was venting her exasperation on me, in order not to offload this onto her patient.

However, over a period of time, it began to dawn on me that my colleague could be missing an important communication, in this attitude which was so regularly being stimulated in her by this patient. The more I thought on this the more convinced I became that there was something else here, in addition to the classical phenomenon of countertransference.

The patient may have been unable to get across what it was about her parents that she was complaining of. Instead, she seemed to have *recreated in her therapist* the kind of attitude towards herself which her parents may have had. Perhaps they (like the therapist) had been blinded by an assumption that they had provided adequately for their daughter; and yet they may have been failing to recognize important ways in which they were shutting themselves off from the unmet needs of this complaining child. In order to communicate this the patient might have been able to touch upon an available countertransference resonance in her therapist, thereby evoking *in her* similar feelings and attitudes to those of her parents. If this really were such a communication, it could be a way of picking up from the patient something of what her parents may have been missing, and which the therapist had been missing too.

So, instead of having to treat this strong response to the patient solely as something belonging elsewhere in the therapist's life (which in one sense it did), it could also be looked upon as conveying an intangible aspect of the patient's relationship to her parents, about which she had been complaining. The parents had been shut off from this patient much as the therapist had come to be. Perhaps, in response to the patient's urgent need to get this across, the therapist had become involved in an unconscious reenactment of the complained-of parents. In his paper "Countertransference and Role-Responsiveness," Sandler was later to describe this process as "actualization" (Sandler 1976).[2]

When I discussed this possibility with my colleague she was able to recognize the interactive communication here, which formerly she had been missing, and she started to listen to her patient differently. In so doing she became less shut off from the patient, and less caught up in her own feelings of intolerance towards her. Heimann (1950) and Little (1951) have both pointed out that the analyst's feeling responses to the patient may contain valuable cues to the patient's unconscious communications. Sandler illustrated how the analyst can be drawn into a behavioral interaction. In "Countertransference and Role-Responsiveness" he writes:

> I believe such "manipulations" to be an important part of object relation-ships in general.... In the transference, in many subtle ways, the patient attempts to prod the analyst into behaving in a particular way and uncon-sciously scans and adapts to his perceptions of the analyst's reaction. (Sandler 1976: 44)

It is all the more important, therefore, that we should be able to distinguish that part of a therapist's responses which offers clues to the patient's unconscious communication from that which is personal to the therapist. In order to make this distinction, at the time of the clinical episode quoted, I suggested we might speak of a "diagnostic response" as compared with a "personal counter-transference" (Casement 1973).

Boredom as Communication

Example 4.2
For some months, in the course of a long analysis, I found myself regularly feeling bored by one particular male patient. I silently explored this as fully as I could to see if my feelings were simply some personal counter-transference to my patient, as a transferential object, thinking here of countertransference in the sense described by Reich (1951). But even after this self-scrutiny, my feelings of boredom continued to occur in many of the sessions with this patient.

When I monitored this boredom more closely, I came to recognize I was responding to the fact that the patient was not relating to me. He seemed to be speaking to himself, as if I were not present; but this was not the whole of it. The patient treated me as physically present but emotion-ally absent. He was assuming that I was not interested, although this was not normally how I felt towards him. I could then see that the quality of his relating to me was as if to someone whose interest he could not engage, or who was unwilling to be engaged. This offered me a fresh clue.

What then stirred in me was a clear image of this patient at the time when he had been in a mental hospital. He had told me how his mother used to visit him regularly. She claimed to be concerned, and yet she continued to rationalize why her son had to remain in hospital. (He would have been allowed home if his parents had been prepared to look after him.)

The patient's presence in hospital was due to a prolonged agitated depression. This in turn was largely activated by the family's readiness to close ranks against this child, who had come to feel that life was not worth living. The parents did not seem to be prepared to let themselves be in touch with, or to be touched by, the patient's depression and despair—or by his need to be allowed home, rather than being left indefinitely in a mental hospital until he was "better." The parents were wanting to ignore the main reason for their son being left there. This was because he had nowhere else to go other than to his home, where his parents felt that they would not be able to cope with him in this chronic state.

With this reactivated memory as my cue, I began to wonder whether my patient might be reenacting with me the empty relating that he had so often sat through while he remained in hospital. He had talked *at* his mother, who had barely listened. His mother, in her turn, had talked *at* him rather than *to* him.

When I began to refocus my listening to the patient, in this new context, I could recognize many other indications which confirmed this impression. I became able to point out to the patient how he was speaking to me, as if he did not expect me really to be interested or to be ready to take seriously anything he said. I wondered whether this may have been how it used to be during his mother's visits to him in the hospital, which sounded as if they had been just as empty of meaningful relating.

Once I had been able to interpret this emptiness in the transference, the patient began to speak to me and to relate to me in a way that began (for the first time) to be invested with meaning. The transference stopped being a shallow relating, as if to a physically present but emotionally absent mother. Instead, the patient began to relate to me as to someone who was emotionally as well as physically present; and I stopped being troubled by boredom when I was with him.

AN EXPERIENCE OF PROJECTIVE IDENTIFICATION

Although I had struggled to understand the concept of projective identification from what I had read about it, as in Klein (1946) and Segal (1964) for example, it was not until I recognized being on the receiving end of this particular form of interactive communication that I began to understand it clinically. I shall again give an example before trying to conceptualize the dynamics illustrated.

Example 4.3
I was asked to see a couple, Mr. and Mrs. T., because of the wife's frigidity.

They were both in their thirties. For the past five years Mrs. T. had been unable to allow intercourse on account of what she described as "gynecological pain." This had been causing great stress in the marriage. There was a serious risk of the couple splitting up.

Medical examinations and tests had revealed nothing, but the referring doctor had mentioned that Mrs. T. had been sterilized three years earlier. He wondered whether this might have left post-operative adhesions. However, the gynecologist thought that it would be pointless to reopen the operation scar, as this would probably only cause fresh adhesions. She could end up no better.

In the initial consultation I saw Mr. and Mrs. T. together, as they had been referred as a couple and had asked to come for help with their marriage. Mr. T. took little part in this consultation. Mrs. T., on the other hand, told me her story. They had been married about ten years, having known each other for several years before that. They had spent the first five years of the marriage getting a house and decorating it, in preparation for beginning a family.

After this introduction, Mrs. T. told me about their two children. They had had a son and a daughter. She then told me the painful details of her discovery that there was something wrong with their first child. When he was six months old he began to scream continuously unless sedated. For nine months she nursed him until he died. Mrs. T. was seven months pregnant with their second child at the time.

After attending the funeral of her son, she "felt tearful but held it in." She had never cried since then. She just felt numb. The second child, a daughter, was also born apparently normal. She died ten months later, of the same constitutional brain disorder as had her brother. It was after this that Mrs. T. was advised to be sterilized.

Internal supervision: What was most striking, during the telling of this terrible sequence of pain and loss, was that Mrs. T.'s face and tone of voice remained wooden and lifeless. Even when she was talking of the children's illness, and slow dying, she showed no feelings at all. But my own feelings, upon listening to her, were nearly overwhelming me. I was literally crying inside.

I wondered about my response. I knew I would be moved by any account of a child's death. Was this some personal countertransference problem, only to do with me? I had to consider this as a real possibility. But, as I looked into this further, I began to realize why I was being so affected. If Mrs. T. had been crying her own tears I would not be feeling so overwhelmed. What was producing this effect upon me had something to do with her inability to show any expression of her own feelings.

I once again called upon my provisional concept of a diagnostic response. I postulated (to myself) that the intolerable pain of losing both her children in this way, followed by the sterilization (losing any chance of having other children of her own), had been too much for her. To survive these intolerable experiences, she may have converted the psychic pain belonging to them into gynecological pain. Perhaps this symptom continued to express, somatically, the repressed feelings related to those unbearable losses, which had been so closely associated with that part of her body.

Mrs. T. did much more than project her feelings onto me. She made *me* feel what *she* could not yet bear to feel consciously within herself. And the manner of this projection was not impossible to identify. I could see that it had been the patient's own lack of emotion that had been having the greatest impact upon me. As a result, I had been feeling in touch with tears which did not altogether belong to me.

> After recognizing this response in myself I was able to draw Mrs. T.'s attention to this. I said to her that there was something rather strange happening in the session. She had been telling me the details of her experience with her two children, but she had shown no feelings about this. I, on the other hand, had felt near to tears *as if for her.* She replied that she frequently needed to talk about the death of her children, but people had begged her not to as it affected them in much the same way as I had just described. She had relied upon not feeling anything about these experiences. It would probably be too painful. Instead she had kept herself active, to keep her mind occupied with other things.

Discussion: I felt sure that, if Mrs. T. could be helped to be in touch with her own crying inside, perhaps to be able to cry openly instead, she would not need her body to continue to be in pain. The subsequent course of her brief therapy fully confirmed this diagnostic impression. As she became able to bear to be in touch with the previously repressed psychic pain, her gynecological pains began to fade away. She was able to enter into the process of mourning which had been so long delayed.

PROJECTIVE IDENTIFICATION AS COMMUNICATION

Unfortunately, it is not easy to get a clear understanding of projective identification from the literature alone, as this concept has become complicated by the varied uses to which it has been put.[3] However, through the above experience and others like it, I became able to recognize clinically a part of what projective identification is about—how it happens and the unconscious purpose of it.

One of the uses of projective identification that many people experience clinically (whether they know it or not) is a form of affective communication.[4] This is especially relevant when what is being communicated is beyond words, relating to unspeakable experiences or to preverbal experience.

In order that therapists (and those in the other helping professions) may be more able to respond therapeutically when they encounter this form of unconscious communication, I shall endeavour to clarify this particular aspect of projective identification. I shall not discuss the other forms of this here, but I refer briefly to these in the footnotes. My description will therefore be incomplete, but I trust that it will be clear enough to encourage therapists to recognize the importance and implications of this key interactional dynamic. With the help of this understanding, it becomes possible to contain some patients who might otherwise remain uncontained. Without it, the meaning of the helper's feelings of stress may be misunderstood, and some patients will not find the help they look for. This frequently results in missed opportunities for better understanding of patients in distress.

I find it helpful to think of projective identification as a more powerful form of projection. It is well known that when projection (simple) is operating, the projector disowns some aspect of the self and attributes this to another. Evidence of that projection is usually to be noticed in the projector relating differently to the other person (or outside world) in terms of what has been projected. The recipient, or observer, may otherwise be quite unaware of any projection operating. What is foremost here is the projector's need to disown some aspect of himself.

When projective identification is used *as a form of affective communication,* the projector has a need (usually unconscious) to make another person aware of what is being communicated and to be responded to. The sequence is roughly as follows: (1) the projector experiences unmanageable feelings, such as an infant might have; (2) there is an unconscious fantasy of putting this unmanageable feeling-state into another person, such as the mother, for this to be disposed of or made manageable; (3) there is an interactional pressure, such as an infant's cry, with the unconscious aim of making the *other* person have these feelings instead of the infant or patient; (4) if this communication by projective identification is successful in reaching the other person, an affective resonance is created in the recipient whose feelings take on a "sameness" based on identification. This affective identification can then be thought of as being brought about projectively by the projector and introjectively by the recipient. There are several different possible results to this unconscious endeavor. If the recipient is open to the impact of the interactional behavior, or other non-verbal pressures from the projector, an affective communication is achieved. What is communicated may be to do with any state of feeling that is experienced as unmanageable by the projector; acute distress, helplessness, fear, rage, contemptuous attack upon the self, etc. The feelings being communicated are felt by the recipient.

What is then needed (for a therapeutic response to be possible) is for the recipient, the mother or the therapist, to be more able to manage being in touch with these feelings than the infant or patient had been. When this response is found, the previously unmanageable feelings become more manageable. They become less terrifying than before, because another person has actually felt them and has been able to tolerate the experience of those feelings. The projector can thereafter take back those feelings, now made more manageable; and along with this can take in something of the recipient's capacity to tolerate being in touch with difficult feelings. The unconscious hope, implied in the use of projective identification as communication, thereby meets a therapeutic response from the mother or therapist.

However, this unconscious hope is not always met. For example, if the recipient remains shut off from this attempt at communication or fails to recognize the interactive pressures as a form of communication, there will be no therapeutic response. The projector then experiences the projection as thrown back; and the unmanageable feelings being projected remain unmanageable. Likewise, if the recipient experiences (but cannot bear being subjected to) the feelings being projected, the projector will experience the recipient as thrown off balance by what is being projected; and the sense of these feelings being unmanageable is traumatically confirmed. Instead of the unconscious hope being met, there is a new state of hopelessness and despair (Bion 1967b: Chapter 9).

In Chapter 7, I present a clinical sequence which illustrates these issues more extensively.

COMMUNICATION THROUGH DEFENSIVE BEHAVIOR

One way of seeking refuge from the pain of being badly treated is to identify with the aggressor and to treat another person in a similar way, thereby inducing in someone else the unwanted pain of that experience (A. Freud 1937). There are times when a patient will unconsciously recreate in a therapist feelings that belong to the experience in question, and which the patient is trying to "get rid of " in this way. It is therefore not only unmanageable feeling-states that come to be evoked in the therapist by means of impact behavior; this may include aspects of the patient's unbearable experience. (Kleinians would probably regard this too as a form of projective identification.)

If a therapist recognizes when he is being subjected to this kind of interactive pressure from a patient, it is often possible to find a clue to such unconscious communication in his own affective response to the patient's behavior (see King 1978).

Example 4.4
A patient, during the early stages of an analysis, noticed that I had been using my library (which is an integral part of my consulting room). I had been looking up references for some work I was doing, and I had not tidied up after pulling out books and journals from the shelves.

The patient said he could not live with his books in such a state of mess. He would want to have the books all in order, and he wondered how I could put up with my shelves like that, day after day.

That evening I thought about the dilemma that I felt placed in. I wanted to tidy my shelves; but if I did this straight away the patient could feel that he had made me tidy them, and I felt uneasy about it looking as if I had obediently done what I had been told to do. Of course, I could avoid that discomfort by leaving everything as it was; but I still wanted to tidy the shelves.

For a while I felt paralyzed by this apparently trivial issue. The only solution was to do what made most sense to me. I tidied the books; but, when I came to the journals that I had not finished using, there remained an element of the same dilemma. Again, I did what suited me. I left the unfinished journals on their side, lying over books on the shelf.

When the patient came to his next session he looked at the changes on the shelves. After some thought, he exploded in a tone of voice quite unlike anything I had heard from him before: "PATHETIC!" After a silence he elaborated further. He thought that I could not have chosen a more ridiculous compromise. He said if I didn't want to feel pushed around by him it would have been better to have left the shelves as they were. Perhaps I liked them like that. If, on the other hand, I actually wanted to tidy them why on earth not finish the job? As it was, he concluded, I had left a few journals not tidied away as a "token gesture of independence." Why hadn't I just done what I wanted to do?

Internal supervision: As I thought about the patient's perception of what he saw as my compromise, I realized I had been in a double-bind[5] after his last session (Bateson et al. 1956). This had seemed insoluble until I chose to resolve it in the only way that allowed me to be free. I had done what had suited me, leaving out the journals I was still working on. The patient expected me to have remained in the double-bind, not able to resolve it. He also assumed that I could not let myself do what I wanted to do.

I began to realize the significance of this interaction. It had already become clear, in the short period of his analysis so far, that this patient had been regularly placed in double-binds by his mother; and he had not been able to find a way out of the paralysis which that behavior induced in him.

> I said I thought the issue was about being in a double-bind, and I told him that I had been aware of being in a dilemma about tidying the shelves. He was right in supposing I wanted to tidy them; but he also assumed I had been unable to do what I wanted. I thought that this assumption was because he had so often not been able to cope with similar double-binds from his mother. He had not found a way out of that through doing what *he* wanted to do.
>
> The patient recognized what I was describing. He said his mother was probably "the double-binding mother of all time." Whatever he did, his mother always found some way of saying it was all wrong. He had never found any way of dealing with this. He also agreed he had been doing to me the kind of thing his mother used to do to him, but he could not see that I had found any way of dealing with his double-binding of me.
>
> I told him I was still using the journals which were not put away, so I had kept these out. Equally, I wanted to tidy the rest and I was glad to have been prompted to get round to this.
>
> What followed helped us to see that the patient had been unconsciously testing me. He was relieved to know I had felt doublebound. He also thought it was no accident he had selected an issue of untidiness. His mother had frequently made him tidy up, or clean; and he could never satisfy her. There was always something his mother would criticize him for, however careful or thorough he was.

Discussion: In this unconscious interaction, the patient had been doing to me the kind of thing his mother had so often done to him. (The defensive behavior here was that of identification with the aggressor.) Through my response to his pressures I had felt something of what he used to feel from his mother. This helped me to recognize what it could have been like for him as a child, with his mother. He was subsequently able to discover that he too could do what made sense to himself, rather than remain constantly paralyzed by trying to please his unpleasable mother; and he began to establish a separateness from her which he had never before dared to attempt.

A COUNTERTRANSFERENCE RESPONSE TO IMMINENT STRESS IN THE ANALYSIS

Example 4.5

A patient, who was leading up to a crisis in her analysis, had been expressing her fear of "going to pieces or going mad," and how she might be left permanently vulnerable because of that experience. Also, she might never really recover from it.

Without recognizing why at the time, I acted upon a countertransference impulse—meaning to help this patient find the courage not to run away from what she was fearing. I mistakenly told her I had found that a lasting strength for me had grown out of daring to face my own deepest fears, even the fears of going to pieces or of going mad.

The patient read my comment (at some level quite correctly) as expressing unconscious anxiety of my own. She took this to mean that I was warning her not to go further into this experience in her analysis

Internal supervision: It would, of course, have been far better if I had continued to analyze the patient's anxiety about whether I could help her through the experience that she feared. By resorting to this non-analytic procedure I am failing to hold her analytically at this moment.

Now, quite apart from any transference implications for the patient, it is likely she will need me to attend to the reality basis for her subsequent fears. She gave me clear confirmation of this need in her next session.

> PATIENT: I had a terrible dream: *I was going up a mountain in a cable-car. Suddenly it broke down and stopped. I was stuck half-way up the mountain, unable to go any further and unable to go back. I was stranded. What made it much worse was that the door of the cable-car kept on swinging open. It was all glass in a metal frame—a casement frame.*

Internal supervision: I was hearing of the patient's journey being in jeopardy from something that had broken down. The day residue referred to in this dream seemed obvious: there was a door swinging open, and the frame of the cable-car was made of glass (too transparent). The frame that she described is (in England) called a "casement frame."

I was immediately reminded of the analytic frame and of what I had told her about myself, in trying to tell her that I was familiar with the kind of experience she feared. I realized this was now causing her to be fearful for her analysis.

> ANALYST: I cannot fail to see the references to what I told you about

myself, and my familiarity with the experience of going to pieces. This has not helped. Instead, it has made you anxious about whether I can cope with what may lie ahead in your analysis—so anxious that you seem to be wondering whether you can even dare to continue your analysis with me.

PATIENT: I feel you are warning me not to go any further towards that experience. In fact, I think you are telling me you might not be able to cope. Perhaps you do feel threatened and need to warn me not to go on. But I also can't go back.

What followed during this session, and the sessions after it, was a period of acute anxiety with the patient having to test and retest my capacity to hold her analytically through whatever was still to come in her analysis. She went into an intensely frightening sequence of sessions, during which she eventually did experience herself as "going to pieces." She also dreamed of her foundations breaking up, as if from an earthquake. But she did not get into this reliving of her childhood experience of disintegration until after we had done the necessary analytic work on her dream, which so clearly showed the implications for her in my attempt at reassuring her and the need for me to recover my analytic holding of the patient.

Discussion: In this sequence, I had to accept that I had provoked what followed in the analysis. But I do not think this accounts for it all.

The patient had already indicated she felt there was a crisis brewing up for her. When she later experienced going to pieces in the analysis, the sense of her foundations being threatened was no doubt linked with what I had introduced in the analysis, by the uncalled-for element of self-exposure. Nevertheless, I do not think this patient would have been able to go on with her analysis if what followed was entirely caused by my break in the analytic frame, which usually preserves the relative anonymity of the analyst from intruding upon the analytic process. The dreaded experience also belonged in her own early life-experience, and had to be lived through in the analysis before she could deal with her own "fear of breakdown" (Winnicott 1970).

Comment: I have noticed that several times, and with different patients, I have fallen into a sequence similar to the one above. There is no doubt that some countertransference is always operating when I deflect a patient, or try to reassure, particularly as I know so well that this does not work. So why does it keep on happening?

It occurred to me during the later session, when this patient told me of her earthquake dream, that I had recently heard about areas in the world where earthquakes are common. Apparently it has been noticed there that animals start to behave strangely, dogs barking and geese cackling, shortly before there is an earthquake. It is the usual practice, in such regions, to seize the children and to get them into the open (for safety) in case there is an earthquake threatening.

Perhaps there is a similar function performed by the counter-transference: but in this case (and in others) I had missed the moment of recognition. I now think that the impulse to reassure is not just an important cue for caution. Sometimes it may also be an early pointer to some kind of earthquake-experience which may be imminent in the analysis or therapy. So, if we could listen to this impulse to reassure, like those people who respond to the early warnings they receive from animals, we could be better prepared for what may follow.

One further encounter with the interactive unconscious that I wish to describe, relates to Winnicott's concept of the patient's use of the analyst's failures. He writes of this in a number of different places (e.g. Winnicott 1958: Chapter 22; 1965b: Chapter 23).

A THERAPIST'S FAILURE AND THE PATIENT'S PAST HISTORY

Example 4.6
A therapist was seeing a patient in three-times-a-week psychotherapy. The patient (whom I shall call Miss G.) had been traumatized as a child by her mother's repeated absences, in hospital with cancer, and (at the age of four) by her mother's death.

From the beginning of this treatment the therapist was kept firmly engaged by this needy patient, even though Miss G. frequently failed to turn up for sessions; and for a long time her silence at the beginning of sessions had exerted an enormous pressure on the therapist to speak first.

In this phase of the treatment the therapist listened closely to what she was thinking and feeling, during these silences or unexplained absences. She realized she was left not knowing what was happening to the patient, and (on some occasions) she even wondered whether she would ever see Miss G. again.

Over a period of time the therapist came to wonder whether her patient was making her feel a sense of abandonment and uncertainty, similar to that which Miss G. had probably felt during her mother's unexplained absences in hospital, and after her eventual death. This is another example of communication by impact, the therapist responding to the powerful effects on her caused by the patient's absences and/or silences.

Listening to what the patient was making her feel in this way, the therapist was able to interpret to Miss G. her awareness of how unbearable it must have been when she was so often left in this state of not knowing what was happening to her mother, and what had later happened when she never saw her again. The patient was gradually able to acknowledge that this made sense to her. It also helped her to forego most of her opening silences in sessions; though, at times of deepest despair, she would again resort to lateness (or absence) now knowing that this would be understood by her therapist as a sign of distress.

Comment: We can see here how Miss G. was able to communicate feelings which were beyond words, but which had been heard and understood because of the impact they made on the therapist. The therapist made good use of her knowledge of the dynamics of projective identification, and the patient remained in therapy even through times of greatest despair. The therapist also understood how important it was to Miss G. that she (the therapist) should be regularly there for the sessions, whether the patient came or not. Regularity, reliability, and on-going constancy were carefully maintained by this therapist for her patient.

One morning the therapist overslept.[6] The patient came to the therapist's consulting room for her early morning session, only to find herself shut out. She remained outside the locked door until the cleaner arrived. For the rest of her session time she was looked after by this cleaner, who expressed particular concern about the therapist's absence as it was "so unlike her not to be here." Inevitably, Miss G. felt something really serious must have happened. Perhaps there had been an accident. Perhaps her therapist was in hospital. Maybe she had died.

Discussion: The patient's experience of separation and her increased need of the absent mother had come to be deeply linked in her mind. So, after her mother's death Miss G. began to believe that it could have been the intensity of her need for her mother that had caused her to leave, and eventually to die. In the therapy itself there had now come to be a dramatic repetition of this same sequence, which clearly demonstrated her fantasy that it might be her dependency and need which "caused" the person she depended upon to be absent, perhaps to have become ill or to have died.

It is uncanny how this therapist unconsciously reproduced a real failure in the therapy which was so close to the experience of her patient's own childhood trauma. How is it, then, that we sometimes fail a patient even when we are so carefully trying not to? When this happens it can threaten the whole therapeutic relationship. And yet, when a patient is confronted by a real issue like this, about which he or she can be genuinely angry with the therapist in the present, it can equally become a pivotal experience in the therapy.

It could be that any recreation of an earlier trauma in the therapy comes about partly through an interplay of personal countertransference and role-responsiveness. Winnicott, however, speaks of a further dimension to this unconscious interaction:

> Corrective provision is never enough. What is it that may be enough for some of our patients to get well ? In the end the patient uses the analyst's failures, often quite small ones, perhaps manoeuvred by the patient ... and we have to put up with being in a limited context misunderstood. The operative factor is that the patient now hates the analyst for the failure that originally came as an environmental factor, outside the infant's area of omnipotent control but that is *now* staged in the transference. So in the end we succeed by failing—failing the patient's way. This is a long distance from the simple theory of cure by corrective experience. (Winnicott 1965b:258)

Later, in relation to his own patient in this paper, Winnicott adds:

> I must not fail in the child-care and infant-care aspects of the treatment until at a later stage when *she will make me fail* in ways determined by her history. (Winnicott 1965b: 258-59)

Miss G. may have unconsciously prompted her therapist to fail her "in ways determined by her history." So, at a time when she was being sensitively and consistently held in the therapeutic relationship (with unconscious reminders of a good holding-relationship that had existed earlier with her mother), this therapist became involved in a real failure of her patient. The nature of this failure had a terrifying similarity for the patient to her own childhood trauma. She consequently experienced, in the present with her therapist, her own obliterating anger that belonged to the original trauma.

The patient was able to find in this experience a real opportunity to *use* her therapist to represent the mother who had "failed" her, who had inexplicably shut her out by not being there. She could now begin to attack her therapist with her own strongest feelings about that earlier (and this present) failure, with her therapist surviving these attacks of rage upon her.

In his paper "Use of an Object and Relating through Identification," Winnicott stresses that the key to this survival is to be found in the patient discovering that the analyst (or therapist) has a strength that is not "created" by the patient's fantasy or projection

(Winnicott 1971: Chapter 6). Miss G. could only begin to modify her unconscious fantasy, that it had been her own anger at her mother's absences which had seemed to have been the cause of her death, through subjecting her therapist to her most intense feelings about that absence with her therapist (ultimately) not retaliating or collapsing, but surviving.

VARIOUS ASPECTS OF COUNTERTRANSFERENCE

If we are to suppose, as I do here, that there is a level of communication which is achieved through some interactive responsiveness between patient and therapist, it is essential that there should be ways of distinguishing between different kinds of response to the patient.

A great deal has been written on this. I shall not, however, endeavor to offer any systematic review of the literature on countertransference. This has been done thoroughly by others.[7] I wish only to outline some of the different ways in which countertransference has been written about, in particular those ways which throw light upon the examples given above.

1. Countertransference can be regarded as "a result of the patient's influence on his [the physician's] unconscious feelings" (Freud 1910: 145), for which the analyst should use self-analysis to resolve or seek further analytic help.

2. M. Balint (1933) (in Balint 1952: Chapter 12) and A. Reich (1951), likewise, both emphasized the fact that there are times when an analyst experiences a *transference response* to the patient. This can occur when a patient comes to represent some unresolved aspect of a significant relationship in the earlier life of the analyst or therapist; and this will threaten therapeutic work with that patient unless it is resolved through further self-analysis of the therapist

3. Winnicott, in his provocative paper "Hate in the Countertransference," refers to a truly objective countertransference. For instance, he says: "A main task of the analyst of any patient—is to maintain objectivity in regard to all that the patient brings, and a special case of this is the analyst's need to be able to hate the patient objectively" (Winnicott 1958: 196). And later he adds:

> The analyst's hate is ordinarily latent and is easily kept so. In analysis of psychotics the analyst is under greater strain to keep his hate latent, and he can only do this by being thoroughly aware of it. I want to add that in certain

stages of certain analyses the analyst's hate is actually sought by the patient, and what is then needed is hate that is objective. If the patient seeks objective or justified hate he must be able to reach it, else he cannot feel he can reach objective love. (Winnicott 1958: 199)

4. Paula Heimann stressed the "counter-" part of countertransference, seeing this as the analyst's response to the patient's transference. She emphasized that: "the analyst's emotional response to his patient within the analytic situation represents one of the most important tools for his work. The analyst's counter-transference is an instrument of research into the patient's unconscious" (Heimann 1950: 81). She later continues:

I would suggest that the analyst along with this freely working attention needs a freely roused emotional sensibility so as to follow the patient's emotional movements and unconscious fantasies. Our basic assumption is that the analyst's unconscious understands that of his patient. This rapport on the deep level comes to the surface in the form of feelings which the analyst notices in response to his patient, in his "counter-transference." This is the most dynamic way in which his patient's voice reaches him. (Heimann 1950: 82)

5. Pearl King, in her paper "Affective Response of the Analyst to the Patient's Communications," tries to get free of the confusingly different uses of countertransference:

It is thus of central importance to distinguish between countertransference as a pathological phenomenon and the affective response of the analyst to the patient's communications, particularly his affective response to the various forms that the patient's transference takes. (King 1978: 330)

WHAT BELONGS TO WHOM?

What most writers agree upon, in their differing ways, is that therapists are affected by their patient's impacts upon them, whether this be due to a patient's personality, a patient's transference, or a patient's manner of being. Often, the therapist's response to this may indicate something that has only to do with the therapist. At times, there may be elements also of unconscious communication from the patient. It cannot always be rigidly defined as countertransference or not, as pathological or not.

Once it is accepted that there can be an interactive communication between patient and therapist, a number of technical issues are immediately raised. I wish to concentrate on problems relating to the question: "whose pathology is operating at any given moment, the patient's or the therapist's, and how can we distinguish one from the other?"

Even after a personal analysis, any therapist is still liable to use the defenses of projection and denial, particularly when under pressure. So, the first step must be to monitor one's feelings, in any therapeutic interaction, for personal countertransference. Even though this may be triggered by something about the patient, a therapist must first accept what belongs to himself. The next step is to determine whether a patient is prompting the therapist to feel or to respond in a given way, and if so how and to what unconscious end might that be?

THE THERAPIST'S RESONANCE TO THE PATIENT

A therapist's receptivity to the patient's unconscious communication becomes manifest in his resonance to interactive pressures. This resonance results from a matching between what is personal to the therapist and what comes from the patient. How responsive a therapist can be to patients, at this interactive level of feeling compared with cognitive understanding, will depend upon two things in particular about the therapist.

First, he or she needs to have access to these unconscious resonances across as wide a range of feeling as possible. Therapists do not have to remain limited to their own experiences, their own ways of being and feeling. It is possible that each person carries the potential to feel all feelings and to resonate to all experiences, however strange or alien these may be to their conscious selves; but, whenever there are unresolved areas of repression or continued disavowal, there will continue to be degrees of feeling that remain deadened and unresponsive. The expanding of a therapist's range of empathic resonance is a major gain from analysis, and this needs to be a continuing process.

Second, every therapist has to learn to be open to the "otherness" of the other—being ready to feel whatever feelings result from being in touch with another person, however different that person is from themselves. Empathic identification is not enough, as it can limit a therapist to seeing what is familiar, or is similar to his own experience. Therapists therefore have to develop an openness to, and respect for, feelings and experiences that are quite unlike their own. The greater freedom they have to resonate to the unfamiliar "keys" or dissonant "harmonics" of others, the more it will enhance their receptivity to these unconsciously interactive cues that are often central to an understanding of patients.

A REVIEW OF THE EXAMPLES

In the examples given we can see different admixtures of what belongs to the therapist and what comes from the patient. The therapist who complained about an ungrateful patient was aware of a similarity between the patient and her daughters. This awareness prompted her to be cautious, but this caution also inhibited her. Once she could recognize that her resonance to the patient's ingratitude was also a response to something from her patient, she could begin to see that her attitude to the patient had become similar to that of her patient's parents.

My boredom, with the second patient, did not lift however much I looked for reasons within myself. Once I recognized a similarity between that analytic relationship and an empty kind of relating in this patient's earlier life, I was able to understand the feelings that this patient had so regularly engendered within me.

When I was with the woman whose children had died, the intensity of my feelings might have belonged only to me. Once again, however, the patient's contribution to my response (in the absence of her own feelings) led me to be confident that there was also an unconscious communication through her evoking those feelings in me.

The fourth example, when I tidied my bookshelves, is different. I was placed in a situation in which I could not do right in the patient's eyes. Here the feeling was of being trapped, or paralyzed, which helped me to recognize that the patient had unconsciously maneuvered me so that, whatever I did, I could not escape criticism—even ridicule. I had a hunch that the patient may have been identifying with his mother, placing me in a situation similar to that which he had experienced in childhood. It was only possible to explore this possibility by sharing with the patient my perception of that experience, and how I had set about resolving it.

One factor which these four examples have in common is that we are able to identify, in each, some contribution from the patient towards the therapist's responses. This is important because, if we can see what evokes these responses to the patient, we are on surer ground when we postulate that there may be some communication being conveyed by means of this interactive behavior.

In the fifth example, when I tried to reassure the patient, I was clearly responding to some unconscious anxiety about what lay ahead in this patient's analysis. This could have been more clearly anticipated if I had recognized the diagnostic element in my countertransference response to the patient. Consciously I felt well equipped and prepared for what lay ahead. Unconsciously I responded like those animals that sense an imminent earthquake.

The last example is more problematic. One view could be to regard this therapist's oversleeping simply as an acting out against the patient. We must not ignore this possibility. My impression, however, is that it becomes more meaningful when this is also considered as a further example of interactive communication. I find Winnicott's theoretical statements about a patient's use of the analyst's failures convincing, but I acknowledge that it would be wrong for any therapist to shelter behind this as a way of denying his own part in failures encountered in an analysis or therapy.

THE ISSUE OF INTENSITY

An interesting idea, which seems to be missed by other writers, arises from this notion of interactive communication. If it is valid to think of patients using communication by impact or projective identification, as a means whereby the unspeakable can be conveyed to the therapist, then there will be times when the feelings involved are going to be very intense. Sometimes it may be the *intensity* that is the main point of the communication. So, if therapists are to be adequately in touch with this, they will find themselves also experiencing feelings with a similar intensity.

In contrast to this, Heimann describes the more usual view when she says:

> Since... violent emotions of any kind, of love or hate, helpfulness or anger, impel towards action rather than towards contemplation and blur a person's capacity to observe and weigh the evidence correctly, it follows that, if the analyst's emotional response is intense, it will defeat its object .... The analyst's emotional sensitivity needs to be extensive rather than intensive, differentiating and mobile. (Heimann 1950: 82)

My experience with patients has led me to disagree with this view. The analyst or therapist has to learn to tolerate being in touch with violent emotions so that they do not "impel towards action," rather than to suppress these feelings. And, when the capacity for clear contemplation or observation is blurred, the possible communication in this too should be looked for when sufficient clarity of thinking has been recovered.

THE USE AND MISUSE OF COUNTERTRANSFERENCE IN INTERPRETATION

Some therapists interpret almost directly from their own feelings about the patient; but if a therapist says to a patient (for example), "You are making me feel...," this can suggest that all responsibility for what the therapist is feeling is being placed upon the patient.

Similarly, it is unwise to subject a patient to samples of self-analysis when trying to understand (or to explain) some erroneous interpretation, or other disturbing activity by the therapist. That should be the therapist's private affair. Heimann therefore said that there should be no confessions by the analyst to the patient. However, she was clear that: "The emotions aroused in the analyst will be of value to his patient, if used as one more source of insight into the patient's unconscious conflicts and defenses" (Heimann 1950: 83–4).

Margaret Little on the other hand, considers that there are occasions when it can be of great benefit to a patient if the analyst is open about *some* of his or her feelings:

> In the later stages of analysis then, when the patient's capacity for objectivity is already increased, the analyst needs especially to be on the look-out for counter-transference manifestations, and for opportunities to interpret it, whether directly or indirectly, as and when the patient reveals it to him. Without it patients may fail to recognize objectively much of the irrational parental behaviour which has been so powerful a factor in the development of the neurosis, for wherever the analyst does behave like the parents, and conceals the fact, there is the point at which continued repression of what might otherwise be recognized is inevitable. (Little 1951: 38)

The above examples illustrate some occasions when a cautious honesty about feelings evoked by a patient can enable the therapeutic process. This is less likely to be intrusive if we can identify the patient's contribution to this, as for instance in Example 4.3 where I told the patient about the suppressed crying.

However, when it is not yet clear whether there is any real communication from the patient in the therapist's responses, the patient should not be burdened with uncalled-for evidence of what the therapist is feeling. I can illustrate this most easily from Example 4.2. There, I did not think it fitting to tell the patient that I was feeling bored. So, rather than interpret direct from the countertransference (which is always inadvisable) I was able to listen more alertly; and from that new alertness I could begin to recognize the empty relating which had been so powerfully acting upon me to evoke this boredom.

It is a sound principle that countertransference should not intrude upon the analytic process; but this should not deter us from using our resonance to the patient to aid our further listening. Any subsequent interpretation that is based upon interactive communication needs to be linked to some identifiable cues from the patient, that he or she can recognize when made aware of them. When we cannot identify these cues, this usually indicates that there are not yet sufficient grounds for an interpretation if it is arrived at solely through the therapist's responses to the patient.

❖5❖

Listening from an Interactional Viewpoint: A Clinical Presentation

In the last chapter I gave an example of a therapist reenacting a traumatic element of the patient's childhood experience (Miss G. in Example 4.6), where it was possible that this reenactment grew out of the therapist's unconscious response to unconscious cues from the patient. I shall give here a more detailed illustration from an analysis in which, during the reported sequence, similar dynamics gradually emerged.

I also use this clinical sequence as a further illustration of learning to use internal supervision. I therefore follow the analytic process at three levels: (1) the analytical dialogue—what the patient and I said, in sequence, in each session; (2) internal supervision— what I was thinking, in the session, and how I arrived at each intervention; (3) hindsight—a commentary on some of what I later realized I had missed at each point in the session. Much of this hindsight occurred to me when writing notes after each session. I selected this particular week for making fuller notes than usual because I knew I was currently having difficulties in this analysis, and I was trying to sort out what was happening.

We will see that I made a number of mistakes in this sequence, which at the time seemed quite inexplicable. Gradually I began to recognize, and to respond to, the patient's unconscious cues which helped me to recover an analytic holding in the analysis. The following day, the patient made a surprising use of this recovery, reexperiencing in the session a very early trauma. With hindsight, some of those "mistakes" could then be understood from a dynamically different perspective.

BACKGROUND TO THE WEEK OF SESSIONS TO BE PRESENTED[1]

Mrs. B. was in the third year of her analysis. (This patient has been referred to already in (Chapter 1, Example 1.5.) She was about thirty when she started treatment, at which time she had not been long married. She had given birth to a son, here called Peter, six months prior to the week that follows. Before her pregnancy with Peter, the analysis had focused mainly on an accident that had occurred when Mrs. B. was eleven months old. She had pulled boiling water onto herself, while her mother was busy elsewhere, and had been severely burned. This experience was worked over repeatedly during the analysis, in dreams and in many sessions, but it had remained as a memory never to be consciously remembered.

After her son's birth Mrs. B. became healthily preoccupied with being a mother, the accident shifting largely into the background of the analysis; and having begun to feel much better, she suggested dropping her Friday sessions. Peter was beginning to wean himself, and (as it seemed) so was she. Mrs. B. also told me she was offering flexibility to Peter, for him to be able to move away from her—with her still there when he needed her. Therefore, when she showed anxiety about losing her fifth session permanently, I wondered if she had been prompting me to offer her a similar flexibility. As a result I offered her a compromise arrangement. I agreed to keep her usual Friday time available for a month or two, during which period she could see how it felt to be coming only four times per week. Then, when Mrs. B. showed concern about my wanting to use that time for another patient, I told her I would be using it for myself, for reading. She seemed pleased and grateful for this offer; but, as soon as she began coming less frequently, her anxiety mounted. The week I shall now present is the fourth week with this reduced frequency of sessions.

Hindsight: We can see that I have interrupted the analytic process in a number of ways. Rather than analysing the unresolved anxiety about dropping this session, I have presented myself in the role of a good mother, offering a flexible weaning. This appears to gratify the patient but it more clearly meets a need of my own. The patient prompts me to reconsider my offer. She could be indicating the inappropriateness of the flexible arrangement, but I fail to recognize her cue. Instead I rationalize my offer by telling her how I plan to use the Friday time. I thereby give her valid grounds for perceiving me as wanting a rest from seeing her so often.

THE CLINICAL SEQUENCE

Monday
The patient began the session by saying she had had a mixed weekend. She felt it was possible she was not yet ready to drop her Friday sessions. (*Pause.*) She had had two dreams. In the first: *a girl was looking after a cat that had had a kitten. She had helped this cat deliver the kitten, which was lying in a pool of blood. The kitten was too weak to survive and died.* In her associations Mrs. B. told me she had a friend whose daughter had the same name as the girl in the dream. (I shall call her Emma.) "Emma has a white kitten. This kitten has a scratch that won't heal." On saying this, Mrs. B. became very distressed. (*Pause.*)

Internal Supervision: The patient seems to identify herself with the kitten in the dream. I note the references to "too weak to survive" and "a scratch that won't heal." I also note that the primary concern seems to have been announced at the beginning of the session when she said she was not yet ready to drop the Friday sessions. I therefore choose to interpret with this issue as my focus.

I said I had the impression she was anxious about dropping the fifth session, partly because she was afraid she might not be inwardly strong enough to cope with the change, and she might be afraid I would assume from such a change that the emotional scars had healed more than perhaps they had. The patient agreed with this interpretation and told me the other dream. *She had been swimming very slowly in a pool.* She had no associations.

Internal Supervision: I believe this dream is offered as confirmation of her need to go slowly, and I prepare to acknowledge that I have heard this.

Hindsight: I am intervening prematurely; it would have been better to formulate a silent hypothesis at this point and to wait for the patient's further thoughts before intervening. I had been selective in my playback of the patient's own words, avoiding any reference to the pool of blood or to there having been a birth and a death in the first dream. The patient now offers a second dream, in which she was swimming in a pool. We cannot be sure whether this is a confirmation of the interpretation offered, as I am assuming in the session, or whether it is an indication by the patient that I have been going too fast. She again gives no associations, as if to highlight the fact that I had interpreted the earlier dream almost on my own. I had responded too quickly and with few associations from her.

I said I thought this second dream stressed her need to go at her own pace. She replied that she was actually "crawling" (doing the crawl) in the dream, and she added that Peter was now experimenting with crawling.

Internal Supervision: I feel these comments are further confirmation of my interpretation that she needed to go at her own pace.

Hindsight: I am too quick to hear confirmation of this interpretation. The concern about the flexible arrangement is not being confronted directly in this session, and I fail to notice the omission. I am still assuming this flexibility to be what the patient needs, so 1 am deaf to any indications to the contrary.

Mrs. B. then told me she wanted to explore the question of the Friday sessions further. I suggested to her she could do one of two things, with regard to Fridays: either she could use her Friday time on a demand-feeding basis, asking for the extra session during those weeks when she felt a need for it, or she could go back to five sessions for as long as needed. I suggested she let me know which way she would like to arrange the Friday sessions when she felt ready to decide.

Hindsight: There has been a further shift away from an analytic approach to the unresolved problem of the Friday sessions. Instead, alternate arrangements are being suggested to her. We also need to note that I have shifted into a manipulative mode. I am directive, making suggestions, and offering solutions to the patient rather than allowing her to be free to find her own. By intervening prematurely, I cut across the patient saying whatever she had just started to say, deflecting her onto the alternative arrangements I am now suggesting to her.

Towards the end of this session, I introduced a new topic, saying I felt it might be related to the matter at hand but I was not certain. I wondered aloud to the patient whether she had needed to emphasize the importance for her of being allowed to go at her own pace. She had, for instance, made sure she did not direct my attention from the baby part of herself either by bringing her actual baby to show me or by bringing a photograph of him.

Hindsight: The possibility that there might be some significance in

Mrs. B.'s never having volunteered to bring her baby to a session had been suggested to me some months earlier when I had attended a clinical presentation by a female analyst who was talking specifically about her experience with patients who had been pregnant during analysis. She had quoted several such cases, in all of which the mother had at some stage brought the baby to a session. When I mentioned I had a patient who had never brought her baby to a session, the patient having been pregnant while in analysis with me, I was told that I may have been blocking her from feeling able to show me her baby; perhaps I had been communicating some jealousy of her relationship with her baby, from which I was excluded. I had not thought so at the time, and I had felt no need to bring this issue up with her until now. For some reason I chose to mention this now, even though it was manifestly quite irrelevant and far removed from the issues that were much more in evidence in this session.

I am still blocking the analytic process by remaining in a manipulative mode of functioning. I say I am not sure whether this new topic relates to the matter at hand. My introduction of this here suggests some unrecognized need (of mine) to direct the patient away from what is disturbing the present state of the analytic relationship. Indications of countertransference are present in the manipulative quality of my intervention and in the implied pressure upon the patient to feel that she "should" bring her baby, or a photograph of him, to show me.

> Mrs. B. replied to this by saying she hadn't felt I needed to see the baby, or a photograph of him, because she had assumed I already knew him so well through her. (This was the end of the session.)

Internal Supervision: I feel reprimanded by the patient. In her response she points out that I should not need to see her baby, or a photograph of him, at least not for the purposes of the analysis. She indicates that she had assumed I knew him well through her, but now she may be wondering whether I do. Her use of the word "need" alerts me to the fact that she is picking up some countertransference interest expressed by me. However, because it is the end of the session, this is not dealt with. Having allowed my internal supervision to lapse in this session, I shall have to be more alert in the future. The unresolved issues are likely to appear as a continuing concern in the next session(s).

Tuesday
The patient arrived six minutes late. This was most unusual for her. She

started the session standing, and offered two photographs to me while I was also still standing.

Internal Supervision: The patient prompts me to see that there is something amiss, by coming unusually late. She also demonstrates, by standing, that the photographs do not belong in the analysis.

Hindsight: We can see a silent protest here along with the patient's compliance, but I fail to use my awareness of this in the current session.

One photograph was of Mrs. B. with her baby when he was a few weeks old, and the other was a more recent photograph of him with both parents. I responded to these by saying "They are lovely," and handed the photos back to her. She lay down on the couch.

After a pause, Mrs. B. repeated what she had said at the end of the previous day's session, that she had felt I already knew her baby and her husband intimately without seeing the photographs; but, outwardly, she seemed pleased I had seen what they look like.

Hindsight: We can note her repetition that I should not have needed to see the photographs. Even though initially I had been alert to this as a break in the normal analytic boundary I fail to deal with it in this session, possibly because there are now several framework issues to be dealt with.

The patient continued by saying she was still not sure about the fifth sessions. She didn't know whether it should be on a demand-feeding basis or not, as she might end up wanting her session on every Friday.

Internal Supervision: This question of the flexible arrangement remains unresolved, and the patient continues to be anxious about it. The idea of demand-feeding had been introduced by me, not by her. The effect of this is to make her feel she would be greedy if she were to ask for a full return to five sessions per week.

Mrs. B. went on to say she didn't want me to assume too many of the Friday times would be available to me for my reading.

Internal Supervision: More errors come home to roost. Mrs. B. specifically picks up the unconscious implications of my earlier self-exposure with regard to the reading. She shows here quite clearly how she is reacting to these implications; that she is anxious I might want the Friday time for me when she could be needing this same time for herself. The offer of a demand-feeding arrangement is not turning out to be as reassuring as it was meant to be. It is making the patient feel criticized, as being "demanding" if she should need her Friday time back. In the guise of seeming to be generous to the patient over the Friday times, I have projected some unacknowledged greediness of my own into the patient.

> I said I felt it had been unhelpful telling her how I planned to use her time, while keeping it available to her. Knowing this, she now saw me as the mother who wanted to be allowed to get on with her own things once the child was beginning to grow up. I was aware of the implications of this for her, because her accident had occurred at a time when her mother was busy elsewhere—and at that time she herself had just recently begun to walk.

Hindsight: There is an attempt here to acknowledge the patient's reality perception before referring to any childhood precedent to it. But, I am still being too quick to pass on to the past from the uncomfortable reality in the present. In effect, I am deflecting the patient away from my own failure in attention to that of her mother. This could be seen by her as a further indication of my sense of discomfort at the recent lapses in the analysis. I do not leave her free to elaborate on this, in her own way or in her own time. I preempt her by doing this for her.

> Mrs. B. replied to this by remembering in some detail how her mother always seemed to be putting housework and cooking before spending time with the children. Her mother always wanted to have the house cleaned, and a good meal prepared, as if all they needed was to be housed and fed, whereas Mrs. B. would have preferred a simple lunch and more time with her mother.

Internal Supervision: The patient seems to be playing back her perception of me as having been preoccupied with getting the recent mess in the analysis cleaned up, and myself reinstated as the good mother ready with a good meal, whereas she would have preferred me to have allowed her to have had more time in the session for her to have used this in her own way.

> Mrs. B. went on to tell me about her nephew (aged nine) and niece (aged seven) who were staying with them at this time. Her niece had been away for the weekend. She had a favorite cookery book that she had brought with her for her stay; and she had also taken this with her for the weekend, so her brother would not use it while she was away. Mrs. B. had let her nephew use one of her own recipes for him to cook with her, which he wanted to do. Half way through making something in the kitchen with

her, he complained that she was not really letting him do the cooking. She was doing too much of it for him.

Internal Supervision: I regard this as unconscious supervision by the patient. I reflect on this and feel she is alerting me to my having done too much for her, in her recent sessions, in relation either to the frequency of the sessions or to the issue of the photographs or both. I prepare to explore each of these in turn.

Hindsight: What I do not recognize here is the theme of *two people wanting the same thing.* The niece wants to keep her cookery book for herself, to prevent her brother using it when she is away. The patient may be alluding to my telling her I would use her time on Fridays for myself when she is away. She could feel I am wanting the time for myself, not wanting her to have it.

I said I felt she needed to confirm that she was being allowed enough freedom for her decision about the Friday sessions to be really her own. Mrs. B. replied to this by saying she didn't feel I was interfering in any way with that. There was then a silence.

Internal Supervision: I note the word "interfering," and again I feel rebuked by the patient. I sense this might be related more directly to the photographs.

I said to Mrs. B. I felt perhaps the missing freedom had more to do with the fact that I, and not she, had raised the issue of the photographs. Although she had complied with my comments, apparently happily, I felt she may have had more reservations about doing so than she had been showing. She picked this up quite readily and said that, although she was pleased I had seen the photographs, she was aware of being anxious I might assume from them that everything was now all right. Everyone looked so well and happy in the photos. She was afraid I might be unaware that, inside herself, she was still having to deal with more distress than she felt able to cope with in four sessions per week.

Internal Supervision: I note the patient is elaborating on her anxiety related to showing me the photos, and she inserts a further reference to the still unresolved question of frequency. I see that I must attend to this now.

I said she was clearly still anxious about the question of the Friday sessions. She replied that she was, and asked if she could (at least) come this week on the Friday. This was agreed to.

Hindsight: The issue of the treatment structure is only partly resolved. It was not until after this week that Mrs. B. made an unreserved request for a return to five times per week, on a regular basis, which was how the analysis continued.

Mrs. B. continued by telling me a dream: *She was holding a container with something valuable in it. There were other people around and they seemed to want their share of what was in the container. She felt as if they had robbed a bank, or something, and she was now carrying the loot for all of them. They were sent to prison, but there was a friendly prison officer who saw to it that she was put into a cell on her own for her protection. She finished her sentence before the others. She was being conducted across the yard towards the gate to freedom when the others set upon her and kicked her head in. She lay dead on the ground.* Mrs. B.'s subsequent associations referred to the analysis, but I could not recall these after the session had ended.

Internal Supervision: I feel flooded by this dream and the associations. I am abstracting the themes in the dream while listening to what the patient is saying. I choose to play back those themes I can recognize as relating to the analysis, and to the current issues regarding it.

Hindsight: There is a further reference to the theme of *other people wanting what she has,* what she is holding in the container, but I miss this and therefore still do not deal with the issue of the Friday time being no longer clearly hers. Also, my not being able to recall the patient's associations indicates a difficulty in following, rather than leading, her in this session.

I said the patient was trying to preserve her analysis, as the container with something valuable in it, from whatever was threatening to take it from her. She needed me to be a protector of it, allowing her to have space to herself, particularly as she may have felt I intruded on her space by my reference to her bringing her baby or a photograph of him. Maybe she saw me as being jealous of her special relationship with her baby, wanting some of it for me too.

Hindsight: This attempt at interpretation is too long. Also I refer ambiguously to two kinds of intrusion by me: (1) into the analytic space, and (2) into her space with her baby. The reference to jealousy is a further carry-over from the comments made by my senior colleague about babies born during an analysis.

Mrs. B. agreed with what I had said (an agreement too easy to be convincing) and added that she thought her reason for not bringing her baby to show me was that she wanted to be allowed to have something all to herself.

Internal Supervision: She picks up what makes most sense to her from what I have been saying, and she adopts the same ambiguity in her response "something all to herself," as I had used. This phrase can refer either to the analytic relationship which she does not want shared with any third party, or to her relationship with her baby which she does not want me to intrude on. I choose to pick up first the matter of the analytic frame.

I replied that this comment is particularly true of her wish to have her analysis to herself, without having other people intrude upon her being allowed to use her sessions in her own way.

Hindsight: I have stopped hiding behind the ambiguity and have acknowledged that the analytic frame requires privacy, not being subjected to suggestion or directives from the analyst. Had I responded to the earlier cues, with regard to the Friday time, I could have been more specific here. She is also wanting the Friday time to be "all to herself."

She said that this was true, and she began to relax in the session for the first time, having been noticeably tense. She remained calm until the end of the session, a few minutes later, without talking.

Internal Supervision: During the silence I begin to realize that the attack upon the patient, in the dream, has not been referred to by me or by her. I have selected only those themes in which I can see myself reflected in a positive light. Because I have ducked the negative references, she could see me as not yet ready to tolerate the more painful perceptions of me.

Wednesday
Mrs. B. arrived eight minutes late. Still standing (again), before moving to the couch, she asked me if she had left the smaller photograph anywhere in my room the previous day. I told her I had not seen it.

Internal Supervision: She is using the same defense of isolation as before (i.e. standing rather than using the couch). She is also late again. I recognize that something is still interfering with the analytic space.

Mrs. B. told me she was late because the car wouldn't start. "There was no light in the battery," and it was only the second time that this had happened with this car. She had then taken her husband's car. She hadn't looked in her own car for the missing photo.

Internal Supervision: I hear of something that has been lost, something to do with her having brought the photographs the previous day. I listen to this, around the current framework issue related to the photos. I try to find a bridge towards dealing with this.

Hindsight: "No light in the battery" is a strange way of referring to a flat battery. English is not the patient's original language, but as she is fluent this expression stands out as unusual for her. There may be a reference to my not having been more enlightened in my recent handling of her sessions. I have become like the car—not working properly.

I said she may have needed to feel that the photo had been lost, for the purpose of this session, so we could look at the implications of this for her. For instance, she could feel (with some justification) that she would not have lost this photo if I hadn't mentioned she might show it to me. She agreed. She then wanted to refer back to the previous day's dream.

Internal Supervision: Again her agreement is too quick. I am left feeling unsure whether this is confirmation. I note, however, the patient's indication that there is something we have not looked at left over from the previous day's dream.

Mrs. B. pointed out to me her passivity in relation to the people threatening her in the dream. She saw them as people from her past. She commented that she could not gain anything if she merely sought protection from them rather than facing them.

Internal Supervision: The patient picks up one of the aspects of the dream I had bypassed in my selective playback of themes from the dream. She also offers a deflection from me onto people from her past. She may have registered that I had previously avoided the negative references to me in the dream. I think she could be expressing a perception of me as needing to be protected from her more negative feelings. I also note her passivity in relation to my comment about the photographs.

Hindsight: We can see how the patient parallels my own defensive maneuver in the previous session, when I deflected her too quickly from my own failure onto the failure of her mother. This could be seen as a further indication to her that I might have been feeling unable to cope with the critical allusions to me in her dream.

> I said it seemed to me that I appeared in two forms in her dream: as the prison officer, who is seen as friendly and who is putting her into protective custody, and I might also be represented in the dream by the people threatening her.

Internal Supervision: This is a clumsy attempt to bring the patient back to the present reality, rather than collude with a possible flight to the past.

Hindsight: I am interpreting without giving the patient time to present me with the material for an interpretation. I am therefore still acting upon my countertransference anxiety at having made so many mistakes recently, one leading to another.

> Mrs. B. seemed puzzled by the second part of my interpretation and asked me how I had arrived at it.

Internal Supervision: The patient points out that I have picked my interpretation out of thin air. Certainly, she has not given me the grounds for this intervention, in the course of this session, so naturally she cannot see where I have got it from. I am in too much hurry to correct my recent errors. I therefore try to remedy this situation by playing back some of the missing ingredients from the dream, hoping to provide a bridge from that to my interpretation.

Hindsight: It would have been better to remain silent and let the patient lead.

> I said I felt we should see how the dream had started. She had been carrying something valuable in a container, which she was trying to protect from the other people in the dream who were seen as wanting to have their share of it. She had also told me she had felt some reluctance about showing me her baby. Nevertheless, she had brought the photos and she had had this dream the following night. At the end of the dream her head is kicked in, possibly a reference to her feeling she had not been allowed to think for herself. She reflected on this and partly agreed with it. She added that she hadn't been conscious of any wish not to bring the photographs; it had merely not crossed her mind to do so.

Internal Supervision: I note that it "had not crossed her mind," in other words it was not her own thinking. I see this as some degree of confirmation, and I feel that perhaps we can now look at the transference elaboration of this experience.

Hindsight: It is evident I remain impatient to move away from the present reality. By not giving her time to continue from here on her own, I am still threatening her space while acknowledging her need for me not to do so.

I said it was possible I had come to represent a bit of her past experience with her mother, in which she had not felt able to stand up to her, or in this instance to me. Instead, it appeared that she had felt a need to please me by bringing the photographs; but this apparent need may have been caused by her seeing me, at the time, as the mother who needed to be pleased. Mrs. B. was nodding as I was making the last part of this interpretation. She went on to tell me about something that happened on "Friday—no, Thursday night" of the previous week.

Internal Supervision: The slip seems obvious. I see this as a reference to the missing Friday sessions.

Hindsight: The Friday issue is dealt with only temporarily here. It is not until after this week that the Friday sessions are reinstated on a regular basis, so in this sense the Fridays are still missing.

Mrs. B. continued by saying that on Thursday evening her husband had been away, so she had invited herself to supper with friends. She told me in detail about a rich sweet dish that she took with her to the supper, how she had eaten too much and had then felt sick. In the night she had been afraid she might be ill the following day and unable to feed Peter, who was still being breast-fed. She therefore made herself vomit; and by the morning she was feeling better and more able to cope.

Internal Supervision: I note the themes: husband absent; feeding herself; making herself feel sick by eating too much; fear of having to interrupt her baby's feeding. I decide to offer a bridge towards dealing with some of this.

I pointed out to Mrs. B. the timing of this experience, prior to the Friday morning when she would not be having her usual session. She agreed it was probably because she was feeling deprived of the Friday session that she had allowed herself to eat too much.

Internal Supervision: She gets to this on her own. I do not need to over-feed her.

She also pointed out that she was aware of having had a choice: either to remain feeling ill and helpless, or to do something about it in order not to have to interrupt her present feeding pattern with her baby.

Internal supervision: She indicates the theme of interruption, which I see as alluding to interruptions of various kinds. I decide not to interrupt here.

She went on to say it would not necessarily have meant having to wean Peter abruptly; but certainly *she* thought it would have meant an unwarranted interruption of the feeding pattern.

Internal Supervision: I note the words "unwarranted interruption." The issue I feel she is highlighting, with her reference to feeding, is that of the Friday sessions—one of which was the previous Friday just referred to.

I said to her she had come to experience the recent interruption of her Friday sessions as unwarranted. On the Monday, in her first session after the sequence she had just described, she had indicated that she wanted to review the decision to drop Friday sessions. She agreed. It was by this time the end of the session.

Internal Supervision: I think it only became possible for Mrs. B. to refer to the dropping of her Friday sessions as an unwarranted interruption once it had been agreed that she could come back to her Friday session, at least for this week. The long-term arrangement has still not been settled.

Thursday

Mrs. B. started the session by telling me about Emma's mother. This mother had said that Emma should stay the night with Mrs. B. and her niece. She had also said in front of Emma: "It would be so nice for me." Mrs. B. felt terrible about this, feeling very sorry for the child and feeling she should have been given a chance to say what *she* wanted. Mrs. B. went on to say it seemed wrong to push Emma out of her own home in this way, to please her mother.

Internal Supervision: I seem to be hearing about a self-interested mother. Listening first for the external realities being alluded to here, I wondered if that incident were being told to me as a further unconscious prompt from the patient. I decide to start with this as a bridge-comment towards exploring the patient's internal reality, which I believe is being indirectly referred to here.

I said to Mrs. B. that here we have an example of a child being separated from her mother, because of wishes of the mother rather than of the child, and the child had not been given a chance to say what she felt about it. Mrs. B. agreed and fell into a distressed silence. After a while she told me that, during the previous night, she had awakened thinking she heard a child calling "Mummy." The older children were both soundly asleep. She went to see Peter but realized (of course) he could not talk yet. She then noticed that the voice had been saying "Mummee," which was how a child would call for a mother in her own childhood language. She relapsed into silence and was noticeably more distressed.

Internal Supervision: There is ample confirmation here of the theme of an *absent mother.* I feel she needs some acknowledgement by me, that I am aware of the meaning of her distress, rather than having me leave her too long in a silence in which I also could be seen as the mother who cannot hear.

I said: "So it was the child in you calling out for your childhood mother." She agreed and heaved a sigh of relief. She added that she could not count on her mother to hear. She went on to ask why it was she still went on and on with the same problems, and again became silent.

Internal Supervision: I reflect that the patient is needing help to deal with feelings about her absent mother, and I feel she is also alerting me to my recent absences (my lapses of analytic attention), which triggered this material. I look for a current focus to this theme of inattention, where I could have been failing her in ways like the mothers she is criticizing (Emma's mother and her own).

After a fairly long silence, I said that what set this off again in her might have been her uncertainty about whether I had been offering her flexibility, with regard to the sessions, to meet *her* needs or whether I was really wanting to get on with my own business. (I was silently bearing in mind that I had told her I would be using her time for myself.) Mrs. B. said that consciously she had been glad I had explained to her about the reading.

Internal Supervision: I note her emphasis on "consciously," so I wonder about the unconscious aspect.

I said I felt that to her unconscious, my having told her about my wish to have time for reading had given her occasion to develop a perception of me as being too much like her mother, wanting to have time to get on with her own things, and like Emma's mother who had behaved in a similar way. Mrs. B. said the child part of her would probably latch onto anything like that to feel anxious about. She said she was wondering whether her need to go back to five times per week had stemmed from a need to be sure that her Friday times would still really be there for her.

Internal Supervision: I see some of this as a confirmatory response, but I find myself wondering about the original dropping of the Friday sessions, whether the arrangement had been such as to allow this to happen too readily.

I said I felt perhaps she had become unsure where she stood with me, once I had offered to let the structure of her sessions become flexible. She might have accepted this change partly because it had been made to appear seductively easy rather than her having been given a chance to work this through, to have her own say on it, to the point of being sufficiently clear in herself to take this step on her own.

Internal Supervision: I am beginning to get hold of the point I had missed until now; it could have been the *flexibility* that had made things so difficult for the patient. The analytic framework had begun to suffer further breaks from that point on.

Mrs. B. replied she didn't know about this; but shortly afterwards she said that she had suddenly developed a splitting headache, and she said it was most unlike her to have headaches.

Internal Supervision: She is telling me there is still a painful conflict around here. I listen for further cues.

After a silence, Mrs. B. began to tell me about feeding Peter. He had a great appetite and at this time happily ate solids during the day, but he continued to be breastfed in the mornings and the evenings. Until recently she had felt she needed to be very careful about what she herself ate, in order to be sure she had an adequate supply of milk and a proper balance in her milk for the baby. She had since discovered that she really didn't need to be so "ultra careful," and her baby had continued to be perfectly all right.

Internal Supervision: I hear further unconscious prompting here. I have been too careful with Mrs. B., in thinking she needs flexibility; so my attempts to hold her particularly carefully around the time of "weaning" in the analysis have made her more anxious and insecure, not less so. As a result, I have lost my balance as analyst and I am still in the process of having to recover this.

I said perhaps she had experienced me as being overly careful with her, offering her such a gradual change from five-times-per-week to four-times, that she felt I was thinking of her as more fragile in this respect than she actually was. Mrs. B. replied with surprise saying her headache had gone now.

Internal Supervision: I take this as confirmation of my interpretation, and so does she. I then reflect upon this theme of my trying to be the over-protective mother, in preparation for my next interpretation.

I said there had been a painful conflict in her. She had been anxious for me to be sensitive to her child needs, in order that my behavior did not appear too similar to the insensitivities she had experienced in her mother; but she also needed me to acknowledge her adult strengths. She agreed that she would feel I was letting her down either way: if I responded only to the child in her or only to the adult.

As the session was ending, and she was about to leave, the patient added that she wondered whether she had pointed out to me she still had the negative of the lost photograph. She had noted to herself that still having the negative meant she could recreate the positive. I said I felt she had needed me to learn from her, in order to recognize what had been a negative experience in the past few sessions, so we could reestablish the positive which had been lost. She nodded and smiled her agreement as she left.

Internal Supervision: The analytic holding seems to have been recovered. The patient has found her own symbolic way of letting me know this.

Comment: It should be noted that my preoccupation with the recent mistakes (although necessary as a step towards resuming the analytic process) was also presenting a degree of interference. This concern over errors is always a hazard if the work of the internal supervisor is allowed to become too active and conscious during a session. It then functions instead as an internalized supervisor, which at times can even become persecutory to the therapist. (This is especially true if the clinical material in question is going to be presented to scrutiny by others, as in a clinical seminar, which was the case here.)

My recent high level of concern is being pointed out by the patient as being "ultra careful." I had been giving her a pain in the head. Even though I do not recognize this particular contribution to her headache, in the current session, her headache lifts when I show that I acknowledge there had been too much carefulness somewhere and, by implication, that I am ready to relax and to allow the analytic process to be resumed.

Friday
The patient arrived slightly late. She referred to the previous Wednesday night, when she had had a dream she had forgotten until that morning.

Internal Supervision: The patient had "forgotten" this dream. Maybe she could not let herself remember it while we were still caught up in other matters. She is also late, so there may be something still holding her back.

In the dream *there was a river. She was lying beside this river, the sides of which were like springtime with new growth all around. She was either very small or was lying on her front as the water seemed to be at eye-level. It had then begun boiling and threatened to destroy everything around. She felt the boiling water was coming straight at her. She wanted to turn away, because she was so frightened, but instead she looked at the water and it became an ordinary river again.* The patient paused in her recounting of the dream and said with amazement: "I was able to stop it boiling."

Internal Supervision: I note the themes in this dream: springtime and new growth; the patient is very small or lying on her front; there is eye-level water; the water begins to boil; it threatens to destroy; it seems to be coming straight at her. I sense that I am being presented with a traumatic memory, or a dream-reconstruction, of the accident. The boiling water had been at eye-level, and it was the patient's front that had been so badly burned. She also seems to indicate a readiness to look at the water. Possibly she is letting me know that the "memory," which had always been too terrible to remember, is close to being consciously recalled. Just possibly she is feeling more secure now we have worked all week on reestablishing the analytic framework. I decide to explore this with her, but being careful not to lead her towards my own thoughts about the dream. She needs to be ready to see the implications of this for herself.

I commented that the river had stopped boiling once she was able to look at it. I also noted she had "forgotten" this dream until she felt safe enough with me to look at it. She replied she hadn't realized until telling me the dream that it so clearly referred to the accident. She then became very distressed and began to experience the accident as happening to her in the session. It was as if the boiling water were pouring onto her and burning her. She cried out loudly in extreme pain and sat up, saying: "When I was lying down it wouldn't stop coming at me." She sobbed for a long time, holding her head in her hands.

Internal Supervision: Her holding of her head in her hands prompts me to see that she needs to feel held. I recall that earlier in the analysis she had told me that, after the accident, the pain only ever felt tolerable when she was being carried by her mother. She had felt as if she had been able to "put" her pain into her mother; but when her mother laid her down again it had been as if the pain were too much for her mother, so it seemed as if she were "putting it back" into the patient.

I cannot but feel under enormous stress, being with the patient now in this session. It is excruciating. I feel a very powerful wish to stop this experience, in any way possible, by trying to reassure her or by trying to divert her: anything seems preferable to remaining witness to her pain. Alongside this impulse to protect myself is a realization that this had been Mrs. B.'s perception of her mother's response. For the patient's sake, therefore, I know I must find some way of staying with her through what is happening, without trying to by-pass it.

> I said I felt she was holding her own head in her hands as a way of telling me that she needed to feel "held" through this experience. Still crying, she replied: "My mother couldn't face it—she had to turn away from it—I couldn't bear it alone."

Internal Supervision: I recall that her mother had in effect caused the accident by not being in the room, where this now mobile child was and where there was water boiling. After the accident her mother had not been able to look at the results of the accident. Mrs. B. had a memory image of her mother dressing the wounds while trying to turn her face away from them. I feel I am being tested by the patient to see if I can bear to see her in such pain. She is telling me she cannot bear this alone.

> I said to her: "You need me to be able to stay with you in your pain and not to have to turn away from it." She looked me straight in the eyes (she was still sitting on the couch) and said: "Can you?" I answered: "I know you need me to bear it with you." After this she lay down, saying: "Let me see if it has stopped now. Before, the boiling water kept coming at me. I could not bear the pain. It is better now." After a while she added: "I never believed I could bear to remember it; but now I have."

Internal Supervision: This is a quite different level of experience from all the earlier allusions to the accident. Mrs. B. had dreamed of the accident a number of times, but it was always more disguised. For instance, the boiling water had often been represented by its opposite, by ice. In one dream it was the movement of the water that was frozen, as it began to fall towards her, like in a photograph. I note the progression.

> I said to Mrs. B. that this was the first time she had let herself experience the accident undisguised. She replied: "This time I let it flow over me; and, even though it burned me, I now find that I am all right." At the end of the session she again looked straight at me and said: "Thank you for staying with me."

AFTERMATH OF THE SEQUENCE

The following week Mrs. B. told me she had realized that she had been singing to herself over the weekend. This was something quite new, and it reminded her of her mother singing to her. She recalled prodding her mother to get her to go on singing when she stopped. This was the first remembered link between a good mother from before the accident and a good mother still there after it.

What followed later was the patient's hating me most intensely, as the mother who had allowed the accident to happen to her and as the analyst who had allowed it to be repeated in the analysis. She also had to test me out extensively to discover whether I could continue to hold her analytically. She expected me to become the mother who could not bear remaining in touch with her pain, or who might retaliate if being in touch with this became unbearable to me. She expected to be left to fall for ever. (Part of that sequence is described in Chapter 7.)

It took a further year before Mrs. B. could begin to find real peace from the unspeakable dread of the anxieties which had come to be so closely associated with her experience of intense dependence on her mother after the accident, and on me as analyst after she had reexperienced the accident in the analysis. Much else, of course, occurred during the next year of treatment, but the experience of the week reported here remained a basic foundation to most of the subsequent progress made in the analysis.

DISCUSSION

The Interactional Viewpoint

As in Chapter 3, this presentation illustrates a number of points that are most clearly observed when the clinical sequence is considered from an interactional viewpoint.

It shows once again how closely a patient monitors the analyst. Mrs. B. not only noted my conscious interventions, and other expressions of myself, but she also monitored for the unconscious implications of my behavior; my intrusions, my deflections, my timing of interventions or failures to intervene, my choice of what I referred to and what I had overlooked, and my capacity to cope with what she needed to be able to present to me or my unreadiness for this.

Also, by a series of cues offered to me, this patient was able to help considerably in the reestablishing of a more secure analytic framework—without which she could not have reexperienced in the analysis the memory which she had felt she might not survive remembering.

Evidence of Indirect Countertransference

One influence affecting this week's work with Mrs. B. was my knowing that I had decided to present it to a clinical seminar, at which a number of senior colleagues would be present. The seminar leader was also known to be rigorous in his criticism.

Having chosen to present whatever happened in this week, with this particular patient, my listening was already less relaxed than I would wish. The work of my internal supervision became tilted away from the more subliminal way of working I wish to advocate, and at times it was more like that of a severe internalized supervisor. I was internalizing the anticipated critical attitude of the seminar leader—"identifying with the aggressor." This intrusive presence of an influence from outside the analytic situation is what has been described as "indirect countertransference" (Racker 1968). To that extent, therefore, this work is not an illustration of how a more autonomous and relaxed process of internal supervision should be.

Countertransference and Role-Responsiveness

There is also evidence that I was responding to the patient with personal countertransference.

At some level, I must have known there was more to be dealt with in this (so far) quite short analysis. Mrs. B's accident had been analytically encountered at various levels, all of them significantly less traumatic than the accident itself. The patient had dreamed about this many times, always with a high degree of "dream-work" disguise (Freud 1900: 461n). But it had never been experienced in the session. I had assumed that so early a trauma could not be really remembered or relived in an analysis. I now recognize I must have hoped this, so that I would not have to be confronted by the impact of this trauma upon myself.

With hindsight, it is also possible to recognize there was a likelihood Mrs. B. would become anxious at the time when she began to feel better because it had been when she was beginning to be a normal lively toddler, exploring the world around her, that the accident had occurred.[2] So, when she felt better and suggested she might be ready to drop one of her sessions, I should have been more alert to the possible significance of this for her. However, it must have suited me unconsciously to collude with the patient's confidence, I too wishing to think we had been through the worst of her analysis already.

When Mrs. B. became anxious, immediately she had begun to do without her fifth session, I was getting early warning signals that all was not as well as it had appeared.

When I introduced the topic of her baby, that she had not brought him or a photograph of him to show me, this looks (at first sight) entirely unaccountable. On reflection, however, it begins to make more sense if we see this in terms of what it did to the analysis. It temporarily deflected the analysis onto the patient's *well baby*, and away from the *unwell baby* in her unconscious memory. She later pointed this out, when she explained her reservations about my seeing how well she looked in the photographs; that I might assume everything to be all right, and I might therefore overlook that there were very difficult things still to be dealt with.

In the process of this accumulation of errors, there began to be an uncanny parallel between how I was behaving with this patient and how her mother had been at the time of the accident. I was too quick to assume her readiness to cope more on her own, when she first said she was feeling much better. I agreed to drop the fifth session without a careful analysis of the implications. I compounded this by telling her how I would be using her time, that I would be using it for my own business. So, by these several stages, I came to represent her mother who had been prematurely absent from her child at the time when she was at risk as a toddler needing more active attention rather than less.

Can this parallel be explained only in terms of personal countertransference? I think there must have been some unconscious role-responsiveness too, which contributed to my becoming so fully involved in this reenactment of the mother who had failed this patient at the time of the original trauma.

The Recovery of Analytic Holding

This patient could not dare to experience her original trauma while the state of the analytic framework and holding continued to be inadequate and therefore insecure.

An essential part of this sequence, in my opinion, emerges through the patient's tenacious cueing of me to see those things that were still not right. By listening to the sequence interactionally, and by gradually recognizing and attending to her anxiety concerning whether I could bear to stay with her pain in the analysis (rather than to divert her), she rediscovered that I could be responsive to her cues. The analytic hold thus came to be restored; and the patient was able to acknowledge this symbolically in the Thursday session.

Reexperiencing the Original Trauma

Before this week of analysis, I was not familiar with Winnicott's notion that the details from early traumatic events are "catalogued" (Winnicott 1958: 247). Elsewhere, he writes:

> One has to include in one's theory of the development of a human being the idea that it is normal and healthy for the individual to be able to defend the self against specific environmental failure by a *freezing of the failure situation*. Along with this goes an unconscious assumption (which can become a conscious hope) that opportunity will occur at a later date for a renewed experience in which the failure situation will be able to be unfrozen and reexperienced, with the individual in a regressed state, in an environment that is making adequate adaptation. (Winnicott 1958: 281)

Mrs. B. unconsciously found her own way back to the moment of trauma, by degrees which were in proportion to her fragile but growing trust in my capacity to hold her through these experiences. Earlier in the analysis she had only been able to enumerate the details as they had been told to her. Later she could let herself dream about them.[3] She needed eventually to experience, in the transference, the "unthinkable anxieties" of her childhood and in particular the "fear of falling" (Winnicott 1965b: 58; 1970).

The analysis gradually moved towards a situation which, in important respects, replicated the earlier experience of failure. Gradually, too, she helped me to represent "an environment that is making adequate adaptation" Only then could she combine in her analysis a representation of the original failure with an unconscious hope that (this time) she could go through the experience in the presence of someone able to stay with her through it, with herself and the other person both able to survive that intensity of feeling.

Here again, as in Example 4.6, "the patient uses the analyst's failures, often quite small ones, perhaps maneuvered by the patient." The patient was then able to use me to represent the mother who had previously failed her. The "failure situation" had become unfrozen, and she could now attack me with the feelings she had first experienced towards her mother, at the time of the accident (Winnicott 1965b: 258). If these dynamics do apply here too, it is remarkable how precisely the details of the original failure were unwittingly repeated in this analysis.

I had to learn how to survive these attacks. What helped most in this was my being able to recognize the unconscious purpose in this sequence, and the cost to the patient if I were to collapse or retaliate.

❖6❖

Key Dynamics of Containment

By using internal supervision, and trial identification in particular, I shall examine some failures to contain. We can then see more clearly the dynamics that are involved in what I am here calling "containment." I shall also illustrate how insight and analytic holding are helped by an awareness of communication by impact as described in Chapter 4.

CONTAINING

There are times when people cannot cope with their own feelings without some assistance. We could then think of these feelings as spilling over towards others. The analytic view on this phenomenon is to recognize this spilling over, or inability to contain, as an unconscious communication to others that there is something amiss, something that is unmanageable without help.

Basically, the help being searched for is always for *a person* to be available to help with these difficult feelings. Often, however, the response from the people around is to treat those feelings as if they were abnormal or dangerous. Medication can subdue them. Referral elsewhere can alleviate the problem for those otherwise most directly exposed to such pressures; but this seldom changes anything for a patient who inwardly still feels victim to powerful feelings.

If anything, these deflective or suppressive measures can add to the sense that there is an intensity of feeling which nobody could manage. If this were really so then suppression, even by addictive means, might appear to be preferable to continuing with a struggle regarded as having no solution.

I am using the notion of containment here as a general term for the management of another person's difficult feelings, which are otherwise uncontained.[1] There is, of course, a proper place for treatment by medication; and for treatment in hospital, which can offer "asylum" to those who need a safe place in which to be ill. Nevertheless, it is important to remain aware that it is usually a personal form of containment that is being looked for.

In more human terms, what is needed is a form of holding, such as a mother gives to her distressed child. There are various ways in which one adult can offer to another this holding (or containment). And it can be crucial for a patient to be thus held in order to recover, or to discover maybe for the first time, a capacity for managing life and life's difficulties without continued avoidance or suppression.

When feelings are "dealt with" through suppression a person can be given a breathing space, during which life's problems may be attended to differently; and for many this is enough to help them through that particular time of stress. This form of help should therefore not be undervalued.

However, there are some people who continue to be gripped by the fantasy that their most difficult feelings can only be dealt with by avoidance. The power to overwhelm, attributed to these unmanageable feelings, is confirmed when others treat them as if they share that assessment of them. It is only when these feelings can be admitted within a relationship that the underlying fantasy can begin to be modified. It is then an altogether different experience (for both patient and therapist) when a patient's attacks upon the therapist are survived knowingly, rather than being deflected because of impervious ignorance. Here it is important that therapists should have insight into what is being reenacted with them. The survival of the therapist, and the understanding of what is being encountered in this experience, are both central to the patient's ultimate recovery.

I shall first give examples of attempts at reassurance that fail, so that we can see why it is they fail.

FAILURES TO CONTAIN

A Misuse of Supportive Action by the Therapist

Example 6.1

A male patient (Mr. S.) was seeing me in twice-a-week therapy, coming on Wednesdays and Fridays.

One Friday he had difficulty in speaking. He sounded extremely depressed. After a while, I noticed that there was a sense of foreboding in the way he spoke and in the tone of his presence during the session. I therefore said to him: "You are not actually referring to suicide, but I am picking up a suicidal feeling in how you are speaking to me to-day." Mr. S. began to cry openly, and agreed that he was finding it extremely difficult to see any future at the moment. He hadn't realized it consciously, but he had been brooding upon suicide. It had been at the back of his mind, but it was definitely there; he had never felt so low.

At this point I misjudged the kind of containment this patient was needing. I found myself thinking about the long break between this Friday session and the next Wednesday. So, I offered to see Mr. S. on the Monday, if he would like to have an extra session. He asked me if he could think about this and let me know. I later had a telephone message saying he would be coming for the extra session.

The Monday session began as follows:

PATIENT: I had a dream last night: *I was in a boat, trying to negotiate rapids in a river that was flowing too fast for me to be able to control the boat. There was a man at the back of the boat, helping to steady it. He was actually in the river, steadying the boat with his hands. We got through these rapids to a point where the river became more manageable, and I was able to start rowing again. But the man was still hanging on at the back. Now, instead of helping, he was making it more difficult for me to steer the boat for myself. (Pause.)* I have come today because I said I would. In actual fact I am feeling better and I now don't feel this extra session to be necessary; but something happened on Friday that was important. You were able to pick up my suicidal feelings without my having to spell these out to you. That helped me to feel not so completely alone, and it helped me to feel that life was not quite impossible after all.

Discussion: Mr. S. had no hesitation in identifying who the man was, at the back of the boat. He knew that what had helped him most on the Friday had been my awareness of how he was feeling. That had been enough. It was what his mother had not been able to do for him. She had been trapped in her own depression when he was small, still mourning the death of a previous baby.

When I had offered the extra session Mr. S. was at first grateful. He later felt obligated even resentful. It was not what he was needing. This sequence therefore helps to illustrate that trying to reassure, or offering extra support, is often motivated by the helper's own need for reassurance because of the anxiety stirred up by a patient's (or client's) distress. Containment is seldom, if ever, achieved by reassuring the patient.

I had initially been in touch with how Mr. S. had been feeling, but my own continuing anxiety led me into being over-active. When I suggested he might come for an extra session, this indicated my doubt that he could find the inner strength he needed. In effect, therefore, I was undermining the strength that he did have. This hindered more than it helped, in his dealing with what lay ahead of him, as if I saw myself as indispensable to his survival. His dream spelled this out with unmistakable clarity.

A Misuse of Reassurance

Example 6.2
A therapist was being severely tested by a patient (Miss G.), who was chronically depressed and despairing. (See also Chapter 4, Example 4.6.)

Miss G.'s mother had died when she was four. Relatives had failed to provide any adequate replacement home. A children's home had done no better. The patient had come to feel there would never be anybody who could cope with how she was feeling. Everyone had either turned away from her when she cried, as if she were too old still to be crying, or they had sent her away to other relatives and (eventually) to the children's home. She remembered herself as often crying, or trying to hide her crying.

PATIENT: I am afraid you must be beginning to despair of me ever getting better.

THERAPIST: If *I* felt that I would not be here.

Discussion: When I heard this brief sequence, during a supervision session, I felt a twinge of anxiety through my trial identification with the patient. It brought to my mind what I had already heard about this patient's experience of people who had stopped being there, particularly when she could not stop herself crying. Her despair had been based upon the experience of no-one being prepared to remain in touch with what she was feeling.

I saw the patient's communication as an unconscious prompt, trying to indicate what her testing out of her therapist was about. It seemed possible, indeed likely, that this patient was still in search of someone who could tolerate being in touch with her unbearable despair.

If Miss G. had been looking for this kind of containment, what she heard could have a very different meaning from what was intended. The therapist meant to reassure Miss G. that she was not despairing of being able to help her. But the patient could easily mishear this as a confirmation of her dread, that not even her therapist would allow herself to be in touch with her despair and be prepared to go on seeing her: "If I felt *that* I would not be here."

The therapist failed to recognize the patient's need to be able to communicate her despair. Had she been more familiar with the unconscious processes operating at the time, she could have tested out her comment before speaking by trial-identifying with the patient. It would have been easier for her to recognize the possibility that Miss G. may have been trying to find out whether her therapist could bear to be in touch with the despair that she herself was feeling.

A principle of interpretation can be drawn from this. Whenever possible, we should interpret what a patient is actually feeling at the time, and not attempt to speak to what we would like the patient to feel instead. Here, Miss G. was feeling despair. A different response could therefore have been along the lines of:

> THERAPIST: I believe you are telling me you are afraid that I might not be able to bear being in touch with your despair. Instead you expect that I might in some way stop seeing you, if you were to succeed in communicating your despair to me so that I could actually be feeling it too.

This form of interpretation would have allowed Miss G. to experience her therapist as really in touch with what she was feeling. Any reassurance to be gained, therefore, could come from being really heard and adequately understood.

When this therapist later overslept (see Chapter 4, Example 4.6), that experience took on a terrifying meaning for Miss G. Did it mean her therapist had begun to feel the patient's despair, and was that why she wasn't there? This dramatic enactment of her worst fear required much reworking in the therapy before Miss G. could begin to realize that she had really been able to communicate her despair to her therapist; and (even though it may have contributed to the oversleeping) this had not resulted in an unresolvable collapse, or retaliation, such as the patient had always previously experienced.

CONTAINMENT BY A PERSON

A Suicidal Patient Seen in Psychotherapy

Example 6.3

I wish now to give an example of a patient (Mrs. F.) who had been regularly dependent upon medication. She had originally turned to this, as a substitute for being "held" by a person, when she began to find that her lifelong self-sufficiency was beginning to crumble. She needed more from a person than anyone seemed able to give her. She therefore became increasingly dependent upon drug substitutes for this. Eventually, she used an overdose of pills in an attempt to kill herself—and (unconsciously) to punish those who had failed to be there for her when she had most needed them.

Mrs. F. (aged 50) was referred to me from hospital after a very determined suicide attempt. She had nearly died. This had occurred at a time when she had been feeling acutely anxious, and she had experienced those around her as refusing to be in touch with what she was feeling.

When she started seeing me, there were said to be practical reasons why she could only come once a week. She was still on medication for her anxiety states and insomnia; and she continued to have difficulty in sleeping. Even when she did sleep she would regularly wake to anxiety, which often reached the point of terror.

In one particular session Mrs. F. pleaded with me to speak to the referring psychiatrist, to have her medication changed or increased, saying she had to have something to dampen these feelings that were again becoming so unbearable. She was convinced that neither Dr. Y. (the referring psychiatrist) nor I had any idea what terrors she was having to go through every day. And nothing was making this any better. She deeply regretted the hospital having succeeded in saving her life.

I agreed to discuss the problem with Dr. Y., but I did not promise any change in her medication. I said that I was not convinced it was more pills she was really needing.

PATIENT: You obviously don't understand. Can't you see it is unbearable? You have got to do something. I just cannot go on with these anxieties and terrors, and not sleeping. I NEED MORE PILLS.

THERAPIST: I can *see there is something you need more of. I don't think it is more pills, but what the pills stand for. I believe there have been times when you needed a person to be more available to you; but you experienced that person as unwilling, or unable, to cope with the intensity of your feelings. So, instead, you have been trying to shut off those feelings with pills*

PATIENT: I cannot go on like this. You have got to ask Dr. Y. for more pills, or stronger pills.

THERAPIST: I will speak to Dr. Y.; but I would also like to suggest that you consider allowing yourself more time here this week. I could see you in three days time if you would be prepared to come then.

Mrs. F. said she would come for the extra session. In the meantime I spoke to Dr. Y., who agreed with me that it would be a backward step to give into Mrs. F.'s demand for stronger medication. It was clear she was dependent upon suppressing her feelings, rather than daring to experience these and to share them with another person in order to understand them.

Three days later Mrs. F. came for her session. She was calmer and was looking rather embarrassed. She explained what had happened.

After her last session a number of things had emerged. She had put out her second sleeping pill, to take after midnight when she still had not got to sleep (which had been her regular habit). In the morning she had woken to find she had slept without it.

She then told me about a period in her childhood, when she had been about three and her mother was busy with her baby sister. Mrs. F. used to go to the local shop, round the corner from where they lived, and the man behind the counter used to let her have a dummy. Her mother objected to her having this and would take it from her; but the man in the shop used to give her another, whenever she asked him.

I suggested to Mrs. F. that the dummies, which the man used to give her, stood for her mother whom she was needing but was having to do without. It seemed that her mother had not responded to the distress signals, which Mrs. F. had been giving to her, when she went in search of dummies as her way of telling her mother she needed more time with her. So, when her mother used to remove the dummies without giving her more attention, Mrs. F. may have come to feel it was more dummies that she needed. Wanting more pills now was like wanting dummies for the anxious child within herself.

Mrs. F. then told me she had been surprised by a memory, during the night when she had slept without the extra sleeping pill: "It was so vivid it had seemed like a real experience in the present." She had a sense of being in bed with her mother (which used sometimes to happen when she was small) and feeling her mother's big strong back, there beside her. This used to be one of her happiest experiences as a child, being able to be close to her mother while her mother slept.

I said it may have been the only time she felt able to lean upon her mother, to make hidden demands upon her presence while she slept, as there was then no fear of her mother disapproving or turning away from her. Mrs. F. agreed, and she began to cry. It then became evident that she found relief from her earlier distress in being able to express this in her crying, in the presence of someone who was prepared to be in touch with what she was feeling.

Discussion: Why was this offer of an extra session different for Mrs. F. from that in the case of Mr. S. in the previous example?

It had been a feature of Mrs. F.'s whole life that she had always been seen as the strong and self-reliant person, upon whom everyone else could lean. She felt she must never let anyone know of her frightened and dependent self. Instead, she usually tried to hide this in order to preserve some contact with others, whom she experienced as leaving her whenever she showed signs of being needy. She had relied on medication to help her in this hiding. When suppression still did not obliterate her feelings, she increased the dose to the point of nearly obliterating herself. Her suicide bid, therefore, was an attempt at finally eliminating those feelings which she could no longer manage alone.

If I had followed Mrs. F.'s own diagnosis, that people could not cope with her when she felt most needy, and that she must therefore have stronger medication, I would have been colluding with her fantasy about the unmanageable quality of her own most difficult feelings. Instead, it made more sense to challenge her limiting of herself to only one session a week. At a time when she most expected me to be unwilling to remain in touch with what she was feeling, I offered to be more available to her. She now had a chance, in her therapy, to reexperience the time of her disowned neediness of childhood with me representing her mother who was still expected to retreat from her. This aroused new memories, to do with her search for substitutes for her mother's presence (the dummies), and her finding a security in her mother's sleeping presence—a secret dependence that felt safe because her mother had been unaware of it.

Mrs. F. gradually dared to draw upon my availability openly, rather than secretly, and the effect of this "relationship-holding" was startling. She began to discover that her own most difficult feelings of distress could be contained within a relationship. Of course we had much further work to do, around this hesitant new move towards allowing herself to rely upon someone else again. Nevertheless, it became (quite clear that my firmness about her need for more time with a person helped her to feel held by me, rather than seeking relief solely through medication.

Over a period of several months, Mrs. F. began to develop a different kind of security, now based upon her use of an outside dependability which she could internalize and consolidate within herself. Her new-found strength was different from her life-long self-sufficiency. Her earlier precocious maturity, arrived at defensively to protect her overburdened mother, could now give place to a more solid maturity that was arrived at differently. This time it could be achieved at her own pace, rather than at the pace of others; and it was more resilient than brittle.

Some years later, when her husband died suddenly, this progress was dramatically confirmed. The patient's GP once again offered Mrs. F. tranquilizers, to alleviate her immediate distress; but she told him quite firmly that she would prefer to arrange a visit to see her therapist. This she did, and allowed herself once again to be analytically held in a relationship in which she felt understood—while she began to mourn this loss she had previously so much dreaded.

CONTAINMENT BY INSIGHT AND INTERPRETATION

A Potential Admission to Mental Hospital

Example 6.4
This example concerns the patient who had been sent away from home by her mother when she had refused to eat. (See also Chapter 1, Example 1.1.)

One day Mrs. P. came to a session in a state of uncontrolled alarm. She began talking to me before she had even left the waiting room. She was talking very fast, with increasing loudness until she was actually screaming. The gist of what she was saying was that things were getting out of control at home. She felt unable to cope. She couldn't go on. Her husband didn't understand. "He just sits there being so bloody calm there doesn't seem to be any way I shall ever get through to him." She then screamed at me (as loud as she was able): "IT NEVER GETS ANY BETTER! WHAT CAN I DO? YOU DON'T CARE EITHER." At this, she picked up a cushion and threw it at me; but she immediately came across to my chair and took it back. She held the cushion close to her and started to cradle and rock it in her arms.

During this episode I was literally sitting on the edge of my chair, wondering what I could do; I felt the patient might need to be hospitalized. However, although she had initially been in a state of uncontrolled desperation and panic, after she began to cradle the cushion in her arms she became calmer.

Internal supervision: I was hearing about the patient not being able to "get through" to someone. I realized she was probably anxious she might be unable to get through to me too. I therefore reviewed what was happening, in the light of what else I knew about Mrs. P., as I knew she had been in a similar agitated state a number of times before.

I recalled that she had been sent to a psychiatric hospital, on a previous occasion. This was after her mother had died: she had then become suddenly overwhelmed by feelings of panic. Her husband had been away. Even when he was called back, her panic had not become any more manageable. The general practitioner had been called in, and he in turn had asked the local mental hospital to provide the containment that seemed impossible at home.

This memory prompted another. As a child, this patient had been sent away from home when she had become very distressed, after her brother was born. She had begun to refuse food, and her mother became unable to cope with this on top of looking after the new baby. She had therefore arranged for Mrs. P. (then aged four) to be looked after in a children's home.

When I remembered this I felt on familiar ground. Mrs. P. had been creating a specific impact on me, which she almost certainly had on others at crucial times such as those I had remembered during this session. Those others may not have been able to cope with what her distress made them feel. Their response in each case had been to send her away.

Mrs. P. had been stirring up in me similar thoughts of sending her away; in fact I was almost sure that she was expecting this. But, after throwing the cushion at me (away from herself), she had quickly retrieved it and was cradling it in her arms (close to herself). As I wondered about that sequence I began to sense an element of hope along with the more immediate despair. Mrs. P. was, in effect, giving me a model of what she was needing from me. She was holding the cushion as a baby would be held. Could I find some way of holding the despairing hurt child in her, so that she did not (this time) have to be sent away?

Once I had recognized these elements of communication in her behavior, I felt an inner conviction which I decided to put into words. She was still rocking but was quieter, so I felt she was ready to let me speak to her.

> THERAPIST: I believe you are showing me what you are most needing just now. You need someone to be in touch with the intensity of those feelings which are making you so afraid. (*Pause.*) I think you are expecting me to send you away, just like other people have done in the past; but I want to continue to help you with what you are feeling—without sending you away. (*Pause.*)
>
> You had to find a way of making me feel how frightening these feelings are to you. Your shouting, and throwing the cushion, were ways of making me feel the anxiety and alarm that you can't bear feeling.

(*Longer pause.*) By holding the cushion close to you now, not leaving it thrown away, I believe you are letting me know that this is what you are needing me to be able to do for you.

The patient, earlier so terrifyingly out of control became calmer and comparatively relaxed. I had been dreading the end of this session, in case she experienced this as a similar sending away. Instead, she collected herself together during the remaining ten minutes, thanked me and said she felt better. She would see me at her next session.

Discussion: In order to find a way of containing this patient, it had been essential that I could recognize the unconscious hope expressed in the patient's behavior. The dynamic operating here was communication through projective identification as I have come to understand it.

If I had not been familiar with this process (which is so often at work in patients who are in search of relationship-holding) it is highly likely that I too would have called in a doctor. But had I done so, under these circumstances, I would have confirmed this patient's fantasy that her distress might always end up being too much for any person to cope with, reinforcing her dread of rejection based on earlier failures to contain. With each similar rejection this fantasy would have become more deeply rooted and difficult to deal with.

The intensity of impact, from patients like this, is often a measure of the frequency with which earlier attempts at finding *containment by a person* have failed. I believe that some mental-hospital patients may be casualties from being too often let down by people who could not contain them, resulting in an assumption that they cannot safely express the intensity of their feelings to any other person. And if someone ever dares such a patient once again to hope, that person can expect to be tested repeatedly for the anticipated failure and rejection.

So, if we are realistically unable to see this kind of patient through the testing times, it is probably better we should not offer to try. It is only when the therapist can survive being tested, to the "bottom of the trough" and out again, that this new experience can begin to expunge the deep impression of past experience.

With some damaged patients we take on a terrible responsibility. We could make things worse for them if we fail to survive at the point when they most need to test our capacity for survival. So we should only offer containment in a relationship, as an alternative to medication or to hospital containment, with a full awareness of the risks that may be involved. We must know what we could be taking on.

A Fear of Violence

Example 6.5

This is an example of a patient using his own particular form of communication by impact, whereby he loudly demonstrated his search for containment and the effects on him of his earlier failures to find this.

Mr. E. came for a consultation after being turned away by a number of other people to whom he had looked for help. He was in his thirties and therefore younger than me. He was also taller (well over six foot) and obviously stronger. So his presence alone had an impact which was soon to be greatly enhanced by his manner.

In the course of telling me about how he had been referred for therapy, he began to shout and to bang the arm of his chair with a barely contained violence. I could, however, sense that what was being expressed was only a part of this man's violent feelings. The greater part was being held in with a fierce control, which was a major feature of this man's life. His thoughts, he had been telling me, were filled with murderous fantasies. His life was being ruined by his need to keep these feelings under constant check.

What follows was all shouted at me; some of it yelled at me:

PATIENT: You are just sitting there. I know. . . You are going to do just the same as everyone else. You don't want to help me. You think that I am incurable. They all say that. They listen to me very politely, just like you, and then they show me the door. They think I am violent. I AM NOT A VIOLENT MAN. I have insight into my problems, but nobody believes me. YOU DON'T BELIEVE ME DO YOU? You think I need pills. They all want me to take pills. I am not going to take pills. I AM NOT GOING TO TAKE PILLS. That's what you want, isn't it? You would like to send me away to someone who will just give me pills. I may have violent fantasies, but that is different. I AM NOT A VIOLENT MAN. No-one believes me when I try to tell them that.

Internal supervision: I could feel myself becoming increasingly anxious. I realized that I was on the receiving end of a powerful projective identification; yet I was not sure what exactly was being put into me. It certainly had to do with violent feelings; but my feelings were not violent—*I felt afraid.*

I knew this patient had made several bids to get treatment without success. He had met with people who reacted to him, as Bion would describe, as if they were "containers afraid of the contained" (Bion 1967b). These repeated rejections must therefore have added to this man's fear of his own violence. Could I cope with it?

After this spate of shouting I interrupted Mr. E.

> THERAPIST: You are thinking and speaking for me, based on what you have experienced with other people. I would like to say for myself what I am thinking. You expect me to send you away; but I am not going to send you away. I am going to offer to take you into therapy. However, I make one condition. I know you have a lot of violent feelings, which you may need to bring into your therapy. You can bring as much violence here as you need to, as long as it is confined to words. If this becomes physical violence, I cannot promise that I will then be able to continue treating you.

> PATIENT: So you are afraid! (*Pause.*)

> THERAPIST: Yes, you are able to make me afraid of your violence; but I believe it may be precisely that which you need me to be in touch with—without having to send you away. I think it is your own fear of your violent feelings that you are needing me to help you with.

Mr. E. began to calm down. He understood what I had said. I think he recognized, even then, that it was true. He allowed me to treat him; and, even though he could only come to see me once a week, it was possible to contain him in therapy without medication.

Discussion: Right from the start the cues were all there for me, if I could but see them. Fortunately I was able to recognize the missing link, when Mr. E. pointed to my being afraid. *I was afraid of his violence and so was he.* I then knew I had to be prepared to be in touch with this fear, if I was going to be able to help him; and he had to find out whether the person he was with could tolerate this. He had tried with other people who may have missed this communication, or had not wished to work with it, but he had not (quite) given up hope that his fear of his own violence might somewhere begin to be contained by another person and found to be manageable.

PSYCHOTIC EPISODES: AN EXTENDED CLINICAL SEQUENCE

Example 6.6
A patient aged twenty-five (Miss W.) was in once-a-week therapy with me. She had been referred to me because her previous therapist was leaving the country, and therefore would be unable to continue seeing her.

That previous therapy had been conducted under supervision. During it Miss W. had experienced a brief psychotic breakdown. On that occasion, she had been hospitalized for six weeks in a mental hospital where her therapist had been allowed to continue to see her. (I shall refer to this as Hospital A.) Although the hospital consultant had wanted to put her on Stelazine he was persuaded by the supervising consultant psychotherapist to maintain Miss W. on Valium alone.

For the following year of that previous therapy, the supervising consultant had recommended that Miss W. might be better contained if her therapy were less intense. This proved to be the case. Therefore, when she was referred to me, I too saw her only once a week.

I had been seeing Miss W. for the whole of the summer term before taking my first holiday break during her therapy with me. I was away for four weeks. When I returned I discovered that she had been admitted to Hospital B, having gone into psychosis during the last week of my absence. Her psychiatrist in this hospital had started her on Stelazine and would not reconsider this, even though I requested that he might consult with Hospital A where it had been shown that Miss W. could be contained on Valium alone.

On this occasion Miss W. was in hospital for four months. Even though I visited her there regularly, I was consistently unable to get through to her at any feeling level. She seemed wooden and lifeless. She said that it seemed as if she were "trying to speak to people through cotton wool."

Towards the end of these four months, I began to feel that I could renew meaningful contact with this patient. She was beginning to have feelings again. When she was about to be discharged, the consultant psychiatrist advised me that this improvement was due to the Stelazine. He reminded me that I am not a doctor, so I would not be able to appreciate Miss W.'s need for this in the way that he could.

When Miss W. saw me back in my consulting room she confided in me that, for six weeks before leaving Hospital B, she had been throwing away her pills instead of taking them. She had felt so removed from other people, while she was still on Stelazine, it seemed to be the only thing she could do. She told me she had not been able to make any use of my visits to her, while she continued to be "fuzzed up" with pills.

After I had continued seeing Miss W. once a week for two years, her mother died. At the time, she coped with this largely by not letting herself feel anything about it, and she continued to manage her everyday life without being noticeably disturbed.

Then, several weeks prior to my next summer holiday break, I received through the post an envelope containing a piece of paper on which was drawn a very small triangle and a single initial beside it. The writing was noticeably shaky, and reminded me of the "Stelazine writing" with which I was familiar from the time when Miss W. had last been in hospital. The post mark was close to Hospital A, and the initial was that of Miss W.'s first name.

Upon telephoning Hospital A, I learned that this patient had been admitted there two days before, in a state of psychosis. I was able to speak to her new consultant, who said she too had started Miss W. on Stelazine, but she readily agreed to have this changed to Valium, and for me to visit.

When I saw Miss W. she clearly knew me, even though she was still in a nightmare world of her own. She talked in bursts of words, not all of which were intelligible or coherent. But from this staccato communication I was able to pick up the following:

PATIENT: Yoga...(*Pause.*) Falling...everything falling...no stopping. (*Pause.*) Being held...Yoga teacher holding me...(*Pause.*) In pieces... They wrote to me...the Yoga class...(*Pause.*) Six months since...hadn't been since...I'm falling again...I can't stop the falling.

Putting together what I could from this, I began to realize that she was telling me of a visit to her Yoga class, the first since her mother died. The returning theme of falling also reminded me of Winnicott's definition of "falling for ever" as one of the "unthinkable anxieties," and "going to pieces" as another (Winnicott 1965b: 58).

With the help of these cues I sensed what may have happened. By going back to the Yoga class, Miss W. had been suddenly hit by an affective realization of her mother's death. This seemed to have thrown her back into a regressed state, in which she became the child who had nobody to hold her. The Yoga teacher had held her physically. She was needing another kind of holding from me. I therefore began to interpret what I believed she was experiencing.

THERAPIST: When you were last at the Yoga class your mother was still alive. You may have been able to delay taking in the fact of her death, until you returned to this class...(*Pause.*) On going back, I think you suddenly realized how your world had changed since your last time there: the person who once held you as a child is no longer there for you now. (*Pause*). Your familiar world, in which there always used to be a mother for you, now feels broken into pieces...This has left you feeling that you are falling, with no-one to stop the falling, and no-one to hold you together.

PATIENT: (*A quiet pause.*) The falling has stopped now...You are there to hold me together...You have stopped the falling.

During the space of half an hour, Miss W. went from hallucinating psychosis to being able to remain in touch with her reality. My hunch, that it could have been the realization of her mother's death, proved to be correct. My being able to interpret what she was feeling helped to provide her with the necessary holding. Through this I was able to get in touch with what she was experiencing, and for her not to be left feeling so alone in this. Her unmanageable experience began to become manageable, and she did not need to *return* to psychosis to avoid the unbearable pain of becoming suddenly aware of being motherless.

Miss W. was kept in hospital for a further ten days, during which time I saw her once more. She was allowed home to her father, for a week's trial period. She then returned to hospital for discharge, and went back to her full-time job. In all, she had been away from her job for only three weeks.

Two days after going back to work Miss W. came to see me. Her father had just died, having had a heart attack. I immediately felt very concerned about her still being able to cope, with so much happening all at once. I recalled the earlier summer break, when she had collapsed into a prolonged psychotic state. We only had two weeks before I would be going away for another summer holiday. All her known supports were being taken from her at once.

I arranged for Miss W. to see me on her way back to her job, after she had been to her father's funeral. When she came I was relieved to see how much more in touch with her feelings she was, compared with the time after her mother's death. She was appropriately upset, and she was able to tolerate being in touch with her feelings. This was quite new.

Because I had earlier been so anxious about how Miss W. might manage during my summer break, I drew her attention to how much better she was coping with this second experience of a death. I told her I had been worried about her having to be alone during the summer, with so much having just happened to her. I told her I now felt she was going to be all right while I was away. I later added that it was almost as if the past few weeks, during which she had come to realize the fact of her mother's death, had in some way prepared her to deal with the death of her father too.

Miss W. came for her last session before my holiday. I soon realized that she was on the edge of psychosis again. I began to wonder what may have triggered this new episode, but she immediately gave me the cue that I needed. She had been feeling quite steady until she had come into my consulting room. She had even been all right at work and in her flat; but she "began to feel wobbly" *on the way to see me.* I felt prompted to reexamine the interaction between myself and this patient.

Internal supervision: Using trial identification, I recalled the patient's last session. I listened to myself trying to reassure her. She may have seen me as not remaining in touch with her precarious state (I wasn't as anxious about her as she was). At the same time I was unconsciously communicating to her my denied anxiety about her capacity to cope on her own (else why would I be trying to reassure her?). This helped me to offer an interpretation.

> THERAPIST: I believe I was unhelpful to you in your last session. I may have put some of my own anxiety into you about whether you would cope during the summer break. When I was trying to be reassuring about this, I think it probably had the opposite effect on you as if I had been trying to brush aside what you were feeling. I know I can only really help you when I am letting myself remain in touch with what you *are* feeling, rather than suggesting you could be feeling some other way."

PATIENT: I am glad you have realized that. I felt you were rather going on about how I would cope; and I wasn't at all sure I could. Then you seemed to be far away from me. It made me feel all alone again. Now I don't feel so alone.

Miss W. returned from the edge of further psychosis. I went on my holiday, and she returned to work and stayed there. She did not find the break in her therapy at this particular point at all easy; and yet she coped with it herself—drawing upon new resources that she had discovered in herself.

Discussion: The state of the analytic holding for this patient, at each critical moment in the sequence, was dependent upon the extent to which I was able to be in touch with her. There were different kinds of obstacle getting in the way. When she was on Stelazine she was contained medically; but she could not be reached emotionally, let alone feel held by insight or by a relationship. The medication had created a barrier to her being in touch with her own feelings, or to my attempts at getting through to her. When she was not on Stelazine, the obstacle that began to get in the way was more to do with my uncertainty about her strengths or my ability to contain her.

While I was behaving in a way that unconsciously communicated my own doubts to the patient, and my distance from what she was feeling, then she naturally felt alone with her anxiety. She only began to cope with this again when I indicated that I had picked up her unconscious prompt to me, communicated so clearly during this last session. Only then could the therapeutic holding be resumed, and not before.

REVIEW OF EXAMPLES

In this chapter I have been giving variations upon a theme. We are taught that "reassurance never reassures." It is an easy principle to remember, but not always so easy to apply. I have therefore given examples to illustrate some of the dynamics which are operating when we give in to this impulse to use reassurance.

At such moments it is also difficult to put into practice another maxim of technique, that "the best containment is a good interpretation." That means being able to make sense of what a patient is saying and feeling, and able to convey this to the patient. It also implies good timing. If an interpretation is accurate in content but poorly timed, it is a bad interpretation; it can even be experienced by the patient as persecutory.

Analytic holding therefore is always based upon a capacity to tolerate being genuinely in touch with what the other person is feeling, even to the extent of feeling those feelings oneself. There must also be some way of making interpretive use of the feelings induced in the therapist by a patient.

However, any interpretation based upon impact should include an awareness of why the patient has needed the therapist to experience what he has been feeling. If it is not yet possible to see this as purposeful communication, there is a serious risk that the therapist will respond unhelpfully by *avoidance* or by behaving in a way that is experienced by the patient as a *retaliation*. The patient is usually expecting one of these responses, based on past failures in relationship.

Patients have taught me that when I allow myself to feel (even to be invaded by) the patient's own unbearable feelings, and if I can experience this (paradoxically) as both unbearable and yet bearable, so that I am still able to find some way of going on, I can begin to "defuse" the dread in a patient's most difficult feelings.

In summary, therapists have to be able to interpret as well as contain. Passive containment is not enough, as it feeds a fantasy of the therapist being made unable to continue functioning as therapist. Interpretation alone is not enough, particularly if it can be experienced as the therapist maintaining a protective distance from what the patient is needing to communicate. Psychotherapeutic technique has to be able to bring together these two functions, in such a way that the patient can experience a real feeling-contact with the therapist and yet find that the therapist is able to continue functioning.

A therapist's capacity to provide a patient with this analytic holding is discovered through the real (and recognized) survival of that which the patient experiences as the worst in himself or herself (Winnicott 1971: Chapter 6).

❖7❖

Analytic Holding under Pressure

I now wish to give a clinical example where containment became an issue of such central importance that the outcome of the analysis depended upon it. As always, it is when an analyst or therapist is under stress that analytic holding comes to be most tested.

When pressure from a patient is extreme there are two pitfalls in particular that need to be avoided. One is for the therapist to look for security in a rigid adherence to the usual rules of technique; but patients do not feel secure with a therapist being defensive in this kind of way. The other is for the therapist to feel justified in stepping outside the analytic framework, in order to accommodate to the special circumstances; and yet patients usually sense a therapist's alarm when extra-ordinary ways of working are resorted to. Occasionally, however, we may have to introduce an exception. When we do, we should anticipate the implications of this for the patient and follow closely the subsequent repercussions (see Eissler 1953).

In order to illustrate this dilemma, I shall present a further sequence from the analysis of Mrs. B., several months after that described in Chapter 5.

BACKGROUND TO THE CLINICAL SEQUENCE

After Mrs. B. had reexperienced the accident (when she had been burned by boiling water), I imagined there could be no worse thing for us to encounter in her analysis. I was thinking of what Winnicott had said: "There is no end unless the bottom of the trough has been reached, unless *the thing feared has been experienced"* (Winnicott 1970: 105).

I did, however, know that Mrs. B. had been operated on at the age of seventeen months, under a local anesthetic, to release growing skin from the dead scar tissue left from her burns. I also knew that the mother had fainted during that operation, leaving her child confronted by the surgeon who continued with the operation regardless. A memory of this experience had suddenly erupted into consciousness, at a time when Mrs. B. had been feeling particularly unsupported in her marriage; and she had recalled thinking that the surgeon was going to kill her with his knife. At the time of the operation she seems to have absented herself from this unmanageable experience by going unconscious. (It had, in fact, been the distress of this memory that had first prompted Mrs. B. to look for psychoanalytic help.)

Even though I knew the details of that early memory, I believed it did not compare with the experience of the accident, which had been brought into the earlier session. I wanted to think we had already negotiated "the bottom of the trough."

THE CLINICAL SEQUENCE[1]

Soon after the summer holiday Mrs. B. presented the following dream. *She had been trying to feed a despairing child. The child was standing and was about ten months old. It wasn't clear whether the child was a boy or a girl.* Mrs. B. wondered about the age of the child. Her son was soon to be ten months old. He was now able to stand. She too would have been standing at ten months. (That would have been before the accident.) "Why is the child in my dream so despairing?" she asked. Her son was a lively child, and she assumed that she too had been a normal happy child until the accident.

I felt prompted to recall how Mrs. B. had clung to an idealized view of her pre-accident childhood. Was she now daring to question this? I therefore commented that maybe she was beginning to wonder about the time before the accident Perhaps not everything had been quite so happy as she had always needed to assume. She immediately held up her hand, signaling me to stop.

During the following silence I wondered why there was this present anxiety. Was the patient still needing not to look at anything from before the accident unless it was seen as perfect? Was the accident itself being used as a screen memory? I thought this probable. After a while, I said she seemed to be afraid of finding any element of bad experience during the time before the accident, as if she still felt the good that had been there before must be kept entirely separate from the bad that had followed. She listened in silence, making no perceptible response for the rest of the session.

The next day, Mrs. B. came to her session with a look of terror on her face. For this session, and the five sessions following, she could not lie on the couch. She explained that when I had gone on talking, after she had signaled me to stop, the couch had "become" the operating table—with me as the surgeon who had gone on operating regardless after her mother had fainted. She now could not lie down "because the experience will go on." Nothing could stop it then, she felt sure.

In one of these sitting-up sessions Mrs. B. showed me a photograph of her holiday house, built into the side of a mountain with high retaining walls. She stressed how essential these walls are, to hold the house from falling. She was afraid of falling for ever. She felt this had happened to her after her mother had fainted.

Mrs. B. had previously recalled thinking her mother had died, when she had fallen out of her sight during the operation. Now, in this session, she told me one part of that experience which she had never mentioned before.

At the start of the operation Mrs. B.'s mother had been holding her hands, and she remembered her terror upon finding her mother's hands slipping away as she fainted and disappeared. She now thought she had been trying to re-find her mother's hands ever since.

Mrs. B. began to stress the importance of physical contact for her. She said she was unable to lie down on the couch again unless she knew that she could if necessary hold my hand, in order to get through this reliving of the operation experience. Would I allow that or would I refuse? If I refused she wasn't sure she could continue with her analysis.

My initial response was to acknowledge to her that she needed me to be "in touch" with the intensity of her anxiety. However she insisted she had to know whether or not I would actually allow her to hold my hand. I felt under increased pressure, due to this being near the end of a Friday session, and I was beginning to fear that the patient might indeed leave the analysis.

My next comment was defensively equivocal. I said that some analysts would not contemplate allowing this, but I realized she might need to have the possibility of holding my hand if it seemed to be the only way for her to get through this experience. She showed some relief upon my saying this.

Over the weekend, I reviewed the implications of this possibility of the patient holding my hand. While reflecting upon my counter-transference around this issue, I came to recognize the following important points: (1) I was in effect offering to be the "better mother," who would remain holding her hand, in contrast to the actual mother who had not been able to bear what was happening; (2) my offer had been partly motivated by my fear of losing the patient; (3) if I were to hold this patient's hand it would almost certainly not, as she assumed, help her to get through a reex-periencing of the original trauma. (A central detail of this had been the *absence* of her mother's hands.) It would instead amount to a bypassing of this key factor of the trauma, and could reinforce the patient's perception of this as something too terrible ever to be fully remembered or to be experienced. I therefore decided that I must review with the patient the implications of this offer, as soon as I had an opportunity to do so.

On the Sunday, I received a hand-delivered letter in which the patient said she had had another dream of the despairing child, but this time there were signs of hope. *The child was crawling towards a motionless figure, with the excited expectation of reaching this figure.*

On the Monday, although she was somewhat reassured by her dream, Mrs. B. remained sitting on the couch. She saw the central figure as me, representing her missing mother. She also stressed she had not wanted me to have to wait to know about the dream. I interpreted her fear that I might not have been able to wait to be reassured, and she agreed. She had been afraid I might have collapsed over the weekend, under the weight of the Friday session, if I had been left until Monday without knowing she was beginning to feel more hopeful.

As this session continued, what emerged was a clear impression that Mrs. B. was seeing the possibility of holding my hand as a "short-cut" to feeling safer. She wanted me to be the motionless figure, controlled by her and not allowed to move, towards whom she could crawl—with the excited expectation that she would even-tually be allowed to touch me. Mrs. B. then reported an image, which was a waking continuation of the written dream. She saw the dream-child reaching the central figure, but as she touched this it had crumbled and collapsed.

With this cue as my lead I told her I had thought very carefully about this, and I had come to the conclusion that this tentative offer of my hand might have appeared to provide a way of her getting through the experience she was so terrified of; but I now realized it would instead become a side-stepping of that experience *as it had been* rather than a living through it. After a pause I continued. I said I knew that, if I seemed to be inviting an avoidance of this central factor of the original experience, I would be failing her as her analyst. I therefore did not think I should leave the possibility of holding my hand still open to her.

Mrs. B. looked stunned. She asked me if I realized what I had just done. I had taken my hand away from her just as her mother had, and she immediately assumed this must be because I too could not bear to remain in touch with what she was going through. Nothing I said could alter her assumption that I was afraid to let her touch me.

The following day, the patient's response to what I had said was devastating. Still sitting on the couch, she told me that her left arm (the one nearest to me) was "steaming." I had burned her. She could not accept any interpretation from me. Only a real physical response from me could do anything about it. She wanted to stop her analysis, to get away from what was happening to her in her sessions. She could never trust me again.

I tried to interpret that her trust in her mother, which had in a fragile way been restored after the accident, seemed to have been finally broken after her mother had fainted. It was this ultimate breach of that trust which had got in the way of her subsequent relationship to her. I felt that it was this she was now in the process of reenacting with me, in order to find that this unresolved breach of trust could be repaired. She listened, and was nodding understanding, but she repeated that it was impossible to repair.

The next day, Mrs. B. raged at me still for what she saw as my withdrawing from her. The possibility of holding my hand had been the same to her as actual holding. She felt sure she would not have abused the offer. It had been vitally important to her that I had been prepared to allow this; but my change of mind had become to her a real dropping away of the hand she needed to hold onto. To her, I *was* now her mother who had become afraid. Her arm seemed to be on fire. To her, I was afraid of being burned too.

Mrs. B. told me that the previous day, immediately after her session with me, she had become "fully suicidal." She had only got out of this by asking a friend if she could go round to see her, at any time, if she felt that she couldn't carry on. She had not ultimately needed to see her friend; it had been her friend's availability which had prevented her from killing herself. She rebuked me with the fact that her friend could get it right. Why couldn't I?

I told her that she did not need from me what she could get from others. She needed something different from me. She needed me not to buy off her anger by offering to be the "better mother." It was important I should not be afraid of her anger, or of her despair, in order that I stay with her throughout the relived experience of not having her mother's hands to hold onto. (*Pause.*) She also needed me to remain analyst, rather than have me as a "pretend" mother. It was therefore crucial I do nothing that could suggest I needed to protect myself from what she was experiencing or was feeling towards me. She listened and became calmer. Then momentarily before leaving the session, she lay down on the couch. She thus resumed the lying position.

I shall now summarize the next two weeks. Mrs. B. dreamed of *being lost and unsafe amongst a strange people with whom she could not find a common language.* I interpreted her anxiety as to whether I could find a common language with her. In one session she had a visual image of a child crying stone tears, which I interpreted as the tears of a petrified child (herself). She dreamed of *a baby being dropped and left to die.* She dreamed of *being very small and being denied the only food she wanted; it was there but a tall person would not let her have it.* In another dream *she was in terror anticipating some kind of explosion.*

Throughout this, she persisted in her conviction that she could never trust me again, and she experienced me as afraid of her. Alongside this, she told me her husband had become very supporting of her continuing her analysis, even though he was getting a lot of "kick-back" from it. This was quite new. I interpreted that, at some level, she was becoming more aware of me as able to take the kick-back from her in her analysis.

Shortly after this Mrs. B. reported the following two dreams in the same session. In the first *she was taking a child every day to meet her mother to get some order into the chaos,* which I interpreted as her bringing her child-self to me, in order to work through the chaos of her feelings towards me as the mother she still could not trust. She agreed with this, but added that she didn't bring the child to me by the hand. She had to drag her child-self by the hair.

In the second dream *she was falling through the air, convinced that she was going to die despite the fact that she was held by a parachute with a helicopter watching over her.*

She could see the contradictions (sure of dying whilst actually being safe) but this did not stop her feeling terrified in the dream, and still terrified of me in the session. She stressed that she did not know if I realized she was still feeling sure she was dying inside.

On the following Monday Mrs. B. told me she had dreamed that

she had come for her last session as she could not go on. She had begun
falling for ever, the couch and the room falling with her. There was no
bottom and no end to it.

The next day the patient felt that she was going insane. She had
dreamed *there was a sheet of glass between herself and me, so that she*
could not touch me or see me clearly. It was like a car windscreen with no
wipers in a storm. I interpreted her inability to feel that I could get
in touch with what she was feeling, because of the barrier between
her and me—created by the storm of her feelings inside her. This
prevented her seeing me clearly, just as it had with her mother. She
agreed and collapsed into uncontrolled crying, twisting on the
couch, tortured with pain. At the end of this session, she became
panicked that I would not be able to tolerate having experienced
this degree of her distress.

On the Friday, she spoke of a new worker in her office. She had
asked him how long he had been trained. She then realized she was
asking him for his credentials. I interpreted her anxiety about my
credentials, and whether I had the necessary experience to be able
to see her through. I added that maybe she used the word
"credentials" because of the allusion to "believe." She replied: "Of
course, credo." She said that she wanted to believe I could see her
through, and to trust me, but she still could not.

The next week, Mrs. B. continued to say she did not think she
could go on. She had had many terrible dreams over the weekend.
The following day she again sat up for the session. Intermittently,
she seemed to be quite deluded—with her awareness of reality
fleeting and tenuous.

For the greater part of the session she was a child. She began by
saying she doesn't just talk to her baby, she picks him up and holds
him. Then, looking straight at me she said: "I am a baby and you
are the person I need to be my mother. I need you to realize this,
because unless you are prepared to hold me I cannot go on. You
have got to understand this." She was putting me under immense
pressure. Finally, she stared accusingly at me and said: "You *are* my
mother and you are *not* holding me."

Throughout this I was aware of the delusional quality of her
perception of me. (I now understand this in terms of the psychic
immediacy of the transference experience.) There was little "as if"
sense left in her experience of me in this session, and at times there
seemed to be none. It was meaningless to her when I attempted to
interpret this as transference, as a reliving of her childhood experience. Not only was I the mother who was not holding her; in
her terror of me I had also become the surgeon with a knife in his

hand, who seemed to be about to kill her. At this point there appeared to be no remaining contact with me as analyst.

Internal supervision: I reflected upon my dilemma. If I did *not* give in to her demands I might permanently lose the patient from the analysis, or she might really go psychotic and need to be hospitalized. If I *did* give in to her I would be colluding with her delusional perception of me, and the avoided elements of the trauma could become encapsulated as too terrible ever to confront. I felt placed in an impossible position. However, once I came to recognize the projective identification process operating here, I began to surface from this feeling of complete helplessness. This enabled me eventually to interpret from the feelings engendered in me by the patient.

Very slowly, and with pauses to check that the patient was following me, I said to her: "You are making me experience in myself the sense of despair, and the impossibility of going on, that you are feeling...I am aware of being in what feels to me like a total paradox...In one sense I am feeling that it is impossible to reach you just now; and yet, in another sense, I feel that my telling you this may be the only way I can reach you."

She followed what I was saying very carefully, and slightly nodded her head. I therefore continued: "Similarly, I feel as if it could be impossible to go on; and yet, I feel that the only way I can help you through this is by my being prepared to tolerate what you are making me feel, and still going on." After a long silence Mrs. B. began to speak to me again as analyst. She said: "For the first time I can believe you, that you *are* in touch with what I have been feeling; and what is so amazing is that you can bear it."

I was then able to interpret to her, that her desperate wish for me to let her touch me had been her way of letting me know that she needed me to be really *in touch* with what she was going through. This time she could agree. She remained in silence for the last ten minutes of this session, and I sensed it was important I should do nothing to interrupt this.

The next day, Mrs. B. told me what had been happening during that silence. She had been able to smell her mother's presence, and she had felt her mother's hands again holding hers. She felt it was her *mother from before the fainting* she had got in touch with, as she had never felt held like that since then.

I commented that she had been able to find the internal mother she had lost touch with, as distinct from the "pretend" mother she had been wanting me to become. We could now see that if I had agreed to hold her physically it would have been a way of shutting off what she was experiencing, not only for her but also for me, as if I really could not bear to remain with her through this. She immediately recognized the implications of what I was saying, and replied: "Yes. You would have become a collapsed analyst. I could not realize it at the time, but I can now see that you would then have become the same as my mother who fainted. I am so glad you did not let that happen."

To conclude, I will summarize part of the last session of this week. Mrs. B. had woken feeling happy and had later found herself singing extracts from the Opera *"Der Freischütz,"* the plot of which (she explained) includes the triumph of light over darkness. She had also dreamed *she was in a car which had got out of control having taken on a life of its own. The car crashed into a barrier which had prevented her from running into the on-coming traffic. The barrier had saved her because it had remained firm. If it had collapsed she would have been killed.* She showed great relief that I had withstood her angry demands. My remaining firm had been able to stop the process which had taken on a life of its own, during which she had felt completely out of control.

The same dream ended with the patient *reaching out to safety through the car windscreen, which had opened to her like two glass doors.*

DISCUSSION

This case illustrates the interplay between various dynamics. My initial offer of possible physical contact was, paradoxically, tantamount to the countertransference withdrawal which the patient later attributed to me in my decision not to leave the offer of the easier option open to her. In terms of Bion's concept of "a projective-identification-rejecting-object" (Bion 1967b: Chapter 9) the countertransference here became the container's fear of the contained.

The resulting sequence can be understood in the interactional terms of Sandler's concept of role-responsiveness (Sandler 1976); or in terms of Winnicott's description of the patient's need to be able to experience in the present, in relation to a real situation between patient and analyst, the extremes of feeling which belonged to an early traumatic experience but which had been "frozen" because they had been too intense for the primitive ego to encompass *at that time* (Winnicott 1958: 281).

There had come to be a real issue between this patient and me, in the withdrawal of my earlier offer of the possibility of holding my hand. In using this to represent the central element of the original trauma, the patient entered into an intensely real experience of the past as she had perceived it. In so doing she was able, as it were, to "join up with" her own feelings, now unfrozen and available to her. The repressed past became, in the present, a conscious psychic reality from which (this time) she did not have to be defensively absent. During this, I had to continue to be the surviving analyst, and not become a collapsed analyst, in order that she could "defuse" the earlier fantasy that it had been the intensity of her need for her mother that had caused her mother to faint.

The eventual interpretive resolution within this session grew out of my awareness of the projective identification process then operating. I sensed that the pressures upon me related to the patient's desperation being unconsciously aimed at evoking in me the unbearable feeling-state which she could not on her own yet contain within herself.

It is a matter for speculation whether I would have been so fully subjected to the necessary impact of this patient's experience had I not first approached the question of possible physical contact as an open issue. Had I gone by the book, following the classical rule of no physical contact under any circumstance, I would certainly have been taking the safer course for me; but I would probably have been accurately perceived by the patient as afraid even to consider such contact. I am not sure that the reliving of this early trauma would have been as real to the patient, or in the end so therapeutically effective, if I had persisted throughout at that safer distance of classical "correctness."

Instead, I acted upon my intuition; and it is uncanny how this allowed the patient to reenact with me the details of this further trauma, which she needed to be able to experience within the analytic relationship and to be genuinely angry about. It is this unconscious responsiveness, to unconscious cues from the patient, to which Sandler refers in his paper "Countertransference and Role-Responsiveness" (Sandler 1976).

With regard to the recovered analytic holding I wish to add one further point. Because this was arrived at experientially with the patient, rather than by rule of thumb, it did more than prove a rightness of the classical position concerning no physical contact. *En route* this had acquired a specificity for the patient, which in my opinion allowed a fuller reliving of this early trauma than might otherwise have been possible.

I conclude with two quotations from Bion's paper "A Theory of Thinking." There he says (my italics):

If the infant *feels* it is dying it can arouse fears that it is dying in the mother. A well-balanced mother can accept these and respond therapeutically: that is to say in a manner that makes the infant feel it is receiving its frightened personality back again but in a form that it can tolerate—the fears are manageable by the infant personality. If the mother cannot tolerate these projections the infant is reduced to continued projective identification carried out with increasing force and frequency. (Bion 1967b: 114–15)

Normal development follows if the relationship between infant and breast permits the infant to project a feeling, say, that it is dying into the mother and to reintroject it after its sojourn in the breast has made it tolerable to the infant psyche. If the projection is not accepted by the mother the infant feels that its feeling that it is dying is stripped of such meaning as it has. It therefore reintrojects, not a fear of dying made tolerable, but a nameless dread. (Bion 1967b: 116)

Bion is here describing an infant's relationship to the breast. A similar process, at a later developmental stage, is illustrated in the clinical sequence I have described. I consider that it was my readiness to preserve the restored psychoanalytical holding, in the face of considerable pressures upon me to relinquish it, which eventually enabled my patient to receive her own frightened personality back again, in a form that she could tolerate. Had I resorted to the physical holding that she demanded the central trauma would have remained frozen, and could have been regarded as perhaps for ever unmanageable. The patient would then have reintrojected not a fear of dying made tolerable, but instead a nameless dread.

❖8❖

Processes of Search and Discovery in the Therapeutic Experience

Since Strachey, it has been widely accepted that the only "mutative interpretation" is a transference interpretation. Strachey says:

> It follows from this that the purely informative "dictionary" type of interpretation will be non-mutative, however useful it may be as a prelude to mutative interpretations. Every mutative interpretation must be emotionally "immediate"; the patient must experience something actual. (Strachey 1934: 150)

While I accept this as true, I believe there are other important dynamics also involved in the process of analytic recovery. In this chapter, therefore, I wish to explore in particular the patient's *unconscious search* for the therapeutic experience that is most needed; and how trial identification and internal supervision help the therapist to distinguish what is healthy in this search from what is pathological.

THE THERAPEUTIC EXPERIENCE

It is my thesis, here, that the nature of a patient's experience of the therapeutic relationship is at least as important a therapeutic factor as any gain in cognitive insight. It is within this relationship that there can be new opportunities for dealing with old conflicts, for recovering what had been lost, for finding what had been missing in earlier relationships.

A patient also has a chance to use the therapist in ways that may not have been possible in other relationships. When, for instance, earlier bad experience is transferred onto a social relationship, the recipient of that transference will usually not understand what is happening. So, instead of being able to offer understanding or containment, the other person is more likely to respond to the transference attitudes being taken personally.

Alexander (1954) recognized that patients frequently use the analytic experience in order to deal with unresolved conflicts under new circumstances. He therefore pointed out that, if the analyst's reactions to a patient are too similar to those of the parents, this can lead to a mutual involvement in the patient's transference neurosis, which (in extreme cases) could develop into a *folie à deux*. He also noted that, when the transference neurosis has developed, the analyst feels himself to be placed in a role of the patient's choosing. He suggested the analyst should consciously choose to respond in ways that are opposite to the manner in which the parents had behaved, arriving at this role by a "principle of contrast." But this deliberate adopting of a role, in relation to the patient, becomes a way of influencing what he or she experiences in the analysis. In that sense it infringes the patient's autonomy and is antithetic to the analytic process.

Winnicott understood this difference very well. He spoke instead of the patient *finding the object* and *using the object* (Winnicott 1971: Chapter 6). He recognized that there is in every patient an unconscious awareness of the experiences which need to be found, to be relived in the transference. Patients therefore look for opportunities in an analysis, to get in touch with previously unmanageable experiences. In the transference, therefore, the analyst is frequently used to represent an earlier relationship, about which there continue to be unresolved feelings. The analyst's mistakes likewise may be used to represent earlier bad experience (see Chapter 5).

THE NATURE OF THE PATIENT'S SEARCH

When patients seek out psychotherapeutic help it is often because parents, or other caretakers, have previously failed to respond adequately to various signals of distress. There is often a continuing unconscious hope of finding somebody able to respond to the patient's indications of search. These cues are similar to those of childhood, some of which may have been unacknowledged or left unheeded.

I believe that clinical experience and infant observation both support a notion that there could be (from birth) an innate search for what is needed for survival, for growth and healthy development.[1] It is when this search is frustrated or interfered with that we encounter "pathological" response; and yet, even in this response there is a healthy pointer to needs which have not been adequately met.

I am here making a distinction between *needs that need to be met* and *wants*. At birth there is no distinction. With the development of a capacity to tolerate increasingly manageable degrees of frustration, growth-needs begin to be differentiated from wants. A small baby "wants" the mother because the mother's presence is needed. As well as expressing libidinal needs to be fed, to suck or to bite etc., there will be growth-needs. Initially these will be very basic, such as the need to be held, to be related to and played with, and to be enjoyed.[2] In meeting these elemental needs the mother is preparing the foundation for her infant's subsequent growth and development.

In due course, an infant's growth-needs begin to include the need to discover manageable degrees of separateness. And later, there comes a time when the growth-need is for confrontation and a firmness that does not lose touch with caring. This will often be tested by tantrums, which aim to reinstate the infant's earlier control over the mother, because a child does not wish to recognize any distinction between needing and wanting. Hence, the intensity of wanting in a tantrum may seem very desperate. But, when the timing is appropriate to a child's growth, there is also a search for a parent who cares enough to be able to tolerate being treated as bad for saying "No" when it could be so much easier to say "Yes" (Casement 1969). Through finding the necessary firmness a child also finds security. When this is not found, a child's demands may be gratified but it is always a hollow triumph. The child is left feeling insecure, and *more* needy not *less*.

Patients reenact these different stages of growth in the course of therapy. The therapist should therefore try to distinguish between libidinal demands, which need to be frustrated, and growth-needs which need to be met. I believe that some therapeutic opportunities are missed when therapists fail to recognize when it is growth-needs which are being presented for necessary attention. For instance, some patients need to have evidence of having had a real impact upon the therapist; or a patient may need confirmation of valid perception of the clinical reality that this perception is not just fantasy or transference. A patient is let down if a therapist dutifully frustrates these needs, thinking that this is automatically required as a matter of analytic technique.

Even though the patient may look for what he or she needs the therapist is usually regarded as the expert, the one who should know best. In one sense he has to accept this responsibility. It is therefore quite usual for the management of therapy to be thought of as being entirely in the therapist's hands, and that it should in no sense be left to the patient. After all (it could be argued) where might it lead if patients were to be allowed their head in how their therapy should be conducted? Might this not result in the therapist falling into a collusion with the patient? Might it not play into a patient's pathology, offering inappropriate gratification rather than insight? And, was it not partly to avoid such pitfalls as these that Freud insisted that an analysis should be conducted in a state of "abstinence" (Freud 1914: 165)? He was well aware of repressed libidinal strivings in every patient. It was these that he insisted should not be gratified in analytic treatment, for in gratifying them the work of analysis is by passed.[3]

In some patients I have encountered a remarkable sense of what it is that they are unconsciously looking for in therapy; but the manner of a patient's search is often not direct or easily identified. Sometimes there are obvious clues to what is needed. At other times, growing despair of finding this may be indicated by a pressure for further substitute gratification, as if this may be all that could be hoped for. Nevertheless, in this pressure it is often possible to recognize what has been missing for the patient.

When there has been a lack of adequate structure, within which a patient could have more securely negotiated key developmental phases of growth, there is a *search for structure* in the therapeutic relationship. When there has been a lack of sufficient responsiveness in the person taking care of an infant, without which the infant's attempts at communicating preverbally were experienced as hopeless or without meaning, there is a *search for responsiveness* in the therapist. When there has been a lack of mental or emotional privacy, within which a child can begin to establish a viable separateness from the mother (or other adults), there is a *search for space*.

For example, patients who have needed privacy and confidentiality will often indicate from the start their fear that this will not be found even in therapy. Or, a patient who has experienced relationships in which there have been inadequate personal boundaries will demonstrate the need for a firmer sense of boundaries in the therapy. This may be communicated directly in the patient's anxiety about not finding this, or indirectly through behavior that would become uncontainable without an adequate firmness from the therapist. Also, when patients' autonomous thinking has been interfered with by others being too ready to think for them, they will often be passively compliant to the therapist's interpretive activity. Conversely, they may demonstrate an anxiety about being "seen into," or their thoughts not being private to themselves even in a silence. In ways like these, patients often demonstrate what they are needing to deal with in the course of therapy, by bringing the effects of earlier pathogenic experience into the therapeutic relationship.

A MISTAKEN USE OF CORRECTIVE EMOTIONAL EXPERIENCE

Some therapists imagine they can provide a patient with better experience, and that this in itself will be therapeutic. This is reminiscent of Alexander's notion of "the corrective emotional experience" (Alexander 1954). But, in doing so, they fail to allow an analytic freedom to use the therapist in those ways that relate to the earlier experience and inner world of the patient. For instance, when a patient has unresolved feelings about failures in parenting, it becomes intrusive (deflective and seductive) if the therapist *actively* offers himself or herself as the "better" parent.

> *Example 8.1*
> A female patient came into analysis having had some therapy before with a female therapist. The problem she presented, in asking for analysis, was that in her work she was unable to cope with people not liking her. She was a social worker, and it was in particular with her clients that she had this difficulty. She would unconsciously deflect anger, or maneuver people back into liking her, and this was getting in the way of her being able to work more effectively.
>
> When this patient had previously entered therapy she had been suicidally depressed. She ended that therapy feeling she had been greatly helped by her warm and encouraging therapist. She had been personally acknowledged and valued. She had also changed her job upon the therapist's recommendation, being persuaded that she would be good at working with people.

Comment: It should be said that this is not analytic psychotherapy. And yet, some people who do work analytically also seem to think that this "benign" leading of the patient might sometimes be appropriate.

The former therapist had met the patient's need for recognition and for being valued, which had been significantly missing in her childhood relationships. However, it had later begun to dawn on the patient that she had never been able to be angry with her therapist. She then realized that, whenever she had begun to get angry with her therapist, she seemed to take this personally, or she would interpret the anger as relating to someone else.

The patient had always had problems with her anger, and with people being angry with her. Now she found herself taking personally any sign of anger from her clients. As a result, she would try to "woo" them into feeling better about themselves or about her. She knew no other way.

What emerged in the course of this patient's analysis was that she needed to find an analyst who did not prevent her treating him in terms of her earlier relationships, and especially those about which she felt most angry. It was important that her transference use of the analyst should not be deflected, because she needed to be able to get as angry with him as she felt—in order to discover whether he could tolerate being on the receiving end of those feelings she had learned to regard as damaging.

Her parents had been the kind of people who could not cope with anger. It had left her feeling her own anger to be in some way bad and dangerous; and her former therapist had left her with that impression unaltered. The underlying problems, to do with her self-image as apparently bad or destructive, had not been attended to.

Discussion: The former therapist had made the patient feel temporarily better, by actively reassuring and encouraging her to feel she was a worthwhile person. This illustrates what has sometimes been called a "countertransference cure." It may have been the therapist's personal feelings for this patient that had made her feel better, in which case this would have been brought about by means of a charismatic influence and not by any analytic process. In so far as the patient had got better *for her therapist* the benefit had not been long-lasting.

In my opinion, if the other therapist had used internal supervision to question the basis of the patient's improvement, it might have highlighted the extent to which this had been achieved through compliance and a "false-self" suppression of the patient's more difficult feelings. It is always necessary to be aware of the possibility of this kind of false recovery.

What is also significant in this example is that the therapist's countertransference (which may have included a need to be liked) seemed to parallel the patient's own difficulty in relationships. This might have been why the patient felt she had not been helped with this particular problem in that earlier therapy.

THE THERAPIST'S NON-INTRUSIVE AVAILABILITY

Patients, given the chance, will find their own form of relating to the therapist. In this sense, we could compare a therapist's availability to the patient with the use of a spatula in Winnicott's child consultations. He regularly demonstrated that, if an infant is allowed a "period of hesitation" to notice and to find an unfamiliar (and potentially interesting) object left within view of the infant and within reach, this object will come to be invested with interest-value. It will eventually be spontaneously reached for. The object that he used happened to be a shiny surgical spatula (Winnicott 1958: Chapter 4).

When an infant is not hurried to find this object, it comes to be invested with such interest or meaning as fits in with the infant's readiness to explore this or to play with it. The spatula may be sucked, bitten, "fed" to the mother, used for banging, for throwing away, for being retrieved by the mother, etc. How this object will be used by an individual infant could not be predicted. Only one thing is certain, that an infant's use of the spatula will never be confined to the use for which it was designed.

If, on the other hand, a child *is* hurried, then this object does not acquire meaning invested in it by the infant. Instead, it remains (or becomes) an alien object belonging to the world of adults, rather than being an object that could be discovered and taken into the infant's world of fantasy and play. Any attempt, therefore, to insert the spatula into an infant's mouth would result in a protest against accepting this intrusive object. The strength of this protest can be regarded as a measure of the healthiness of the child. A less healthy response would be for the spatula to be accepted with passive compliance, or only a token resistance.

If therapists are to avoid being experienced by the patient as an "impinging object," as with the spatula, it is important that they should be ready to wait for relating and understanding to emerge in the patient's own time. This includes waiting for the transference to develop, through the patient's investment of this unknown person with such meaning as belongs to the patient's internal world. The therapist is there to be "found" by the patient. If, however, the therapist's way of being with the patient is overactive or intrusive, then interpretation and the therapist's presence can each become an impingement for the patient.

The evolution of the therapeutic process will only be a creation of the patient, which it needs to be, if the therapy is set up from the beginning with minimum influence or preconception from the therapist. To that end the therapist tries to keep himself (as a person) as little in evidence as can be in keeping with this aim of preserving the therapeutic space, as neutral and therefore free to be used in whatever way belongs to the therapeutic needs of the patient.

A PATIENT'S USE OF THE THERAPIST'S AVAILABILITY

Example 8.2
A female patient came for her first session after a holiday break. She arrived ten minutes late, and explained to her therapist (a man) that there had been a lot of traffic on the way which had held her up. She poured out details of what had happened to her since her last session. She had been feeling unsupported by her husband, having had to cope with the demands of the children on her own and they had been very difficult.

Internal supervision: The therapist sensed that the patient was alerting him to the possible impact upon her of the holiday break. Because of the pressure to talk, which was the most obvious aspect of her communication, he continued to listen.

The patient gave further examples of feeling alone, having no-one to turn to, feeling cold, etc. There were still no pauses in her narrative.

Internal supervision: The therapist was beginning to feel redundant in the session, in that the patient was not leaving any room for comment, and he wondered whether he should intervene to make his presence felt. But, lacking any clearer cue from the patient, he chose to remain silent.

After further out-pouring of holiday details the patient began to describe an incident with her husband. He had been depressed recently and unresponsive. She was feeling in particular need of his support one night, but he didn't reach out to her—even when she was crying. After a pause she added: "He didn't even speak to me."

There was a slight pause in the flow of talk from the patient at this point. The therapist, therefore, took his cue from her silence and used the themes presented to provide a bridge towards eventual interpretation.

> THERAPIST: You have been telling me details of what you have been dealing with since your last session. You now tell me about somebody who has been depressed, who did not respond to you; and you add that he didn't even speak to you."

Comment: The therapist is replying to the patient from a position of unfocused listening. He therefore does not focus the patient's anxiety immediately upon himself; that would be preemptive. Instead, he leaves room for the patient to make her own reference to him, if she is ready for this. The potential link to the therapist is left, like the spatula, within reach of the patient for her to use this in her own way or to ignore it. This guards against a transference interpretation being thrust at her.

> PATIENT: I was beginning to wonder why you weren't saying anything. It occurred to me that perhaps you were sorry to be back at work, or you might be feeling depressed.
>
> THERAPIST: I realized you were anxious, but I was waiting to see if you could let me know more about this. (*Pause.*) I think you may have been trying to let me know about your own depression, which you have been needing somebody to be in touch with; and the holiday break has added to your sense of being left to deal with this alone.

The patient began to cry: the flood of her talking had stopped. After a while she began telling the therapist about her mother's moods, when she was small. There had been times when the patient could not find any way to get through to her mother, who had been too preoccupied with her own depression.

> THERAPIST: I think you may have experienced my absence during the holiday, and my silence in this session, as reminders of being with your mother—her distance from you and your difficulty in being able to get through to her.

The patient recalled more about her relationship to her mother, and began to get angry with the therapist for being like her. By the end of the session, however, the patient was able to notice that her therapist was not being defensive or retaliatory in response to this anger. Her closing comment was: "I expected you to object to my being so angry with you."

Discussion: Here we have an example of a therapist who is prepared to wait, to be found by the patient in whatever way that happens. The patient is therefore not prevented from making use of him to represent a bad experience in childhood. Having attacked him for being like her mother she finds that he has remained unchanged by this.

So, through this non-retaliatory survival of her treating him as a "bad object" she rediscovers the therapist as a "good object."

It is all too easy to cut across a patient's spontaneous finding of the therapist's presence by intervening too quickly. A similar error is to bring the patient's communications to a premature focus onto the therapist, which is often done in the name of transference. This deadens the experience by lessening the sense of immediacy in the transference. By not allowing more time for this to develop in the session, a patient can be blocked from arriving at the more specific details that are often contained in a patient's further associations (if these are not interrupted).

It also deflects from the patient's *experience of feelings* towards *thinking about feelings,* before the actual experience has been more fully entered into. This invites the patient to intellectualize and can also be evidence of a countertransference defensiveness on the part of the therapist. When this happens, patients will often respond to this as a cue from the therapist to avoid what may have been difficult for the therapist to stay in touch with for longer.

PATIENTS' DIFFERING NEEDS

When therapists discover their patients' capacity for sharing in the therapeutic process, they have much to gain from learning to recognize the different levels of prompt. This does not mean that a therapist merely follows where patients lead, nor does it mean that patients are simply given what they ask for (or demand). It also does not mean that all such demands should be systematically frustrated, as if these were always pathological. Neither therapist nor patient alone can know what is best or what is needed. This is jointly discovered as the therapeutic process unfolds.

Therapists, therefore, must learn to distinguish between a patient's healthy strivings in the therapeutic process and pathological resistance to this. And they have to be able to recognize when a patient's perception is valid, even when this is critical of the therapist. It might not just be a further manifestation of projection or transference.

A discipline which I find useful, in listening to what a patient communicates, is to scan for what I might *least* want to hear as well as hearing what I may be anticipating. This helps to counterbalance the residual effects of preconception. It also helps to highlight precisely those issues which countertransference anxiety may prompt me not to recognize.

MISTAKES AND CORRECTIVE CUES

When something happens in a session that does not fit in with a patient's unconscious sense of what he or she needs to find in the therapy, there are various ways in which this may be indicated. This can be thought of as a "countertransference interpretation" by the patient (Little 1951: 39), as the patient's "potential therapeutic initiative" (Searles 1975: 97), as the patient's "unconscious supervision" of the therapist (Langs 1978), or as unconscious prompts. It can become a central issue to an analysis or therapy, to what extent a therapist is able to be responsive to these unconscious cues from the patient.

Inevitably, any analyst or therapist is going to make mistakes. It is therefore important to be able to recognize when this is happening; and it is a function of internal supervision to help in precisely this. When a therapist regularly uses trial identification to review his own part in a session, or in the therapy as a whole, he will discover how often patients give unconscious cues that indicate when something is wrong in the therapy. However, what is more important than a mistake having been made is coming to realize this and doing something about it. How a therapist deals with the effects of his own mistake(s) can become an important part of the therapeutic process itself. If a therapist fails to recognize when he is making mistakes, the patient comes to be cut off from his or her part in this process.

It is, therefore, a tragic loss when patients offer corrective cues to a therapist, but find these thrown back unrecognized for what they are. Some therapists are too ready to interpret all communications from a patient in terms of assumed pathology (in the patient) or as resistance to insight (as given by themselves). The patient's unconscious endeavor to help the therapist can then be defensively ignored.

FORMS OF PROMPTING

Some patients are quite clear when things do not feel right in the therapy, and they are able to point this out consciously and directly. Other patients communicate their criticism of the therapy less consciously.

There are several ways in which unconscious criticism is communicated. Perhaps the most familiar is through a patient's use of *displacement.* Some other person such as a parent, a figure of authority or a person who should know better, may be criticized. Often this can be recognized as alluding to a recent issue in the therapy.

Another form of unconscious prompt is when a patient uses what could be regarded as *criticism by contrast.* It may be that another professional is described as having done a careful job, in the context of the therapist having been unwittingly careless. The patient may be unconsciously holding up a model of better functioning, which it behooves the therapist to recognize as a possible cue to some area of his own poor functioning. Therapist and patient alike can benefit from adaptive responses by the therapist to this kind of corrective cue from the patient.

One other form of unconscious prompt, that is more difficult to recognize (or easier to overlook), is when a patient uses *introjective reference* as a more concealed form of unconscious criticism. By introjectively identifying with an aspect of the therapist, the patient blames himself for something which can be more meaningfully understood as referring to the therapist.

The patient described in Chapter 3 demonstrated each of these forms of unconscious prompting, in the course of the sequence described.

THE ABSENCE OF PRESSURES UPON THE PATIENT

Even though it is generally accepted that the analytic space should be preserved as far as possible from any kind of personal influence, or other pressures, there remains an element of unacknowledged pressure in the application of the "basic rule" which is often applied in analytic psychotherapy. Therapists are usually taught to explain to patients *there is only one rule, that of free association:* that a patient is to say whatever comes to mind, regardless of what it is. When the patient fails to comply with this rule it is frequently interpreted as "resistance." It can easily be overlooked that this resistance is sometimes a response to the basic rule.

It is interesting that traces of Freud's earlier "pressure technique" remain in his use of the "rule" of free association. Although this was regarded as the only rule, it nevertheless contains an implied pressure—in saying to patients that they should learn to use free association, and at the same time suggesting that this "free" association should itself be subject to a pressure to

speak and to say all. Some patients become stuck on exactly this
issue, particularly those patients who have been denied a sense of
separateness and privacy in childhood. It can therefore be a
growth-promoting experience for a patient to find a mental and
emotional space (within a relationship) that is genuinely free from
external pressures. A patient's inability to be free in this way can
sometimes be a prompt for the therapist to reconsider the application of this "basic rule," and the notion of resistance in relation to
this.[4]

There are many other forms of pressure that can be introduced
by the therapist, and patients frequently give unconscious cues that
relate to this. I shall give some examples below (see Examples 8.5,
8.6 and 8.7).

ESTABLISHING THE THERAPEUTIC BOUNDARIES

Example 8.3

When a patient (aged twenty-two) came for her initial consultation she
immediately poured out an account of her life till then. Throughout this,
there was a repeating theme to do with people who did not respect the
personal boundaries of others. Her parents had been intrusively controlling of her life; her uncle had made sexual advances to her as a child; her
doctor was a family friend, and had a reputation of flirting with his
patients. While saying this, the patient became anxious and reached for a
cigarette. She found that she did not have any matches and asked me
whether I could give her a light.

I felt alerted by what the patient had already told me. I therefore said
that I realized she was anxious, and might want to use a cigarette as a way
of dispelling some of her difficult feelings, but there were other issues at
stake. For instance, she had been telling me about people who had failed
to keep to the boundaries necessary to each of the relationships she had
been describing. Most recently there had been this doctor-friend who
flirted with his patients. So, I felt she may be unconsciously checking out
something about me, whether I could maintain a professional relationship
without this being blurred by gestures that could be confused with a more
social kind of relationship.

Once this patient had started therapy it became clear how important to her it had been that I made this stand right at the
beginning. She often referred back to this as basic to her eventual
trust in me. This was all the more crucial to her at times when
she was needing to use me to represent those others who had
misused her.

MAINTAINING THE BOUNDARIES

Example 8.4
A patient (Mr. H.) had started therapy some months before a summer holiday. He had not mentioned having his own holiday already arranged; but when the time approached for my holiday he told me he would be leaving a week earlier than me. This presented me with a dilemma. When I am making the initial arrangements for therapy I also give my holiday dates: if these clash with arrangements already made by the patient, this is usually discussed at the time. We had not discussed this overlap of dates.

I knew that Mr. H. had felt deserted by his previous therapist, who had become ill during a holiday break and had not resumed therapy with the patient. He might, therefore, need to have a clearer sense of continuity over the first break in this therapy—particularly as it was going to be extended by his prior absence. I decided to explore the patient's feelings about this, and to clarify the fee arrangement for his missed week of therapy.

> THERAPIST: I would not normally charge you for sessions missed because of arrangements made prior to starting therapy; but I realize you may have feelings about your sessions being kept for you while you are away. I am therefore wondering what you would like us to do about the three sessions you will miss.

> PATIENT: I would like to have those sessions before I go away.

Internal supervision: I was reminded that when Mr. H. first came to see me he had been wondering about having four sessions per week, but had started with three. Was he perhaps wanting to come more frequently, prior to going on holiday, as a way of helping him to decide whether to shift his therapy to four sessions a week on a more permanent basis? I prepared to explore this possibility.

> THERAPIST: I am not yet sure I will be able to make that arrangement, but we could look into the possibilities and the implications.

Mr. H. thanked me. After a short pause he told me about a previous job he had been at, where it had been necessary to take holidays by a certain fixed date in the year or you would miss your holiday. He added the comment: It was inconvenient in some ways, but at least you knew where you were.

He went on to emphasize his need for regularity in his life, and illustrated this by saying his ulcer usually comes back when that stability has been lacking. He is careful what he eats and has to eat regularly.

Internal supervision: I felt I was being cued to recognize the implications for Mr. H., if I were to offer him those extra sessions as suggested.

> THERAPIST: I think you are pointing out to me that, even if I were able to see you for the extra sessions before you go away, it could be a mixed blessing. You seemed grateful at my offer, but you have since been pointing out to me that you become anxious, even unwell, when there is a lack of stability in your life. A shift in the arrangements concerning your therapy could have exactly that sort of effect upon you.

Mr. H. was thoughtful, and then agreed he needed to know where he was with me. This was more important, in the long run, than having extra sessions.

A THERAPIST BECOMES INTRUSIVE WITH A PREMATURE INTERPRETATION RELATING TO HIMSELF

Example 8.5
A female patient, who was seeing a male therapist, had missed several sessions without explanation or getting in touch.

Upon returning, the patient said she had really not missed the sessions at all; she had been too busy with other things. She hadn't missed her ex-boyfriend either; she felt better off without him. He just wasn't important to her any more.

> THERAPIST: I think you may be wondering how important I am at this moment in your life too.

> PATIENT: No, you are very important. I couldn't do without you at the moment. I have had more important things to do recently, so I have had to give therapy a lower priority. That's all. (*Pause.*)
> I got very angry with someone I hardly know recently. This guy came back to our flat after a party. I was irritated with the way he kept butting in on our conversation. It wasn't as if he had really been invited; he had just tagged on when we left the party, and when he did not get the attention he was wanting he had the nerve to change the TV channel without even asking. I then just blew my top.

Discussion: The therapist arrives at his comment without a firm link between what the patient had been saying and any possible reference to the therapy. He presumes to know what the patient is thinking, so his interpretation becomes an intrusive intervention.

If we trial-identify with the therapist here, he might be feeling badly treated, perhaps even wondering how important he was to the patient. What he says comes across as if he had arrived at this interpretation from his countertransference feelings, and it sounds like a projection of his own doubts. Similarly, if we trial-identify with the patient, we can recognize that the analytic space is being intruded upon by the therapist, who appears not to want to be ignored by the patient.

The patient's response is two-fold. She first reassures the therapist that he need not doubt his importance in the patient's life. She then speaks of an incident where someone (else) had been intrusive. We may be hearing an unconscious commentary (Langs 1978) from the patient, upon the nature of the therapist's intervention as perceived by the patient, and an account of irritation and anger felt towards him.

Although the sequence described by the patient had occurred before this session, the timing in the session (i.e. when she thinks of it) is telling. The therapist was able to recognize himself being rebuked here by the patient, and could acknowledge his awareness of this later in the session. This is a good example of unconscious supervision by the patient. See also below.

A THERAPIST BECOMES INAPPROPRIATELY DIRECTIVE

Example 8.6
The patient, a girl aged twenty-five, was being treated by a female therapist.

PATIENT: I cannot stand the pressures at work. I think I may have to find another job.

THERAPIST: Have you ever thought of going to a careers advice center?

PATIENT: I was thinking about that myself, but I don't think I should need to be given advice about what to do with my life. I ought to be able to get in touch with that within myself. (*Pause.*) I only came back to London after the summer holiday because of you, but I now feel angry with you for some reason. (*Pause.*) My boss will be back tomorrow. I know what it will be like: he will be constantly telling me what to do interfering pressure all the time. He never seems to see me as able to do things for myself.

Discussion: We can see here an example that is filled with corrective cues from the patient. She did not need the therapist to be thinking for her. She also feels that she does not need to be given advice, as she ought to be able to get in touch with her own sense of direction from within herself. That is what the patient has been used to getting in her therapy, and here she feels the therapist is out of role. The patient then appears to change the subject, and we hear about somebody (referred to as her boss) who will be telling the patient what to do. The patient is assumed to be unable to do things for herself.

If we apply unfocused listening to this it is not difficult to pick up the displaced criticism. She is angry with her therapist, for becoming too like other people in her past (and present). She needs to be allowed to use the analytic space more freely than that.

DIFFICULTIES IN GETTING THROUGH TO THE THERAPIST

Example 8.7
A female patient aged thirty was seeing a male therapist.

> PATIENT: I am having difficulties in communicating. I feel lonely even when I am with other people. I feel at a distance from David (her husband). I was angry with him today, but we then made love. That was just before I set out to come here. I didn't actually want sex; I have difficulty in saying "No" or in showing how I am really feeling. It helped to push my angry feelings down, but they don't go away. (*Pause.*) I miss my old boss. I only had to raise my eyebrows and she would realize when I needed to speak to her (*Pause.*) Why do you think I have these difficulties?

> THERAPIST: It probably goes back to your childhood.

> PATIENT: Which relationship? Do you mean my parents? (*Lots of childhood details then followed.*)

Discussion: The themes here include various references to difficulties in relating. The patient feels distant and lonely, even when she is in company. (In the session she is with the therapist.) There is anger, and there is an example of anger being by-passed (having sex). There seems to have been a need to get rid of this anger (or sexual feelings?) before coming to her session. There may also be an example of criticism by contrast when the patient refers to another person (her previous boss), who would respond even to a raised eyebrow—picking up indications of need in the patient. The session ends with another example of a flight to the past being introduced by the therapist.

In this session, the therapist could have played back the main themes, in some not yet specific way, in preparation for dealing with the anxieties indicated. He could have said something like:

> "You have been telling me about feeling not understood and feeling at a distance from the person you are with. You also tell me about feelings that you tried to get rid of before coming here today.

I think there may be some anxiety about whether I am able to understand you, and what feels safe for you to bring to your therapy."

The reason for remaining nonspecific, in this playback of themes, is that we do not know more precisely what this patient is anxious about bringing to her therapy. It may be her feelings of criticism for her therapist. It may be her sense of not being understood. It may be her anger, or her sexual feelings. She allows her husband to deflect her anger: she may be anxious to find out whether her therapist is also someone who feels a need to deflect difficult feelings, or whether he can cope with these being more clearly directed at him.

The therapist's first comment in this session is in response to a direct question. He may have given the patient the impression that he needs more than a raised eyebrow for him to respond. When he then deflects the patient to her childhood, this is likely to confirm her anxiety about the effect of her difficult feelings upon other people. So, when the patient compliantly examines her childhood relationships, at the safe distance of time-past, she may well be reflecting her perception of the therapist. He could be seen as defending himself from the difficult allusions to him in the opening part of this session.

(A few weeks after the sequence given here this patient left her therapy.)

In this chapter I have tried to illustrate some of the many ways in which patients contribute towards the shaping of their therapy, and towards helping the therapist to provide the kind of therapeutic experience which they are needing to be able to discover. And when things are going wrong, patients offer many unconscious cues to the therapist to draw attention to this—for the analytic hold to be reestablished and the analytic process resumed.

Therapists need to recognize the element of healthy searching within a patient's unconscious. If they can adequately distinguish between growth-needs and pathological striving, then they may discover the gradual process whereby a patient unwittingly guides the therapist towards what is unconsciously looked for within the therapeutic relationship. It is in this kind of way, when something is amiss in the therapy, that patients will often nudge the therapist back towards ways of working that are nearer to what is needed by that patient, at that moment in that therapy.

❖9❖

The Search for Space: An Issue of Boundaries[1]

I now wish to illustrate more extensively the part played by a patient's unconscious cues, and how these contributed to the effectiveness of the resulting analysis.

I had to discover how to read the cues of this patient, which I did by trial-identifying with her or with the objects of her relating. From this way of listening it was possible to recognize what the patient was needing that she had not been finding. She dramatically demonstrated her need for clear boundaries to the analytic relationship, and for a genuinely neutral space in which she could become autonomously herself.

INTRODUCTION

Miss K. (as I shall call the patient) was aged twenty-seven when she was referred to me. She had suffered for years with compulsive eating.

For the greater part of her short analysis (twenty months) Miss K. subjected me to severe testing, acting out with others what I would not enter into with her. Outside the analysis she continued to be engaged in attempts at getting alternative help, all of them alien to the analysis. I had to maintain a difficult balance between trying to contain this acting out (which I could only do if I were to interpret this as attacks upon the analysis) and having to be careful not to get caught into repeating the responses of those who had previously been trying to control this patient's life.

Miss K. gave me many unconscious cues for handling her analysis. These were given in the account of her past life, and in the details of her acting out. It was very clear to me what had not helped her, and what was still not helping her. By contrast, I could sense what she was most deeply searching for. I therefore tolerated the acting out (not that I had much option) and I continued to seek an understanding of it through interpretation. This meant, however, that I had often to tolerate being put into a position of apparent analytic impotence, with the analysis seeming to be quite chaotic.

What emerged, after many months of this near annihilation of the analysis, was that it was in my non-retaliatory survival of this testing by the patient that the potency of the analysis ultimately lay. She came to discover that the analysis continued to offer her an unbiased relationship-space in which she could begin to become her "own version of herself." (This phrase occurred in one particular interpretation and was adopted by the patient as a central theme of her analysis.) She did not have to offer a compliance to please. Neither did she have to maintain, indefinitely, her protest against the pressures that had always been upon her to comply.

Having found this neutral space in the analysis, Miss K. began to use it in preparation for how she would be later. For the first time in her life, she was able to own herself and find an independent life apart from the family's expectations of her. The duration of this analysis had to be time-limited due to visa restrictions on the patient's length of stay in this country. Nevertheless the progress made has been maintained since, already over a number of years.

PRACTICAL LIMITATIONS ON THE ANALYSIS

Because of the uncertainty about her length of stay in this country, I felt that I could not offer Miss K. five-times-a-week analysis immediately even though she was asking for this. I therefore waited until it was known how long she could remain here.

I originally saw Miss K. in twice-weekly therapy. This was increased to four times per week once it became clear that she earnestly wished to have analysis as the treatment of choice rather than just "having more." I had to be careful that it did not become another form of compulsive eating, having everything that was available in order to gratify her insatiable hunger. I eventually agreed that analysis, even short-term, could give her the optimum chance of finding the help she needed.

I saw Miss K. for four sessions a week during most of her first year of treatment with me. When her visa position was clarified she knew she could stay for a maximum of a further eight months. For the remaining time I saw her five times per week.

It was during this latter period that Miss K. began to use her analysis in a quite different way; whereas, throughout the first year, there had always been a possibility she might have to leave the country at short notice. She had therefore been constantly fighting against letting herself experience yet another relationship with any degree of dependence, knowing how difficult she had always found separation in the past. She was afraid there could again be an abrupt ending, without time to work through her feelings about it.

THE FAMILY BACKGROUND

In the early part of her analysis the patient poured out details of unhappy relationships and experiences. She came from a moderately well-off Jewish family, which she described as dominated by the mother who was said to be manipulative and intrusive. The patient has a sister two years younger than herself.

Miss K. spoke of her relationship with her father as one of close mutual attachment. She recalled being alarmed when her mother began threatening to leave him, because she was going to take the children with her. She experienced her mother as "stifling," choosing her friends and preventing her from having any real independence. Her father, a businessman, had died suddenly from a heart attack when Miss K. was seventeen. This event was followed by the patient's first period of over-eating.

Miss K. had been breastfed until after she had cut her first teeth. My impression was that her mother may have wished to prolong the breastfeeding, and it could have been the biting that prevented this. Later, it seemed as if the mother felt that *she* had been deprived by the separateness achieved through this weaning, and it may have accounted for some of the pressures upon Miss K. to behave in her habitually placatory (and compensatory) way towards her mother—trying to make her feel all right. It would also throw some light upon the importance of biting in the patient's subsequent attempts to establish a fuller separation from her mother.

There had been a natural predisposition toward an oral fixation, probably encouraged by her mother's flamboyant enjoyment of breastfeeding. She had openly boasted that this had been more satisfying to her than any part of her marriage relationship.

When Miss K. was just two years old she had to give up her mother to a baby sister. There was some suggestion that her mother may have been depressed after the sister's birth. At any rate, the mother withdrew from the home "for a rest after the birth," leaving both children with a nanny.

Miss K. became gripped by jealousy towards her younger sister and regularly turned to her father for comfort. He seems to have received her overintimately. For instance, when she was distressed he would get into her bed to comfort her, and I was told he continued this up until he died. Miss K. felt bereft and empty after her father's death. It was then that she first turned to regular overeating, in an attempt to deal with her grief and depression.

This quasisexual attachment to her father (tinged as it was with a sense of "Oedipal triumph" over her mother) had in no way been resolved before he died. Instead, that experience became a prototype for her relationships to men. She therefore regarded her sexuality as uncontainable, as if this had been responsible for destroying the much needed structure of her parents' marriage. Equally, she saw her sexuality as overwhelming to any object of her love, even life-threatening, and therefore to be avoided. She expected men to retreat from her. The first important boyfriend who did not immediately retreat also had a heart condition.

To add to this confusion about her sexuality, her mother had also behaved seductively towards her daughters. I was told that when Miss K. and her sister had reached puberty her mother would make them lie in bed with her, and she would stroke their developed breasts. She had taunted Miss K. by laughing at her and saying "You're a lesbian."

Her mother's own sexual orientation sounded confused and confusing. She had started an affair with another man before the father had died, but this affair, like the marriage, had been unstable. When her mother was upset by this she would turn to Miss K. for solace. There had also been a strange "aunt," during the patient's early adolescence, with whom her mother would go on holiday without the children. Miss K. wondered whether this woman was a lesbian, and it left her wondering whether her mother had been bisexual.

Miss K. described her difficulties in forming relationships with boyfriends, discovering herself to be manipulative and possessive like her mother. Whenever she was attracted to a man, she became overwhelmed by her feelings and would crave to be loved. She also found that her boyfriends became impotent with her, blaming this on her. At least one boyfriend had described her as "devouring." She had again turned to food in an attempt to deflect this relation-ship-hunger, which she regarded as being too much for any person to satisfy. For most of her analysis, it was precisely this anxiety that I was having to cope with in her relationship to me.

ISSUES RELATING TO OVEREATING

Because the eating problem was so overdetermined, it will simplify my account of this if I consider it in relation to various aspects of the patient's life.

The mother's ambition for her daughter was for her to be "slim and beautiful" and to get married. Outwardly, Miss K. accepted these goals as her own, but there was a much stronger wish to thwart her mother's ambitions. She felt that if she allowed herself to remain thin, which she had been during her early puberty, it would be tantamount to her ceasing to be a separate person. Her mother seemed to "own" her, as if trying to live vicariously through her.

Miss K. discovered that overeating was one way of demonstrating a separateness over which her mother could have no control. This provoked active concern (even wailing) in her mother, that gratified Miss K.'s ambivalent wish to be demonstrably separate from her and yet still the center of her mother's interest. However, she did not see the dynamics of this rebellion against the mother until she was in analysis.

In her mother's company Miss K. usually found she was unable to be angry. Instead, she became desperate to please, and fearful that her mother might prefer her younger sister to herself. Even when Miss K. was in England, away from her mother, she would frequently write placatory letters or telephone her—often daily. At the same time she felt her mother to be like a "cancerous growth" inside, of which she felt she could never rid herself.

The mother was skilled in putting on an act of being hurt: "How could you do this to me after all I have done for you?" etc., and she became very upset if Miss K. ever hinted that her mother might not be the most loving mother possible. Miss K., therefore, could only express her angry feelings by turning these against herself and the internalized mother. When she overate she quite specifically chose to eat "rubbish food," experiencing a sadistic pleasure in "throwing all that garbage at my mother inside."

Because of the highly sexualized relationship with her father, who seemed to have given her little sense of appropriate parent/child boundaries, Miss K. had come to experience any physical contact with a man as incestuous. Her mental image of any boyfriend easily merged with that of her father. She therefore felt guilty about heterosexual physical contact, and one function of her eating was to make herself "physically repulsive" (her own phrase). By thus discouraging the sexual contact, which consciously she craved for, she managed to avoid this incest guilt.

Miss K. also wondered if she could more successfully avoid feeling guilty in a homosexual relationship, but even there she felt trapped by the incestuous implications of her mother's sensual seductiveness towards her. The way felt blocked for her in either direction. She could not allow herself to be genitally sexual without feeling guilty, so she would set up forms of self-punishment—with the unconscious hope that she could thereby allay her guilt about having any sexual feelings at all. For a long time, eating had offered her some kind of compromise and compensation for this lack of genital satisfaction.

The patient had only once or twice experienced orgasm in intercourse, partly due to her infrequent experience of intercourse, and partly because her boyfriends so quickly became impotent with her. She assumed this was because they could not face her insatiable demands. In fact she expected everyone, including me, to retreat from the intensity of her demands upon them.

I never got a clear picture of the patient's sexual life. She did not spontaneously offer to speak of this, and I deliberately chose not to question her.

By putting on a lot of weight, Miss K. could simulate the appearance of being pregnant, and she would fantasize to herself that she was. The significance of this first emerged consciously during the middle part of her analysis, at which time her sister came with her doctor husband to live and work in England. The sister was already four or five months pregnant. Miss K. was invited to live with them. She did, and there were frequent outbursts of jealousy and envy towards the sister and her pregnancy.

Her sister's marriage was already the object of much envy, her sister having "got a husband" whereas the patient regarded herself as too fat and unlikable ever to marry. The pregnancy added a further dimension to the tension, with roots which we were able to trace back to the time of her mother's pregnancy with this sister. Miss K. remembered her mother telling her how she, as a small child, had tried to attack her mother's pregnant belly. She had been violently jealous of her sister as soon as she was born. For a long time after the birth she had refused to eat food prepared by her mother, and at times she could only be fed by her father or by someone else not her mother.

During the course of her sister's pregnancy, Miss K. put on weight in parallel with the growth in the pregnancy. To a large extent she succeeded in making herself look as pregnant as her sister, but inwardly she seethed with envy towards her sister's live baby which mocked the sterile fullness of her own belly.

THE PATIENT DEMONSTRATES HER NEED FOR BOUNDARIES

Miss K. originally came to England, from her home in west-coast America, in pursuit of her former therapist (Dr. Z.). She had been in twice-weekly private psychotherapy, with this doctor in America, for nearly two years. That therapy was abruptly terminated when Dr. Z. accepted an opportunity to work in Europe. There had been no time to work through that interruption of her therapy.

Miss K. continued to be in touch with Dr. Z. during the intervening two years, by letter and by telephone. Her journey to England was a last bid to persuade him to let her resume therapy with him. She telephoned him from London begging him to allow this. She was wanting to find accommodation and work in the town he had moved to. Only then did she accept that Dr. Z. was not going to let her resume treatment with him. Instead, he recommended she try group therapy. Miss K. told me that he had explained this recommendation saying: "the transference to a single therapist would be unmanageably strong." She felt hurt and rejected by this, but she was not deterred from her search for further individual therapy. She was ultimately referred to me.

During the opening phase of her analysis I heard a lot about Dr. Z. At the time of her previous therapy he had been a psychiatric registrar. From the patient's account of that therapy, I gathered that he conditioned her with praise and encouragement. She felt erotically attached to him, and was gratified and excited by his interest in her body. She found that she could manipulate this interest in her, through focusing upon her body-weight. Dr. Z. would weigh her every time she went for a session, and he praised her for each loss in weight. He offered further encouragement by describing the kind of clothes which would set off her figure to best advantage, even to the detail of the best kind of bra. Miss K. described one occasion when Dr. Z. got her to strip to the waist, to show him how her bust was coming along as a result of the loss of weight (helped by the recommended bra).

The overt relationship focus during that previous therapy was around Miss K.'s boyfriend of the time. She described her therapist as "masterminding" her relationship with this boyfriend, and she was able to satisfy by these means her wish to be allowed to be "absolutely dependent" on Dr. Z. He even let her telephone him to ask what she should do next in relation to her boyfriend, and Dr. Z. would tell her.

Towards the end of her treatment with Dr. Z., Miss K. rewarded him by losing a lot of weight; and with his frequent advice and guidance she set about trying to get her boyfriend to propose. It was around this time that Dr. Z. told her he was leaving America to work in Europe.

The impending loss of her relationship to this therapist exposed the extent of her eroticized attachment to him, and he continued to gratify her demands beyond the time when the treatment relationship "officially ended." Apparently, in order to ameliorate her desolation upon losing him, Dr. Z. allowed Miss K. to visit him in his family home. She saw him there several times, during the month remaining before he left for Europe, and she told me she stayed overnight on more than one occasion. Being in the spare room next to the main bedroom, she claimed to have listened to Dr. Z. having intercourse with his wife.

Comment: A number of points need to be made clear about the patient's account of this previous therapy and of her other activities outside the consulting room.

What she was describing was her perception of those experiences. In her relationship with Dr. Z., for instance, we have to bear in mind how her wish to be erotically involved with him would color her perception of that experience, and how she remembered it. So, should we regard this only as an account of the patient's internal world, and as evidence of an unresolved eroticized transference with the distortions of wish-fulfillment? We can certainly see transference elements; but it cannot all be dismissed as transference if the therapist had in reality been gratifying the patient's seductiveness with seductive behavior of his own. We therefore should not describe the interaction between this patient and her former therapist as "*just* transference" (Leites 1977).

Also, the patient's own basic truthfulness, which was a feature of her analysis, should be taken into consideration. Although she did hide some things from me at first, in her acting out of those feelings which she initially split off and kept separate from the analysis, I found she was always in the end prepared to face the details of her own truth—however painful it might be. Miss K. gave me the impression that she never consciously ducked the truth about herself or distorted this by exaggeration.

Miss K. felt utterly shattered when Dr. Z. refused to take her back into therapy. She had been counting on resuming her relationship with him, particularly as she had lost weight "entirely for him." She reverted to massive overeating, and had put on some forty pounds in the last few months before being referred to me. This gain in weight, at that time, was largely motivated by her wish to revenge herself upon Dr. Z.

Miss K. continued to be obsessed with her unfinished relationship to Dr. Z.; she felt herself to be in love with him. Compared with this, her unhappy relationship with the boyfriend in America (which had since broken down) paled into insignificance. In her revengeful eating she had reached the point where she felt no longer able to control her eating at all. She frequently felt desperate, and close to breakdown. She sometimes felt suicidal, but did not think that she had the courage to be actively suicidal.

ISSUES RELATED TO BOUNDARIES

Miss K.'s way of using Dr. Z's first name made it sound as if she were speaking of a boyfriend rather than a therapist, and this was actually how she felt about him. Dr. Z. was kept on a pedestal, and the patient would say: "At least he showed he cared," whereas I was seen as coldly distant and uncaring.

The psychiatrist who referred Miss K. to me had told her that she needed clear analytic boundaries, if she were to have any chance of making better use of further therapy. Being desperate for help, she gave me (from the start) an outward compliance with the conditions of treatment. She never telephoned me and she never asked for extra time. However, towards other people she continued to express the manipulative and demanding side of herself.

I interpreted this as her way of trying to spare me the intensity of her feelings; and when I was able to see how she was pressurizing others I could see what it was that she was protecting me from. It was also her way of being the good and obedient child, in her relationship to me, with the assumption that she would be rejected if she brought to me those other aspects of herself she was expressing elsewhere.

However, I soon discovered that Miss K. had a strong tendency to provoke others into offering her alternative forms of treatment, in parallel to her seeing me. I therefore had to make an early decision on how to handle this.

I felt the patient was trying to provoke me to adopt a non-psychoanalytic role, so that I might try stopping this acting out against the analysis. By trial-identifying with the patient, to consider this option, I recognized that if I responded in any way aimed at controlling her, she might experience me as repeating a traumatic factor of her relationship with her mother. This convinced me that I would not be able to interpret her experience of me as transference, if she could realistically see me as actually behaving like her mother. I sensed that Miss K. was unconsciously provoking me to reenact with her the role of an intrusive mother.

Whilst I had to be alert to this splitting of the transference, and ready to interpret it as such, I realized how quickly this patient used all interpretations as if they were attempts by me to manipulate her, to direct her, or in some way to run her life for her. For a long time, she would react to interpretations as if these were disguised directions.

It gradually became clear that Miss K. had virtually no experience of any relationship between two people in which one person was not actively trying to manipulate the other. This soon became a central aspect of her analytic experience. I had to help her to find a personal space in which to discover her own thoughts and feelings, and eventually her own sense of direction, rather than play into her addictive dependence upon others to provide direction for her.

For a time Miss K. found it exceedingly difficult to believe she had any capacity for inner-directedness, and she fought against my frustration of her demands to have her life controlled for her. For instance, she frequently went outside the analytic relationship to get others to give her the advice I refrained from giving. By successfully manipulating others into a directive role towards her, she could bypass the firmness of my stand upon this.

Most particularly, Miss K. was using her brother-in-law (a doctor) as an alternative therapist. He regularly advised her, and arranged other forms of treatment—all of which were expressions of his opposition to psychoanalysis. Her acceptance of these other treatments also expressed her disowned attacks on the analysis.

The first attempts at alternative treatment were through medication. Initially this was prescribed by the GP; but, after her brother-in-law came to England, Miss K. began to accept medication from him. This included anti-depressants as well as appetite suppressants. I was not told about her use of medication until some time afterwards.

The next major attempt by the brother-in-law was to have the patient's jaws wired. This was regarded as an ultimate prevention against her compulsive eating. Miss K. was to have her teeth locked together, so that no food could be chewed, and she would only be able to take in liquid foods. She first told me about this when she had already been to a dentist to have impressions made, in preparation for having this dental procedure.

As with Miss K.'s earlier attempts to provoke me into trying to prevent her acting out against the analysis, I was here put into yet another dilemma. If I tried to interpret this as a further attack upon the analysis which it so clearly was, it was certain she would hear this as a poorly concealed maneuver by me to stop her having her jaws wired. If I had tried then to interpret her assumption that I was trying to control her (as if this were only based upon her other relationship experiences i.e. as transference) this would have carried little conviction. As I really did want to stop her, I had to be even more careful to let Miss K. make her own decision, whether or not to proceed with the plans already made, without indicating my preference either way.

Miss K. came to her next session with her teeth already wired together. As with her earlier use of medication I was faced with another *fait accompli*. I privately wondered whether she could use this "contraption" in her mouth (which is how she spoke of it) as something transitional between an external relationship controlling her and the beginnings of an internalized capacity for self-control. When I explored this with her it turned out that she could not.

The dentist's device came to be experienced by Miss K. as an embodiment of her intrusive mother. She felt this object (once fixed in her mouth) to be persecuting her, in trying to force a control upon her, as her mother had. It also became something to be defeated by any means possible.

Miss K. experienced the same kind of hate towards this object as she had often felt for her mother. It intensified her wish to defeat her mother's designs for her, and the designs of anybody else who seemed to be aligned with her mother through their attempts at controlling her.

Even though the wiring of her jaws made it impossible for her to bite anything, she became ingenious in finding ways of bypassing this restriction. She crushed up fattening foods, and would suck the resulting mixture through a wide tube. She continued to put on weight; and I used to hear a note of triumph in her complaints of depression at the failure of this last-resort method of her eating being controlled for her.

Nevertheless, a new discovery emerged, that biting played a key part in her pleasure of eating. Deprived of the direct satisfaction of biting into food, Miss K. became much more openly violent in her biting sarcasm, and her angry snapping attacks upon people who angered her. Much of this was directed towards the brother-in-law, who had advised her to have her teeth wired. Some of it was also aimed at me, as I had not stopped her taking his advice.

During the four months that her teeth remained wired together, Miss K.'s sister gave birth to a daughter. This aroused intense jealousy, and envy of the closeness between the mother and baby. Miss K. only felt able to alleviate this by taking over the baby from her sister, whenever possible. She would thereby come between the baby and the real mother, pretending the baby to be her own. We could see here a remembering, through reexperiencing, of the early fantasies which she had around the time when her mother had given birth to her sister. This also confirmed our earlier interpretive work, concerning the patient's childhood feelings of exclusion from her parent's relationship and from her mother's relationship to her sister.

This acting out of the past in the present was further exemplified when Miss K.'s mother visited England to see her first grandchild. Miss K. became jealous of any attention given by her mother to her sister, or to the baby. She frequently resorted to eating as an attempt to suppress these feelings, but indirectly also to express them.

At about this time the brother-in-law, who had come to regard himself as principally in charge of Miss K's treatment, referred her to a behavior therapist. This other therapist insisted she should immediately have her teeth unwired, and Miss K. offered herself into his hands for yet another version of being told what to do.

Miss K. was able to act out, in her relationship with this behavior therapist (whom I shall call Mr. R.), her wish for physical closeness from which she unconsciously assumed I needed to be protected.

She was able to repeat with him many aspects of her earlier relationship with Dr. Z.

Mr. R., like Dr. Z., took an increasingly physical interest in the weight problem and in Miss K's body as a whole. He also changed from seeing her in his daytime office to seeing her in the sitting room of his home. The rationale behind the treatment that he was offering was to condition Miss K. against certain forms of eating. He also said he wanted her to feel better about her body generally. I shall give two examples.

1. Mr. R. got the patient to lie on the floor (in his home) while he put his fingers in her mouth. He was quoted as saying: "Now imagine that my fingers are a Mars Bar." He then encouraged Miss K. to develop fantasies around having a Mars Bar in her mouth, with the excited anticipation of eating this. After this he inserted his fingers further down her throat to make her "gag." The intention here was to create a conditioned-reflex link between eating Mars Bars and an impulse to vomit. What Miss K. did not tell him, however, was that she found the insertion of his fingers into her mouth sexually arousing. She did not want him to stop doing it.

2. On one occasion Mr. R. told the patient she needed to get more used to being touched physically. He apparently proceeded to stroke her body, while she lay on the floor, concentrating mainly upon her breasts. This episode was also in his home. His wife was somewhere around but not in the room. He said that his wife "fully understood" the necessity for his patients to have this kind of treatment.

The patient told me she found the whole episode both exciting and frightening. She was subsequently in a state of acute conflict over returning to see Mr. R. for further treatment. She did not really want him to help her with her eating problems. If she went back, she knew it would be for the sexual arousal involved in it for her. She fantasized about him as a continuation of her relationship with Dr. Z. Eventually however, after much hesitation, she made her own decision to stop seeing this latest alternative therapist.

I interpreted mainly in terms of the patient enacting with other people those aspects of her wished-for relationship with me, which she kept isolated from the consulting room. By getting her brother-in-law to act like the intrusive mother, and the dentist with his "contraption" as an actualization of that, she could keep me as the idealized and therefore non-intrusive mother. Equally, by setting up a quasi-sexual encounter with the behavior therapist, Miss K. was able to keep me as a safe and non-sexual father.

It was not easy to help Miss K. recognize the multiple ways in which she contributed towards setting up these situations. She would complain about people who would keep telling her what to do, how they would manipulate her life and intrude upon it. However, it was clear to me that in some way she was addictively attached to this kind of relationship. In the analysis too she put pressure on me to offer her active advice and direction, as if this might be the only way for her to cope with the problems of her life. She would go through the motions of complaining about pressures from other people, and trying to fight these off, but she would still use her evident helplessness as a way of eliciting futile attempts at helping her. She could then make these attempts fail, and she would tell me of each failure with unmistakable enjoyment—again with a note of triumph in her voice.

ESTABLISHING BOUNDARIES

When her mother was in this country, Miss K. at first fell back into the kind of relationship which she and the mother had always been used to. This involved an oscillation between the patient's compliant wish to please and outbursts of anger. These would be followed by regrets and self-recrimination, wishing to patch up the appearance of a good relationship with the mother.

In the course of this visit, however, the patient discovered the extent to which this pattern of relating was based upon a fantasy that her mother needed to be protected from Miss K.'s murderous feelings towards her. She was seeing her mother as not able to let her become fully separate. It gradually became clear that this was her way of trying to hide from herself her own fear of being rejected by her mother. Both mother and daughter were obsessively trying to deny any bad feelings towards the other. As a result one could become separate from the other.

However, during her mother's stay here, Miss K. dared to challenge this relationship and the shared fantasy that separation could not be tolerated. She spoke her mind to her mother in ways she had never previously imagined possible. To her surprise the mother survived this, and did not revert to a manipulative use of hurt feelings. There was, for the first time, a lot of straight speaking by the patient to her mother. This helped to establish a sense of psychological distance between them. She could then point out to her mother some of the occasions when she was still being intrusive; when, for instance, she was expecting to know everything the patient was doing and thinking or feeling.

Miss K. also became more aware of the ways in which she had habitually invited others to become intrusive. She began to see that she did not have to remain the helpless victim of other people's intrusion. Being more in touch with the ways in which she evoked intrusion, she discovered she could modify her own part in this with correspondingly different responses from those around her.

By the time her mother left England, after a visit of about six weeks, Miss K. had started to establish herself as a separate person. Her mother had responded to this and had begun to see this daughter differently. The relationship between them, which before had been so symbiotic and confused, began to become differentiated. In particular, personal boundaries were established between mother and daughter where before there had been none.

We then moved into the final stage of Miss K.'s treatment with me. Once she learned exactly when her visa was due to expire she was able to finalize her plans to emigrate to another country. We had four months' notice of her departure. This precipitated the patient into a new earnestness, wishing to get from her analysis what she needed before she had to leave.

During these remaining months, Miss K. began to realize that her eating had lost a great deal of its earlier compulsive quality. She felt she would eat normally once she had left England, but she deliberately continued to maintain her overweight while she was still here. She did not want her family, particularly her mother and brother-in-law, to think that any visible progress was in any way due to their pressures upon her if she allowed herself to lose weight while she was still living within their orbit and influence. She regarded this awareness, that her overeating was beginning to become a redundant habit, as a secret which she shared only with me.

Miss K. decided to leave her analysis the week before she left England. This was a deliberate choice, her wanting to have the experience of knowing she could have had more sessions (during the remaining week) but knowing she had chosen for herself not to. In this way she was able to give to her leaving an important element of her own choosing. It was not just passively accepted, as a time set for her by the authorities around the expiration of her visa; nor was it simply the patient preempting the end, though it was that too.

Miss K. used her last session sitting in a chair face to face with me. During this last hour she reviewed what she had gained from her analysis. The statement which stood out most particularly was: "I am becoming my own version of myself." She also spoke about the importance of discovering the space between people. She had experienced this for herself and she was confident that she would never forget it.

DISCUSSION OF THE ROLE OF THE ANALYST

The Decision to Offer Analysis

When I began seeing Miss K., and was hearing the account of her earlier therapy, I had urgently to find ways of understanding the responses which she evoked in me. For instance, it was impossible not to feel the impact of her demanding neediness, and I knew that I too might experience this as overwhelming particularly if I could not find some way of understanding it. Eventually, however, I became convinced that there were important cues here for the management of this patient's analysis.

In reviewing what Miss K. had told me of herself, I could see she had never felt securely contained by her previous therapist, who had probably been subjected to the same kind of pressures as I was experiencing. There was also something about the intensity of the transference which Dr. Z. expected to be too much for one person. Miss K. expected this too, so I knew I must keep firmly to my own personal and professional boundaries, holding on to the familiar framework of analysis, and expect a severe testing-out. In this sense I was forewarned.

Another warning cue was evident in the patient being so compliantly good for my benefit. She was careful not to step over any of the more obvious boundaries, the transgression of which had been such a feature in her previous therapy. As already indicated, she never telephoned; she was always ready to leave at the end of each session: there was no asking for extra contact or any manipulation for this. However, as I listened beyond her compliance, I sensed this to be seductive in order to please, and that it might be an unconscious reminder to me of her need for firmness.

Miss K. seemed never to have experienced anyone prepared, or able, to stand up to her manipulative pressures. It was therefore not surprising that she regarded herself as having something uncontrollable about her. She was still in search of a containing relationship able to withstand these pressures from her. I felt, therefore, that my task was primarily to be that of surviving her manipulations of me, in whatever form these were to come. If I could do that I believed something could be achieved.

My original offer was restricted to twice a week, in order to give me a chance to see how Miss K. and I managed in her sessions. I also needed to decide whether I could realistically risk offering her more intensive therapy, bearing in mind the short time available for her to have therapy in this country. However, once I sensed there was sufficient ego-strength in this patient, and that she was not poised on the edge of an uncontainable regression, I decided she could use analysis.

Feeling Intruded Upon and/or Manipulated

By using two-way trial identification, I was able to learn a lot about Miss K.'s experience of intrusiveness in relationships. For instance, when I listened to my feelings "in the shoes" of the previous therapist, I picked up an impression of being massively intruded upon by the patient. Dr. Z. had frequently been contacted out of session times, and he had agreed to extra sessions. He had also allowed the patient to visit him socially. The patient therefore had an image of a therapist who could be invaded, manipulated and seduced.

Likewise, by trial identifying with the patient, I could recognize that Miss K. must have been similarly subjected to unmanageable intrusion and manipulation; and it was likely that her previous experience of therapy would have confirmed her worst fears about herself. It was inevitable that these issues would be around with me too.

My Role in Relation to the Acting Out

On many occasions Miss K. made me feel helpless, in relation to her acting out—around and against the analysis. Whenever I felt inclined to restrain this by interpretation (as I might with other patients), my trial identification regularly alerted me to the likelihood that she would see me as trying to control her. Her life had been full of other people trying to run her life, so I felt it would be counter-productive if I took on a role which she could realistically see as similar or the same.

I was also alerted by her initial compliance in the analysis, to expect that she was splitting off a healthier but disowned noncompliance. If this were so, that protesting would probably continue to be expressed outside of her relationship to me until we had adequately understood her need to use these defensive ways of relating to me.

I was faced with an acute technical dilemma. I could, of course, still interpret the acting out. Furthermore, I could interpret (in terms of transference) any misunderstanding of my motives for that interpreting, if she assumed I was trying to control her just like everyone else. However, when I did interpret in this way it had little effect. Instead, I had to accept finding myself a helpless witness to the analysis being constantly threatened, perhaps even destroyed, through the various attempts at alternative treatment which were set in motion around it. I knew that it would not help the patient if my motive for trying to control her acting out was mainly in order to reduce my own feelings of discomfort. I also knew that nothing would be gained by getting her to comply with any covert directiveness in my interpretations, aimed at controlling her. That could only result in a facade of change, arrived at falsely. This debate with myself helped me to adopt a different stance in the analysis.

I felt that Miss K. had her own unconscious need for this acting out, chiefly to have a real experience of my letting her run her own life without interference or intrusion from me. I learned to be watchful for any wish of my own to direct her life, whether through word or attitude or manner of expression—however indirectly. We thus came upon her search for space, and her need for me to respect this at whatever cost to me or to my view of myself as analyst.

I had to learn to be ready to accept being made to feel professionally impotent, without having to counter this by attempts to prove otherwise. Only time could tell whether this would be effective or not. I was therefore relieved to find, later in the analysis, that I could resume my interpretation of her unconscious motives behind this acting out, without this becoming a reenactment of the manipulation of her by others.

Splitting of the Transference

During the early part of the analysis Miss K.'s former therapist, like her father, had been persistently idealized. Later, Miss K. came to see for herself that, in important ways, she had not been helped either by her former therapist or by her father because of the lack of boundaries in each relationship. For a while, this awareness led to a shift in the earlier idealization of Dr. Z. She then began to idealize her relationship with me, apparently still accepting the boundaries which I adhered to. That idealization of me in the transference could only be modified through my steady interpretation of the patient's acting out, as her disowned attacks upon me, which unconsciously she expected me to be unable to cope with.

From the start, Miss K. appeared to be using her analysis. I thought she was glad of the opportunity to experience a relationship in which there was a clear framework. Meanwhile she was actively attacking the analysis through her acting out against it. Consciously she was not aware of this as an attack, but the unconscious intent became abundantly clear.

As the analysis continued, Miss K. presented me with one alternative treatment after another, each already entered into or set-up. Rather than being put into a position of trying to influence her, concerning these alternative treatments, I chose to go along with her decisions about these—being careful not to evaluate them.

My survival of this testing out gradually emerged in contrast to the background of advice from others. Miss K.'s appreciation of my part in her recovery became apparent quite suddenly during the final period of her analysis, when she was coming five times a week—knowing exactly when she would be leaving England. My survival had opened up a neutral space for her in which she could experiment with how she felt, and how she really wished to be.

For the first time, Miss. K did not have to comply with someone else's wishes. The potency of this was surprising. She was at first incredulous that I had really been able to withstand her pressures on me, which were aimed at making me become directive and controlling of her like everyone else in her life. She then began to relax into a new calm. She had discovered something of vital significance. Her life could be her own, and she did not have to spend all her life proving this. The long-term effects of that realization can be measured by feedback from the patient, three years later, described in the followup below.

Winnicott's Notion of the "Use of an Object"

From the experience of this analysis, the patient and I each learned much. The patient arrived at a real awareness of my separateness, external to her and not controlled by her. She could therefore begin to discover within herself a comparable separateness from me, and from others. She also discovered the creative potential of a relationship-space wherein she could arrive at a new freedom to be herself.

To this end the patient needed me to have an independent reality of my own, and for her to discover this in her own way. It would not have been enough for her if I had just been a passive container for her projections. She needed the assurance, which only experience could give her, that I had my own capacity to survive her attacks and that I did not need her to protect me from them.

I in my turn discovered more about the importance of *space* in a relationship, and I began to appreciate the clinical importance of Winnicott's concept of "the use of an object" (Winnicott 1971: Chapter 6). Miss K. had been able to make creative use of her own destructiveness, in order to discover that the survival of the other was not dependent upon her.

Once Miss K. had discovered that the other could exist and survive, as an entity in its own right, she was able to discover the possibility of a real separateness. She did not have to remain forever merged with her mother (or another). Nor did she always have to preserve the person she was relating to, and trying to be separate from, by constantly redirecting her destructive feelings onto others or against herself. It was by inwardly (in fantasy) "destroying" me as analyst, and the analysis, through her acting out that this patient could eventually discover my otherness from her. She had anticipated either collapse or retaliation, as the only imaginable responses to those aspects of herself which she had come to regard as uncontrollable, and therefore assumed to be omnipotently dangerous.

Winnicott says of this:

> At the point of development that is under survey the subject is creating the object in the sense of finding externality itself, and it has to be added that this experience depends on the object's capacity to survive. (It is important that survive, in this context, means not retaliate.) If it is in an analysis that these matters are taking place, then the analyst, the analytic technique, and the analytic setting all come in as surviving or not surviving the patient's destructive attacks. (Winnicott 1971: 91)

I was often tempted to interpret, just to reassure myself that I was still able to think and to function in the session when things seemed most chaotic, but I had to learn to refrain. However, once the acting out had subsided it became possible to interpret this without a sense of wishing to control the patient. Much of the patient's understanding of her acting out was therefore arrived at retrospectively, rather than at the time. It was reassuring to find that Winnicott had written of this too:

> The analyst feels like interpreting, but this can spoil the process, and for the patient can seem like a kind of self-defense, the analyst parrying the patient's attack. Better to wait till after the phase is over, and then discuss with the patient what has been happening. (Winnicott 1971: 92)

It was only with hindsight that I could understand where I had been in this analysis, and why. When, in the end, the patient was able to realize I had continued to survive her attacks upon the analysis, and upon me, she began to discover it was safe for her to become more fully alive in herself . When she ended, she left her analysis freely. This time she left looking forward, not back.

FOLLOW-UP

I was very cautious about the possibility of Miss K. writing to me after the end of her analysis. She had already shown how she had used letters in order to hold onto Dr. Z., after ending that therapy. However, I also felt that Miss K. should have some way in which she could let me know what she was doing with her life, rather than imagine that her separation from me could only be dealt with by some artificial, almost surgical, cut-off from me. It was therefore agreed that she could write to me some time after she had been through the initial stages of coping with her leaving.

Miss K. wrote me a "progress report" after four months. Three months later she was passing through London and asked to see me for a single session. I agreed to this. The person who then came to see me was quite different from the patient who had been in analysis with me. She had lost a significant amount of weight, but this was the least of the changes in her. She had a new poise about her. She had been through various personal difficulties, including a relationship disappointment, which previously would have thrown her back to the use of food for revenge and self-comfort. She had not resorted to any of those old ways of escape from conflict. She had dealt with the problems of life with a new maturity.

Miss K. had also come across people from her past, closely linked with her family, who had tried to get her back into the vicious circle of regarding marriage as the only meaningful goal in life, with losing weight to that end as an associated goal. This time she had found enough confidence in herself to be content to make something of her own life in her own way, whether or not this resulted in marriage. She had really begun to find ways of becoming her own self. She had outgrown the former dependence upon her mother and upon her sister and brother-in-law

Her last comment to me, before she left, was that she had only become able to deal with her weight problem once she had begun to see herself differently. Before, her weight used to express a self which she had assumed to be ugly and unlovable. Feeling different about herself *inwardly* she could now allow herself to express that difference *outwardly* in how she looked. She looked good.

Three years later Miss K. let me know how she had continued to benefit from her analysis. Her new-found confidence in herself had remained with her, and she was finding new satisfactions in life. She had rediscovered the creative side of herself and was beginning once again to sing and to paint. She had developed a full and fulfilling life, and was finding herself able to sustain a close and mutually respecting relationship with a man. Incidentally, too, she had regained a normal weight having lost about sixty pounds since leaving her analysis. The strength and wish for this had come from within. She had achieved this for herself.

❖ 10 ❖

Theory Rediscovered

We shall not cease from exploration
And the end of all our exploring
Will be to arrive where we started
And know the place for the first time.

(T.S. ELIOT: "Little Gidding")

This book has been about psychoanalytic technique rather than theory. In particular it has been about using internal supervision, and trial identification with the patient, to enable us to distinguish better what helps the analytic process from what hinders it. I have therefore expected a lot from the reader, either to be already familiar with psychoanalytic theory or to be patient while the threads of this emerge from the clinical examples.

Although I have emphasized the therapeutic use of not-knowing, I do not want to give the impression that analytic therapy can be undertaken by learning from the patient alone. A therapist has to be "held" by the structure provided by theory, and by familiarity with his own unconscious, if he is not to become overwhelmed by a patient's pathology or be retreating into "head-sight" to avoid being overwhelmed.

For those already well versed in psychoanalytic theory, it will have been clear that much of the work described in this book would have been impossible had the therapist or analyst not been familiar with the complex processes of the unconscious: the mechanisms of defense, the dynamics of growth and development, and the various forms of unconscious interaction that can occur in any relationship.

Because unconscious speaks to unconscious it is essential that a therapist should have maximal access to this deepest level of interactive communication via his own unconscious responses to the patient. It is for this reason that analysts and therapists have to be analyzed; and it is that experience, combined with a knowledge of theory, that helps most to make sense of a therapist's unconscious resonance to what is being communicated by the patient. Without personal analysis there is a limit to how much therapeutic use can be made of these elusive levels of unconscious communication.

Nevertheless, there are numbers of talented social workers, counselors and others, who demonstrate that (with the help of good supervision) they are able to make valuable use of their knowledge of psychodynamic theory. The therapeutic contribution of that work, even though it is different from psychotherapy, should not be discounted. It should be more readily acknowledged and encouraged.

I have tried to illustrate how patients lead the therapist back to what he already knows—or further on to what he still has to find and understand. The essential factor in this process lies in the therapist's willingness to be led by the patient: he has to recognize when he is being prompted and cued, unconsciously supervised or having aspects of himself mirrored by the patient. In ways like this, the therapist not only rediscovers theory; he also discovers how to follow the analytic process. Winnicott says of this:

> Analysis is not only a technical exercise. It is something that we become able to do when we have reached a stage in acquiring a basic technique. What we become able to do enables us to cooperate with the patient in following the *process*, that which in each patient has its own pace and which follows its own course; all the important features of this process derive from the patient and not from ourselves as analysts. (Winnicott 1958: 278)

Unfortunately, even though every student analyst or therapist is taught to follow the patient and not to lead, many still become too sure; and this tendency often remains after qualification. What may then develop is a style of interpreting which is more a matter of *telling* the patient than of *finding out with* the patient. The contrast here is between analytic work which becomes dogmatic and that which draws upon the patient's own creativity.

Many therapists quote examples of their clinical work in which they have made statements that imply a surprising degree of certainty. "I told the patient...," "I then showed the patient that..." and "no doubt this was because...": all are phrases which are common in the literature. Why is this so? Is it because psychoanalytic theory has become so refined, and the body of shared clinical experience so convincing, that analysts can now work with a theoretical sureness that would have been impossible to the early explorers in this field of the human psyche? Or is there something else here to do with a need to appear competent, perhaps linked with a self-expectation that one should know? Might there, sometimes, also be an unconscious collusion between the patient's search for certainty and a clinical stance of the therapist appearing to offer it?

I find these questions troubling. If theory is to remain alive, rather than being repeatedly demonstrated in relation to each patient, there has to be adequate room for the patient to play with what is around in the session. It is important, therefore, that the therapist does not dominate the analytic work or monopolize insight in the therapy.

If too much certainty is employed by a therapist, this offers a patient what appears to be a short-cut to "knowing." The dangers here are that insight is intellectualized, that understanding rests on a false basis, and that the therapist appears more all-knowing than anyone really can be. There are no short-cuts to psychoanalytic experience. There is no other path to it than patience, the therapist holding onto the caution of still not-knowing—alongside the dawning sense of beginning to understand.

When a patient is ready to recognize the unconscious implications of what is being communicated, or being experienced in the session, the therapist can begin to draw the patient's attention to the evidence that points to possible unconscious meaning. For this reason, I prefer to speak more in terms of "maybe" or "perhaps," which I believe to be the natural language of potential space. I have also suggested that therapists should develop the art of finding a halfway step toward insight. This does not foreclose on the patient's options, and it allows mental space for him to play with the therapist's comments when these are offered tentatively. They can then be altered, added to or dismissed—by patient or therapist. Instead of insight being given to the patient it can be *discovered* by patient and therapist together. Interpretation does not then become an impingement.

Of course there are many occasions when the therapist should be more sure than merely tentative; when he can offer interpretation with conviction based on the work already done with the patient, or when he has to deal with clear unconscious resistance from the patient. But that sureness of interpretation, if it is to be personal to the patient (not a cliché-response), still has to be arrived at from the patient's own cues and not just from being familiar with psychoanalytic theory. The most obvious time when a firm under-standing is necessary is when a patient feels in crisis and needs containment.

A patient in ferment is like a wine in the making. There is life in the fermentation, to contain which the container must be able to respond to the pressures of growth. Each patient unconsciously looks for a therapist who can be in touch with that growth, be responsive to it, and able to be firm without being rigid. Borrowed insight can never serve that function. What is needed, but is not always offered by the therapist, is insight that is discovered with this patient in this session of this therapy.

No one can *make* another person grow. One can only inhibit growth or enable it. Therapists therefore need to understand the processes of growth and the dynamics of what inhibits this. Trial identification will often expose those times when a therapist is blocking a patient's experience, and the opportunity for new growth. Often, this blocking is caused by a therapist preempting the patient with premature interpretation, implicitly directing the patient to proceed along the anticipated lines of regression, or transference etc., as already extensively described in the literature.

There is a temptation, rooted in the acquired knowledge of psychoanalytic theory, for analysts and therapists to try to master-mind the analytic process rather than to follow it. As with infants, the process of analytic growth has its own impetus. Infants whose natural growth is not interfered with usually wean themselves, and can toilet train themselves too, *when they are ready*. Patients will likewise often resist a therapist's premature application of theoreti-cal knowledge, and preconceived ideas about them, in order to reinstate the necessary "period of hesitation" (Winnicott 1958: 53). Without the space created by this hesitation there can be no room for analytic discovery or play. With it there is room, in every analysis and therapy treatment, for theory to be rediscovered and renewed.

I have described clinical issues as I have found them. I have offered my own understanding of these, but I make no claim for the rightness of how I handled them. The extended clinical ex-amples have been recorded, as far as possible, as they happened. They are offered for learning from and for teaching; they are not meant to be used in any way as a model for others. The reader will find that I have often failed to follow my own ideas on technique. This is partly because my thinking about technique has been influenced by my reflection on the many things that I wish I had done differently. It is also easier to be wise after the event than when caught up in the immediacy of the session itself.

I leave much unanswered; but to have recognized some of the questions is at least a beginning.

> I am a part of all that I have met;
> Yet all experience is an arch wherethro'
> Gleams that untravell'd world, whose margin fades
> For ever and for ever when I move.
>
> (TENNYSON: *Ulysses* 1842)

The Analytic Space
and Process

Introduction

In Part One I focused on the interactional processes in the analytic relationship in order to illustrate the patient's unconscious contributions to the analytic work and to show that theory is not just applied in clinical work—it is also rediscovered. In Part Two I continue to look at issues of technique from the patient's point of view in order to highlight further benefits from using this viewpoint. For instance, it can help the analyst to recognize more easily when some interpretations have ceased to be effective with a particular patient because they have become too familiar. Instead, when working more specifically with the individual patient, insight can be arrived at freshly.

Two themes in particular emerge from the clinical work described here: the importance of analytic space (that makes analytic understanding possible) and the analytic process. With the help of these two reference points the analyst or therapist can be guided towards working more effectively, monitoring the analytic space for what may be intruding upon it and the analytic process for what could disturb it.

When we follow the analytic process with an open mind (not burdened by preconception) it becomes easier to see how this process points towards what is being looked for—for recovery and for health. And what is needed often turns out to be quite different from anything that theory alone might have anticipated or common sense imagined. It then becomes clear how different is the process of analysis from Alexander's notion of the corrective emotional response.

The first patient I ever worked with already showed in striking ways how her unconscious search for the help she needed was expressed in symptomatic behavior. That patient happened to be a child (Chapter 13). I have since come to wonder about the dynamics of the unconscious search for what is needed, which again raises the issue of meeting a patient's needs (or not) in analysis and analytic psychotherapy. This eventually prompted me to suggest the notion of unconscious hope (Chapter 17).

An examination of the interrelationship between inner and outer reality further highlights the issue of "environmental provision," whether in childhood or in the consulting room, so that analysts should allow for effects that *they* are having upon the analytic process—for good or for ill. This again emphasizes the need for self-monitoring, so I suggest a number of ways in which internal supervision can be developed—to help in following the analytic interaction and in recognizing the implications for the patient of the analyst's ways of working (Chapter 19). This then leads me back to the theme of Part Two: "The analytic space and process."

As a link with Part One I offer an outline in Chapter 11 of the influences that lie behind the writing of the two books incorporated in this volume.

❖11❖

Beyond Dogma[1]

Because of the interest shown in my earlier book On Learning from the Patient *(see Part One), I was asked by the editorial board of the* British Journal of Psychotherapy *to outline the process of writing it and where the ideas came from. Prompted by that invitation, I describe here the principal influences that lie behind that first volume (and this) and some of the ideas that form the basis from which I am starting here, before I proceed further into the mysteries, challenges, and discoveries that are inherent in the analytic encounter.*

THE SEARCH FOR MEANING

Quite early in my life I had noticed two apparently contradictory forces operating within me. On the one hand I felt that I had to question everything–particularly anything that was presented to me as a dogmatic "given"; on the other hand I was looking for certainty. In those days I thought of security in terms of being sure–knowing rather than not-knowing.

For a while I tried belonging to a group of fundamentalist Christians. They actively fostered a belief that they could offer the certainty I was then looking for; and, by contrast, all error and doubt could be relegated to others. (In those days I did not know about projection.) I therefore planned to read theology with a view to becoming a priest.

However, in my first year at university I studied anthropology. This helped to open my eyes to the incredible diversity of life; and I began to discover the "otherness" of others–far beyond my previous imaginings. I also began to realize that, in any attempt to

understand other societies—and people different from ourselves—
we have to approach that task without preconception. If too much
weight is given to what is already known, then the unknown
remains elusive and our attempts at understanding introduce their
own distortions to what is being studied. I thus came to realize that
"received truth" obstructs the study of what is new and different:
a balance has to be found between what is already known and what
is yet to be discovered.

When, after that, I still proceeded to read theology it was from
a very altered viewpoint. I was once again challenging everything;
but, this time, I was prepared to stay with my own doubts. I became
a questioning agnostic.

Dogma and Schism

In the course of studying theology I also read a lot of church
history. Here another theme came to my notice, the paradox that
human truth is never onesided—nor can it ever be fully defined.

In my very first publication, an article entitled "The Paradox of
Unity," I wrote:

> Man's mind recoils from paradox, and tries to find some escape from this
> tension either in a form of absolutism or in compromise.... Much of our
> present theological disunity may be attributable to a natural insistence upon
> the unity of truth. But truth . . . may not always be reducible to a single
> dimension. To see the wholeness of truth we may need to see the obverse
> side to that aspect which we can [more easily] see, and contain the two
> aspects in paradoxical tension. (Casement 1963: 8)

What has since fascinated and concerned me is the discovery that
psychoanalysts too can get caught up in this search for certainty,
and in the tendency to regard their own dogma as the criterion by
which the views of all others should be assessed: those who disagree
are then assumed to be in error. Not all of the divisions between
schools of psychoanalysis are because one school has a truth that
another has not; some of these dogmatic differences derive from
the persisting belief that truth can be defined and will prove to be
unified. Truth is bound to be more complex. But we cannot always
stand, or understand, it being so.

Polarization and schism inevitably follow from any dogmatic
claim to the singular correctness of one's own views, and these
tendencies abound in quite different spheres of life: in religion, in
politics, and in psychoanalysis. It has also interested me to find that,
even though psychoanalysis espouses the openmindedness of

anthropology, and is suspicious of religious belief as the illusion that it may be, some psychoanalysts defend their chosen dogma with nothing short of a religious fervor. And sometimes they expect others to have the open minds that they do not always manage to sustain within themselves.

For years now I have held to a questioning agnosticism— unburdened by the "certainty" of either the believer or the committed atheist. My first attempt at articulating this was in an article entitled "False security?" I tried to warn against the seductiveness of certainty, which (I now realize) applies as much to analysts in relation to their chosen "gods" as to any religious person. In that article I say:

> We must search our hearts, be ready to be stripped of any comfort in believing, and be prepared to look beyond our idea of God lest it be no more than our own projection.... Faith must know that it can never know, and must be aware of the guile of its own need to believe. (Casement 1964: 30)

In relation to psychoanalysis, I would wish now to add that dogmatic certainty will always constrict an analyst's capacity to think imaginatively about the patient. It also constricts the analytic space, without which (as I intend to show in Chapter 20) patients cannot grow most fully into the richness of their own creative potential.

UNDERSTANDING THEORY THROUGH EXPERIENCE

When (during my social work training) I was first required to learn about unconscious processes and psychodynamic theory, I remained very skeptical about all of this. Too much seemed to be taken for granted—without (I thought) sufficient evidence to support it. However, when I started seeing social work clients I began to discover my own clinical data; and bits of analytic theory did begin to make some sense. But I still could not accept the idea of interpreting to a client/patient on the basis of theory alone. The anthropologist in me rebelled against putting ideas into someone else's mind. (This reluctance shows most clearly in my work with a child that I describe in Chapter 13.) I therefore preferred to discover with clients and patients—in their own terms—what made sense to them. Even though it might take longer this way, I felt that such meaning as could be found made more sense to a client/patient if I did not insist upon taking the short-cut of applying theory too directly.

Learning about Transference and Countertransference

Having developed a resistance to dogmatism I naturally had difficulty with some of the more extreme attitudes that I came across in the course of my training in psychotherapy, and later in psychoanalysis. For instance, I could not accept that everything said by a patient necessarily represented unconscious communication, or that the process of every session was determined by patients transferring past attitudes on to the analyst. So, how could one justify the technique of interpreting everything in terms of the transference? This seemed to me to be a convenient way for therapists and analysts to ignore those elements of a patient's communication that could be directly about themselves and might sometimes be all too accurate.

I began to feel that the external realities in the analytic relationship should also be taken into account. Here we will often find what has triggered a transference reaction—because of a similarity between an element of present reality and some key experience in the patient's past. The patient then treats this element in the present as if it were the same as something experienced before. But, it should be remembered, that current reality is not always external: it can also be a sense of similarity (to something from the past) that is created through what the patient is feeling; this too can lead into a transference experience.

The above view of transference helped me to see it as more understandable—to myself and to the patient—because less mysterious in how it comes about (see Chapter 1). And the purpose in these transference responses, which emerges through trying to understand them, eventually led me to think that transference could also be thought of as an expression of "unconscious hope" by which the patient signals to the external world that there is conflict needing attention.

For a long time after I had trained as a psychotherapist I questioned the use that some people made of such concepts as countertransference and projective identification.

Countertransference had acquired many different meanings (see pp. 80–81) and, even in the 1970s, some analysts still seemed to regard any affective response to the patient as evidence of something unresolved in the mind of the analyst/therapist: a transference to the patient of some emotional significance that belonged elsewhere in the therapist's own past experience—not therefore to be confused with any communication from the patient. But sometimes, it seemed to me, a therapist was being unconsciously prompted by the patient *to become like* the person with whom the patient was reliving earlier difficulties. If that were so, then I believed it necessary to postulate a distinction between "personal countertransference" (what has to do with the therapist) and "diagnostic response"—that indicates something about the patient (Casement 1973).

It was several years later that Sandler gave us the notion of unconscious role-responsiveness, through which the patient unconsciously prods the analyst to "actualize" a key object-relationship from the patient's earlier life (Sandler 1976). Pearl King added a further perspective on the patient's impact upon the analyst in her paper "Affective response of the analyst to the patient's communications," pointing out how a patient sometimes places the analyst in the role of victim whilst the patient acts out an identification with the aggressor—thereby communicating to the analyst something of the patient's own earlier experience of having been treated in ways similar to how the patient is now treating the analyst (King 1978). I believe that these particular writings have greatly helped to clarify what many analysts and therapists had found in their clinical work without having had an authoritative explanation to support their intuitive impressions. Such is the process of learning from the patient.

Projective identification was even more difficult for me to understand.[2] How did this communication come about, and how could one make interpretive use of it without seeming to understand the patient magically? (I had never been able to accept interpretations being given to patients that seemed to be based solely upon the therapist's feelings about the patient.) I began to understand this process only when I had the experience of being in the presence of a patient whose absence of appropriate feelings had been deeply affecting me: I then realized that I had been picking up a sense of the patient's unshed tears which, for years, she had regarded as too much for her to bear (see pp. 68–70). Only then could I see that it was through her blank manner of telling me about her babies both dying that she was unconsciously communicating to me those feelings she could not manage within herself alone. I then began to understand what was meant by projective identification and why it can be such an important (and powerful) form of communication. (I return in Chapter 14 to discuss the technical issues involved in interpreting from what the analyst is feeling.)

Discovering the Value of Trial Identification

In Chapter 2 I wrote of my experience of working (as a social worker) with someone in a near-catatonic withdrawal. I illustrate there how it was useful to imagine myself in the shoes of the other person in order to monitor how he/she may be experiencing the session and the therapeutic relationship. I then changed how I was trying to relate to him: no longer trying to get *into* his mind but beginning to appreciate why he had so much needed to keep me (and everyone else) *out*. Encouraged by that particular patient's dramatic response to my new approach to the problem of communicating with him, I began to explore other ways in which we can "trial-identify" with the patient—and the value of it. Since then I have also found this type of self-monitoring to be useful in sifting out what we might say in a session from what we do not say.

The Need for an Internal Supervisor

I learned a lot else too, whilst I was still a social worker, that I later adopted in my subsequent work as a psychotherapist and analyst. For example, when supervising social workers, it came to my notice that (all too often) something I had said by way of comment or suggestion would be relayed to a client in the next interview—not always appropriately. This borrowed thinking did not properly belong to the process going on between the social worker and the client, but was a left-over from what had been happening between the social worker and the supervisor. Something more directly related to what was currently happening was clearly needed. I therefore began to advise supervisees that they should aim to establish their own process of supervision (an internal supervisor) that could help to guide them when in the presence of the client or patient (see Chapter 2; also Chapter 19 below, where I discuss more fully the development of this process of internal supervision).

An internal supervisor is *not* an internalized supervisor: these are different kinds of resource for the therapist (or analyst). Drawing upon an internalized supervisor means using someone else's thinking that may then tend to be superimposed upon what is happening in the session. Instead of facilitating the analytic process this will often impede it. By contrast, internal supervision—being more autonomous—can help us to respond to the immediacy of the present moment in a session, in ways that are more appropriate to it.

Discovering the Value of Not-Knowing

On one occasion, whilst I was still supervising social workers, I found a student frantically reading up about marital therapy in preparation for his first meeting with a couple who were seeking help with their marriage. I advised him that it is "all right not to know—and to find out with the client."

For some time I continued to regard this formula as appropriate advice for students, because they could not yet be expected to know everything: I was then thinking of this as "permissible ignorance." It only later began to dawn on me that therapeutic skill does not depend upon knowledge as opposed to ignorance. Rather, there is an important difference between the attempt to understand something from a position of not-knowing and the tendency to prompt, or to direct, which goes with knowing too well. Gradually, therefore, I came to realize that there is real value in keeping to one side what we think we know, in order to leave room for fresh understanding. I then found that Bion had advocated starting every session "without memory, desire or understanding"—his antidote to those intrusive influences that otherwise threaten to distort the analytic process (Bion 1967a; 1970: 45–54).

I have come to understand this saying of Bion to mean that he was warning against such interferences as: the overactive use of what is remembered from an earlier session (or from the patient's history), the wish to find evidence to support a particular view of the patient (often dictated by theory) or even the wish to make the patient better in a particular way, and the attempt at understanding the patient of today in any way that is not found within the session of today. I have found Bion's advice most helpful in preserving the analytic space from such avoidable impingements and the analytic process from influences that will distort it.

Beyond "Corrective Emotional Experience"

When I began to train as a psychotherapist I came to think that, in effect, what we might be providing for our patients was a "corrective emotional experience"—as outlined by Alexander (1954). Clinical experience has gradually made me realize that this is far from the case.

Of course, we do try to offer a reliability that may well be better than patients had previously experienced. But we also provide a freedom for patients to use us in whatever ways belong to their own experience; and we are by no means always put in the role of the "better parent." Instead, our patients frequently demonstrate a need to use the analyst to represent earlier "bad objects." They can then get in touch with the feelings that could not be expressed (or worked through) with the original object(s). My experience with the patient I described in Chapter 7 taught me very clearly the difference between trying to be a better parent and being used by the patient to represent *traumatic experience as it had been.*

Following the Patient

Donald Winnicott, more than any other analyst known to me, was able to remain close to clinical experience, even when writing about theory. And, when I did not at first understand his more difficult papers, I often had the surprise of discovering that I had later stumbled upon what he had been writing about in my own clinical work. I was therefore naturally drawn to his ways of thinking about psychoanalytic experience.

There are some clear examples of re-finding Winnicott in the earlier clinical chapters (Chapters 5, 7, and 9). Repeatedly I had to struggle with what was immediately present, in whatever way I could. Only afterwards was I able to recognize where I had been. This was especially true when I had been involved in a sequence during which the patient had been using my mistakes to represent earlier "environmental failure" as described by Winnicott (1965: 258-9). It was in my work with the patient I discuss in Chapter 5 that I first recognized this link between my own "failure" (mistakes I was making at a time when I was trying most particularly not to fail her) and environmental failure in her early life. That patient was then able to direct at me, most powerfully, the feelings which had belonged to those early experiences of trauma.

Another most valuable thing I learned from Winnicott is the value of playing (see Winnicott 1971). This has prompted me to "play" with clinical material, in supervision or in clinical seminars, and to explore the different meanings that are potentially present within a session.

I have also found it helpful to play with some of Winnicott's own ideas, and to use them differently. For instance, I think of the *analyst's presence* being potentially available—like the spatula—to be found and to be used in whatever way belongs to the patient at that particular moment.[3]

Likewise, I believe that the transference experience is more convincing when a patient has really been allowed time to invest the analyst with transference significance. The analyst can then be discovered, as an object that has become meaningful to the patient, in the patient's own way and the patient's own time. However, some transference interpretations do seem to be given by the analyst as if these were being pushed down the patient's throat, like a spatula being used (as originally designed) by a forceful physician. It is almost as if this were thought to be what the transference interpretation had been designed for!

As for interpretation in general, I have found it useful to think of Winnicott's "squiggle game" in his child consultations (Winnicott 1958: Chapter 9). He would draw a shape and invite the child to make something of it; or, conversely, the child would draw a shape for Winnicott to do something with. I believe that there is an important place for these incomplete "shapes" in our work with patients; and this is what has led me to think of offering a *halfway step to interpretation*—for the patient to do something with rather than the analyst monopolizing insight in a session.

There are many other parallels between Winnicott's clinical observations and my own work, and it is to him that I am most indebted.

Mutuality between Patient and Analyst

I have already given some references (above) to some of the writings on the unconscious interactions between analyst and patient (e.g. Sandler and King). In addition, I was much influenced by the earlier writings of those other British analysts who had already drawn attention to an unconscious mutuality between patient and analyst. For instance, Paula Heimann had said: "The analyst's countertransference is not only part and parcel of the analytic relationship, but it is the patient's *creation*, is part of the patient's personality" (Heimann 1950: 83). And Margaret Little introduces yet another quite new idea: "We often hear of the mirror which the analyst holds up to the patient, but the patient holds one up to the analyst too" (Little 1951: 37). This brings us back to the importance of the analyst becoming aware of his/her own contribution to the analytic encounter and the need to monitor the effects of this on the analytic process.

British analysts (and many others from abroad) have been deeply influenced by the work and teaching of Rosenfeld who increasingly focused upon the analyst's contribution to what was happening in the analysis—in particular in the event of analyst and patient getting into an impasse (Rosenfeld 1987). This view of the analytic relationship has long been acknowledged in the clinical practice of British analysts even though it was never systematized (except recently by Rosenfeld) in any way comparable to the comprehensive development of an interactional viewpoint *per se* that is found in the writings of Langs.

Resisting Dogmatic Certainty

When I first read one of Langs' books, *The Listening Process* (1978), I recognized many parallels between his way of working and what I had been evolving over the previous ten years. For a while, therefore, I tried (albeit rather self-consciously) to apply his ways of thinking to my clinical work, and I give examples of that endeavor in Chapters 3 and 5. But I began to feel uncomfortable about the incisiveness with which Langs evaluates the clinical work of others. It appears as if he thinks that there is only one right way of working analytically. Ironically, I am now sure that it was precisely the dogmatic certainty of his approach that had first attracted me (without my realizing it) to Langs' views—and it was this also that later turned me away from his own use of them.

I began to understand there was something wrong here, for me at least, when I noticed that my own internal supervision was becoming self-persecutory (see Chapters 3 and 5). This amounted to a resurgence of an *internalized supervisor*, which was contrary to the style of work I had been developing before, and it prompted me to realize that my readiness to adopt some of Langs' sureness showed a regressive manifestation of my own earlier wish for dogmatic certainty.

It was inevitable, therefore, that I later moved away from the influence of Langs. Nevertheless, despite these points of disagreement, I readily acknowledge my indebtedness to him in the earlier volume; and I still regard his concept of "unconscious supervision by the patient" (an imaginative extension of Little's notion of the patient as mirror) as one of the most productive new insights into psychoanalytic technique that has come to light in recent years.

In the remainder of Part One (and here in Part Two) I try to show a more playful use of internal supervision, wanting to create the atmosphere of a sandpit (playing with different shapes) rather than that of a court-room; but a continuing tension between these two attitudes is still evident in Part One. Outgrowing a longstanding wish to be more sure can only be achieved gradually and with difficulty.

REMAINING AN INDEPENDENT ANALYST[4]

It has been interesting to find that a number of reviewers of Part One felt it necessary to locate the author theoretically. As a result, I was variously labelled as a "disciple of Winnicott," "a pupil of Bion," or as "primarily indebted to Langs"; and why am I not a self-psychologist? This probably reflects my training as a member of the independent group of the British Psycho-Analytical Society. From that position, in a society which has been able to hold together differing viewpoints within a creative tension, it was possible for me to draw upon whichever ideas have most helped to develop my clinical work. My interest therefore has come to focus upon the patient, and what makes sense with a particular patient in a given session, rather than upon any one theoretical position. I think that this more open minded approach to clinical work is not easy for everyone to stomach, particularly for those who closely identify themselves with one school of psychoanalysis as *opposed* to others.

Because of this insistence upon an openminded approach to understanding the individual, one of the criticisms leveled at the independent psychoanalysts in the British Society is that they are said to be "woolly minded." However, J. B. Priestley had his own strong views on what some people choose to call "woolly mindedness":

> Both the fanatical believers and the fixed-attitude people are loud in their scorn of what they call "woolly minds." I have defended woolly minds before, and will now do so again. It is the woolly mind that combines skepticism of everything with credulity about everything. Being woolly it has no hard edges. It is easy, pliant, yet it has its own toughness. Because it bends, it does not break.... The woolly mind realizes that we live in an unimaginable gigantic, complicated, mysterious universe. To try to stuff the vast bewildering creation into a few neat pigeon-holes is absurd. We don't know enough, and to pretend we do is mere intellectual conceit. (Almost all men who like to refer scornfully to woolly minds suffer from this conceit.) The best we can do is to keep looking out for clues, for anything that will light us a step or two into the dark.... The woolly mind can be silly at times, but even so, it finds out more and enjoys more than the rat-trap intelligence. Second-rate scientists are never woolly-minded whereas great scientists let their minds go woolly between experiments. (Priestley 1972: 30–1)

SOME OTHER REACTIONS TO PART ONE

Some regret has been expressed that I did not give a fuller theoretical framework. But in neither volume have I been trying to write a book that would be complete in itself. Each is intended to be accessible to a wider readership than a more theoretical book would be. I therefore rely upon the reader either being familiar with the theoretical frames that I refer to, or take for granted, or upon the reader's readiness to seek a fuller description of these elsewhere.

It also seems that, in Part One, I did not make it clear at which level I think the process of internal supervision takes place. For instance, do I really wish to suggest that it should all be at a conscious level—as it would appear from some examples I gave in the text? No! I would wish to advocate something more nearly preconscious; but the act of writing about it inevitably shifts the focus away from the more subliminal level at which this process most usually needs to function.

I offered in Part One a series of statements about clinical issues that I believe to be important, but I chose to leave them incomplete—rather like Winnicott's squiggles. These were for others to interact with, to complete in their own ways or to challenge, according to their own thinking and experience. I therefore made no attempt there to resolve the dissonances between established theory and some of the therapeutic practices that I described. Instead, I left evidence around there (as I shall here in Part Two) of a continuing tussle within myself on both clinical and theoretical issues.

I make no apology for leaving the reader with some continuing uncertainty, as I regard this to be an essential basis for a healthy questioning of what analysts and therapists are trying to do. I also believe that psychotherapy students and others can be better helped in discovering that they are not alone in being so much less than certain in their own clinical work. This conflict, between a search for certainty and a need to remain open to the experience of still not-knowing, can become the source of a patient's greatest potential for change and creativity.

Part Two describes further clinical encounters in which individuals wrestle to become free from the influences of the past—helped by the analytic process, which (when followed) can lead both analyst and patient towards what the patient most needs to find in the course of the analytic encounter.

❖12❖

Interpretation: Fresh Insight or Cliché?[1]

In this chapter I try to show how a too dogmatic application of analytic interpretation can become absurd or sterile. There are times when it is more fruitful to work in a way that leaves room for insight to become a genuine experience of discovery, for the analyst as well as for the patient.

When we find ourselves using similar forms of interpretation with several different patients, it is probable that we are becoming stereotyped and repetitive. And when this repetition develops into cliché interpreting, it is likely to promote an intellectualization of the analytic experience. How then can we recover that freshness of insight which alone can promote therapeutic change?

Typical examples of cliché interpretation might be: "You are really talking about me"; "You are seeing me as your mother"; "You are experiencing separation anxiety"; "You are rendering me impotent"; "You are experiencing castration anxiety"; "You are making envious attacks upon my understanding." Examples like these are common in the analytic literature, which makes me wonder how frequently they may be used in the consulting-room.

We cannot always avoid interpreting in ways that have been frequently used before (by others or by ourselves) but the effectiveness of such interpretations is easily dulled through overuse. Also, when we rely on what has come to be regarded as universal truths, we can lose touch with the individual. Therefore, when some stereotyped interpretation is foremost in our thinking, it is often better to delay before speaking and to look for some less focused comment that can lead towards subsequent interpretation. The patient will frequently lead us to insight that is more specific and often quite new.

Example 12.1
I once pointed out to a patient a recurring theme that he, as a child and since, had become preoccupied with protecting his penis against some expected hurt or threat. (The interpretation that I was not making is quite obvious here.) He replied: "I am afraid of it being broken off." Let us notice how much more telling is his own description of castration anxiety. The threat was not just to the penis but to the excited penis. It cannot be thought of as being broken off unless it is erect.

I am not thinking only of the danger that actual interpretations become clichés because of their familiar form. I am also concerned with the stereotyped thinking that engenders this: for instance, the notion that everything in a session should be interpreted in terms of the transference, or in terms of the patient's current regression in the transference relationship. The danger then is that we will notice only what our theoretical assumptions prompt us to look for, and our preconceptions begin to be imposed upon what we see.

I came across a salutary warning of this, when I was reading anthropology, in a book about the sexual symbolism of musical instruments. The author, captivated by his reading of Freud, argued that every musical instrument is symbolically male or female. Having got carried away by the shape of violins and cellos he noticed that they are played on with long thin things called bows. These, he claimed, are phallic symbols. He then proceeded to go through the entire orchestra; and how could anyone argue with him?

He pointed out all those other long thin instruments that people put into their mouths; the shape of those wooden drumsticks; and those other drumsticks with large woolly balls; and, what's more, these drumsticks are beaten against the stretched skin of the drums, which (he said) represents the hymen. And what about those inviting hollows at the end of all the brass instruments; and the triangle, which is set ringing by a very small phallic symbol? And so on! After reading all of this, some joker had written in the margin: "If Sir Malcolm Sargent knew what is really going on in front of him, and what he is waving around in his own hand, he would never conduct another concert!"

What I am trying to illustrate in this caricature of analytic interpretation is that, when any psychoanalytic assumption is held to be beyond question, interpretations can too easily be imposed upon whatever appears to fit in with that assumption. Clinically, we must always be wary of this tendency to think that we are seeing evidence of what we are expecting to find, particularly as we are all inclined to relate to the familiar as if it were universal.

I would like to suggest that some of our stereotyped thinking is due to a mistaken response to the patient's communications. This response could be described as a *transferential attitude to elements of the clinical situation* (see pp. 13–16). In ways similar to the processes of transference, we can find ourselves responding to a patient in terms of our familiarity with analytic theory or other clinical experience. We then transfer on to the patient the understanding that we have gleaned elsewhere, even though it may not apply to this particular patient.[2] This is what I mean by cliché-thinking.

I believe that we are most likely to engage in these repetitive forms of interpreting when we feel insecure about our clinical understanding. By prematurely imagining that we recognize what the patient is communicating, even if we don't, we can preserve the appearance (at least to ourselves) of being competent. There is then a danger that we interpret on the basis of similarity rather than from a more genuine process of analytic discovery.

The pitfalls of preconception are a hazard not only for the novice. A similar danger lies in wait for the experienced therapist. The authority of experience can tempt the practitioner to become lazy in his thinking, or too sure. And it is often tempting to use shortcuts to insight, based upon what has already made sense with other patients.

In the following vignette I was fortunate that my patient prompted me to reorientate my thinking.

Example 12.2

In a session some time during the first year of analysis, a patient began to be distressed about her hair going gray. At first I thought I was hearing about vanity, particularly when I noticed that I could not see gray hairs. I tried looking closer, peering over the back of the couch, but I still couldn't see any gray. However, when I wondered about this shift in my position— from sitting normally in my chair to leaning towards the patient—I thought that I was being maneuvered into getting physically closer to her. I therefore mistook this interaction to be evidence of some hysterical manipulation.

When I interpreted this as the patient trying to get me to be closer to her, she became much more distressed. She began crying from deep inside herself. Only then did I recognize that the patient had been trying to tell me about how she felt inside herself, where the scars of her childhood experiences made her feel that she was growing prematurely old. Part of the problem was that her emotional scars were not visible—and yet she needed me to be aware of them.[3]

My reorientation here was possible only when I recognized that the patient's response to my first interpretation was not due to resistance, as I had been tempted to think. Her increased distress contained an unconscious cue for me to listen to the deeper meaning in her communication. She needed me to be prepared to be in touch with the pain of her *internal* world.

In my initial failure to look beneath the surface appearance I had become like her mother. The patient then felt left alone with her distress, as she had been as a child. But, through a reorientation of my listening, I was able to arrive at a quite different understanding of this sequence. Moreover, the patient was also able to discover that her capacity to cue the other person had not after all been lost to her for ever. That is how it had seemed to her after she had been badly burned at the age of eleven months. After that trauma her mother had seemed to be no longer able to respond to her inner pain; she had concentrated instead on the healing of the external scars from the burning.

It is not easy for a patient to question, let alone to reorientate the therapist unless the patient is unusually tenacious—as with the patient I have just described. So, what happens if we let ourselves become dogmatic in our interpreting? One thing at least is certain: that we will become less receptive to correction from a patient.

Also, let us wonder what is happening when our theoretical orientation becomes obtrusively evident in what we are saying to a patient. Are we imposing our theory upon what we are hearing? I think of this as "jelly-moulding," giving a shape to clinical material that does not inherently belong to it.

The next example comes from the work of a foreign colleague. I think that the style of interpreting here would be described as a caricature. Similar caricatures can be found in all schools of psychoanalysis.

Example 12.3
At a clinical workshop I heard a case presentation given by a therapist who is bilingual, in English and the language of her mother-tongue. The patient she described is a man whom she had been seeing in three-times-a-week therapy. The sessions were reported in English but the therapy was being conducted in the patient's own language.

It was soon evident that this therapist's style of work is one of quite unusual sureness about her understanding of the patient. Then, in one session that was described in detail, the patient reported a dream. He said: "I had a dream last night in which my head was being squashed by someone sitting on my face."

What followed, after the patient had failed to free associate, was a product of the therapist's silent working over of this dream in the context of her assumptions about the patient's state of regression in the therapy. He was regarded as still at the breast. But in the dream, where there should have been a mouth/breast relationship, there was a face pressed against buttocks. The therapist was therefore able to argue to herself that this must have been derived from a distortion of the feeding relationship. She therefore offered the following interpretation: "Because of your envy, you are unable to take in the good milk of my interpretations. Instead you take in my words as poisonous faeces."

The patient's response to this interpretation was to remain silent, and then to appear to change the subject. He eventually came out of his silence with the following statement: "I am going to America for my holiday, but I don't speak English. This will make me very vulnerable because it means that I will have to be totally dependent on my wife to explain to me everything that is being said." The therapist then proceeded to interpret the patient's separation anxiety.

This material was from sessions during the month prior to a summer break, so it was not surprising to hear the therapist refer to reactions to separation when the patient had spoken about his summer holiday. Indeed, at some level, these interpretations may have had their own truth. But what if the patient is not simply regressed to an infant/breast relationship? What if the patient is also responding to the therapist's style of working? We might be hearing examples of *unconscious supervision by the patient* (Langs 1978).

If we go over the material once more, using trial identification with the patient to help us to look at *the patient's view of the therapist*, we gain a different position from which to listen to this interaction.

The patient may be feeling battered by his over-sure therapist. If so, the dream might allude to the experience of not being allowed his own thoughts. Someone was squashing the patient's head—perhaps making thinking impossible. It could therefore be an unconscious prompt to the therapist to reconsider her dogmatic way of interpreting.

The therapist, however, seems to be unaware of any prompting by the patient. She proceeds to interpret this dream no less dogmatically; and she regards the ensuing silence to be an acceptance by him of the interpretation. She also assumes that the change of subject has been determined by the impending holiday break. Her interpretations therefore seem to be superimposed upon what the patient is saying: they do not develop from within the session itself.

Let us again trial-identify with the patient. Where does the notion of "poisonous faeces" come from in this session? Surely not out of the patient's own thinking but from the therapist's theoretical orientation. Maybe, then, the patient's next statements are more directly related to this interpretation. As well as referring to the holiday break, the patient could be saying: "I can't understand your language. If you can't use mine it could make me totally dependent upon you to explain to me what you are saying."

The communication here is, of course, bound to be overdetermined—having several levels of meaning at the same time. We may also be hearing references to the transference, in that we know the therapist to be fluent in more than one language and it is quite likely that the patient knows that too.

Holiday breaks are one of many stimuli for cliché interpretations. We might consider some other clinical phenomena that can trigger what I am calling here a transferential attitude to familiar clinical experience.

Lateness may be an expression of resistance, or of some angry feelings towards the therapist. But it can be other things too. For instance, it is sometimes a token bid for the session to start in the patient's own time—not the therapist's. And that does not always have to be seen in terms of a wish to control the therapist. Patients quite often endeavor to "own" the analytic space, and the time of a session; and it is important that they can find ways to establish this as truly theirs. Too often, lateness is listened to only for its negative connotations.

This may also apply to *silence*. We encounter many different kinds of silence in the clinical setting, but some therapists are prone to fall back upon stereotyped thinking when trying to deal with prolonged silences. One of these stereotypes is to hold too strongly to the notion that the patient should always be left to speak first. There are occasions when we need to recognize that the *patient has already started the session*—with silence. We are less likely to get into a sterile game of waiting if we learn to "read" a patient's silence, and sometimes to respond tentatively to what we sense as the underlying communication which is being conveyed in this. Silence does not always have to be withholding or resisting.

A similar stalemate sometimes develops around the issue of a patient's *anger*. Not infrequently we notice that a patient has difficulty in expressing anger—particularly in the session. It is then

talked about as something that happens only outside the consulting-room, or as something that seems not to happen at all because
of the patient's inhibition of anger.

Example 12.4
One therapist, whom I supervised, quite often interpreted the *absence of
anger* in her patient's life—as paralleled in her relationship to the therapist.
It was known that, throughout her life, the patient had been unable to give
expression to her angry feelings; and this could be understood as an
inhibition linked with her mother's frequent absences in hospital, and her
eventual death when the patient was not yet four years old. Maybe she was
afraid that her therapist would be harmed, even killed, by the murderous
anger that still brooded in the patient's unconscious, most particularly
towards those upon whom she depended and who were too often absent
when she needed them.

  Gradually the patient began to agree with her therapist that it would be
a relief if she could let herself be angry in her sessions; and she had a lot
to be angry about. The therapist was of course absent between sessions,
and away for holidays. And these absences were experienced by the patient
as a desertion of her by the therapist, as by the mother who had often been
away in hospital—and who then had died.[4]

In supervision I began to hear details of how this therapist felt in
response to the patient's frequent lateness and occasional missing
of sessions, and her regular silences at the beginning of every
session. I had, in fact, encouraged the therapist to make a point of
starting every session on time—with or without the patient. In this way
she came to be most directly exposed to the impact of the patient's
various kinds of absence. The therapist had then noticed that she
felt badly treated by the patient. She sometimes felt abandoned; or
she felt suspended in a state of not knowing where the patient was
in a session whilst she remained in prolonged silences; or not
knowing what had happened to her patient when she missed a
session without telephoning.

  Out of this monitoring of the therapist's responses to these
silences, or absences, it began to become clear that we had been
missing an important point. It was far from true that the patient
was unable to express her anger in the sessions. She was doing this
nearly all the time—*but it was not being recognized as anger.*

  It then began to be possible to rethink the communication
conveyed in the unconscious interaction here between this patient
and her therapist; and it seemed possible that the therapist was
being unconsciously tested to see if she could be aware of the
murderous anger being expressed in this behavior.

  Surviving that silent aggression unwittingly, whilst speaking of the absence of the patient's anger in sessions, may therefore have been experienced by the patient as evidence that the therapist was actually afraid of her anger—and that she was unconsciously retreating from this by not letting herself be aware of it. This was exactly how adults had responded to her when she was a child. They too had not been able to cope with her angry feelings around the time of her mother's death and after it. She had eventually been sent away to a children's home when nobody felt able to manage this distressed child, who had also become very withdrawn. Important changes in the therapy grew out of this new awareness that the patient's anger had been in the session all along, and particularly during her absence.

In this example we can see a shift from cliché-thinking to fresh insight. Silences and absences had been mistaken for resistance. But these could be understood quite differently once the therapist had begun to monitor her affective responses to the patient. It then became possible to see that the patient was "communicating by impact" (Chapter 4). She was evoking in the therapist, by means of projective identification, a resonance to her own difficult feelings, which she could not communicate in other ways. The therapist could thereby begin to recognize important aspects of the patient's own unmanageable experiences, such as being confronted by her mother's unexplained absences, and not knowing where she was or what was happening to her. But a reorientation in listening had been necessary before this understanding of the patient's non-verbal communication became possible.

As an exercise in differentiating between clinically similar situations, I shall describe a case in which I too was having to struggle with silences in a session.

Example 12.5
A patient (whom I shall call Mrs. D.) would frequently fall into silences during which she was in evident distress. But when I tried to interpret from my own reading of her distress (in the way I have just been suggesting) it didn't help. Equally, if I left her in silence, that didn't help. Either way she experienced me as putting her under a pressure to speak; and I experienced myself as being in a double bind. Whatever I did was wrong.

One day the patient stammered out of her silence: "I am sorry, but I can't help being difficult like this." She was now experiencing a pressure to apologize. But she was also prompting me to look at her distressed silence differently. I was hearing about something called "being difficult." I took this as an unconscious cue.

I was reminded by this that Mrs. D.'s mother would often accuse her of "being difficult." She had previously told me that, when she was upset as a child, she could never speak to her mother about what she was feeling. Her mother used to regard this reluctance to speak as perverse and would accuse her of "being difficult." But if Mrs. D. then tried to speak about what she was feeling her mother would turn away from her, saying that she was "now being impossible." Her mother could not bear being made to feel upset, as a result of which the patient was made to feel that she was always in the wrong. I had already been aware of this double-binding by the mother. But in this session I was able to hear the patient in a new way.

> I replied: "Perhaps it is precisely this difficulty, in communicating what you are feeling, that you need to convey to me now; but you expect me not to be prepared to stay with you if I actually experience some of that difficulty, so you feel that you must apologize."
>
> The patient then told me more about her fear of being upset in the presence of her mother. She had frequently been rejected by her for expecting emotional help which was not forthcoming. To avoid this she would shut herself away in her bedroom, in despair of ever finding help with her distress.

Mrs. D. had to find out whether I could bear to be affected by her difficulty in communicating, without finding her "impossible." She also needed to discover whether I could recognize, and find ways of dealing with, her experience of being double-bound; and she had been able to communicate this by double-binding me.

Patients, as well as therapists, may use their familiarity with analytic theory to fall into cliché-thinking, and this will be just as detrimental to real insight. In these situations much of what we might normally be able to say to a patient, without it sounding stereotyped, is heard as cliché by the patient who then says: "Oh, I thought you would say that." Other patients seize upon any stereotyped interpretation to further their intellectualization of the analytic process. In either case real experience in the analysis is warded off.

In the following example the patient was constantly ready to make a defensive use of any predictable insight.

Example 12.6
Mrs. E. came to me for therapy when she was nearly thirty. She had a long history of depression, and now her second marriage was in a state of

breakdown. She was analytically sophisticated, anticipating much of what I interpreted to her in the early months of her therapy with me. (She had previously been in treatment with a psychiatrist who seems to have been prone to giving her "wild" analytic interpretations.)

This patient, born in a Mediterranean country, had been brought up as a Roman Catholic. She first married when she was seventeen. After three years her husband left her, accusing her of frigidity. She felt guilty about sex without knowing why, and she told me that her head would become "filled with accusing nuns" if ever she began to enjoy sex.

After her first husband had left her she became promiscuous, and began to think of herself as no better than a prostitute. Subsequently she married a much older man. But she so often provoked him to jealousy, by flirting with other men, that he too was threatening to leave. She now felt that she could not stop herself being sexual towards any man who interested her.

Her history revealed an alarming degree of self-destructiveness. This included a car crash from which she had nearly died. Intermittently she had been actively preoccupied with thoughts of suicide. She had also had two abortions. Her relationships with each member of her family were difficult. From early adolescence her father used to beat her, or shut her up in her room, if she ever showed interest in boys. Her mother was also fiercely critical of her. She had a brother four years younger than herself of whom she was intensely jealous.

Much of the detail of this patient's history lent itself readily to a familiar theoretical formulation. For example: I could postulate that Mrs. E. had been Oedipally attached to her father, particularly looking to him for love when her mother turned to the new baby; that she felt a fierce rivalry from her mother; that her persecutory superego (an introjection of this critical mother) was later represented by the accusing nuns; and that she had come to experience her sexuality as bad—to be totally inhibited or punished lest it became uncontrollable. In addition, there was evidence that she tried to deal with this self-destructively, or to get others to punish her in relation to her sexual interest in men. This interaction may well have originated with her father.

However, this was all based on theory or on other clinical experience. It had not yet grown out of my analytic work with this patient. Some of it had been postulated by the patient herself, based on what she had read, thus forestalling a deeper analytic experience. In addition, it was noticeable that Mrs. E. displayed an excited expectation that I would be interpreting her Oedipus complex, as her psychiatrist used to do. I therefore chose to defer further interpretation of this.

Gradually the patient's own preconceptions began to fade—as I was not exciting her with sexual interpretations. The therapy moved into other areas, with my own theoretical formulations falling into the background of my thinking and listening. And I stopped looking for, or thinking that I saw, the most obvious things that my analytic training had led me to expect.

> In the second year of this three-times-a-week therapy Mrs. E. told me a dream. She said: "I was in a bathroom with Kojak. There were many baths—side by side in a row." She had no associations. After a while I commented: "I don't understand this dream yet, but I do wonder why there were many baths." (I was trying to help her to free associate without directing her to say more.) Mrs. E. had no thoughts about this. After a pause I added: "I wonder if there could be an unconscious metaphor here for some kind of frequency." (I was thinking aloud about this strange detail in the dream, knowing that I still could not interpret.) She made nothing more of this so we left it.
>
> In a session two weeks later Mrs. E. said: "I dreamed about Kojak again last night. He was with me in my parents' bedroom. He was being sexual with me and I was feeling very excited. We were about to get into bed to make love when I woke up." This time Mrs. E. freely offered associations to her dream. She recognized the bedroom because this had been in a house where they had lived when she was four. She remembered it well, as her family had lived there during the year that her brother had been born. About Kojak, she said: "I really fancy that man. He sucks lollipops like a child and yet he is ever so sexy."

Here, I felt, I should be especially careful not to preempt the patient's discovery in what she was beginning to tell me. I therefore looked for a neutral way of providing a halfway step to insight in order to keep her options open.

> After a pause, I offered the comment: "I notice that you have recently had two dreams about Kojak." (At least there was nothing directive about that!) Mrs. E. began to wonder about this: "I think it has something to do with his bald head. It fascinates and excites me—I can't think why."
>
> I used a form of stereotyped response here; but, fortunately, it did not lead to the intellectualizing reply that it could have done. I said: "Perhaps Kojak is not the only person with a bald head who has fascinated or excited you."
>
> "No," she replied, "I don't know any bald men—at least not intimately." After a pause she cried out, in alarm and disbelief: "My God! it can't be . . . But yes . . . My father!" (Pause.) "My father used to wear a wig. I only ever saw him without it once, when I was very little. He was asleep and it had slipped off. He was totally bald; and I had completely forgotten that until now."
>
> Mrs. E. then poured out a memory that horrified and shocked her. She was in the bathroom with her father. She was four. Her father was playing with her naked upon his lap, when her mother came in. Her mother started

screaming, plunging her into the bath and washing her viciously all over. Her mother was screaming at her father (or was it at her?) whilst looking closely at her vagina.

In the following sessions many other details emerged that related to this experience. Mrs. E. was convinced that her father had actually abused her sexually; and not only on this occasion but frequently before this too. (Perhaps that was what had been alluded to in the dream detail of the many baths.)

I learned that her parents' marriage had collapsed about that time. Her father, she was eventually told, had turned instead to prostitutes. Could that have been why she had later come to identify herself with prostitutes? And her father punishing her, as a teenager, for being sexual; had she been provoking her second husband to treat her in a similar way?

Psychoanalytic theory, in this case, was discovered to be vividly borne out by clinical experience. But, for it to be clinically useful it had to be rediscovered, not merely applied. It would have served only to increase the patient's defenses against remembering if I had anticipated this eruption of unconscious memory by interpreting earlier. Instead, I had to preserve the analytic space from my own preconceptions—and hers. Insight, when it was arrived at, was no cliché. It was discovered when the patient was emotionally ready for this; and she could be ready only when she felt analytically secure enough to remember.

What was then necessary in this therapy was a careful working through of this new insight in the transference. During this phase of the therapy, the patient was only gradually able to allow herself to realize that her manner of relating to me was also clearly sexual—as with "any man who interested her." For a long time previously she had believed that it was only by her keeping all sexuality isolated from the therapeutic relationship that this had been kept safe. It therefore became an entirely new experience for her to discover that her sexuality could be acknowledged by me without being exploited, that it could be affirmed, not ignored or run away from. Only thus could she begin to see her sexuality as containable and therefore as benign, as neither bad nor destructive.

CONCLUSION

We do not have to be so quick to use old insights when we can learn to tolerate longer exposure to what we do not yet understand. And, when we do think we recognize something familiar from a patient, we need still to be receptive to that which is different and new.

> There is . . .
> At best, only a limited value
> In the knowledge derived from experience.
> The knowledge imposes a pattern, and falsifies,
> For the pattern is new in every moment
> And every moment is a new and shocking
> Valuation of all that we have been.
> ("East Coker")

> . . . Last season's fruit is eaten
> And the fullfed beast shall kick the empty pail.
> For last year's words belong to last year's language
> And next year's words await another voice.
> ("Little Gidding")
> (T.S.Eliot *Four Quartets*)

In psychoanalysis and psychotherapy our task is to find, in the patient and in ourselves, that other voice.

❖ 13 ❖

A Child Leads the Way

A key theme in Part Two is that of the unconscious search for what is needed, whereby children and patients give unconscious cues that indicate what they are looking for in key relationships.

My first analytic work of any kind was with a child. From my detailed notes we can follow the process whereby this child gradually prompted me, first to provide the therapeutic setting she needed and then to put into words the anxieties that had been blocking her learning. Eventually she made me overcome my reluctance to interpret, and she began to make significant progress when I did.

INTRODUCTION

I have already indicated, in the previous chapter, that one time when therapists are most likely to fall into using the stereotyped thinking of others is when they are feeling insecure about their own clinical understanding. The choice then seems to be either to interpret as others might or to trust in the patient's unconscious to lead the way. But this latter choice presupposes a positive potential in the analytic process which can safely be followed. I was fortunate to have had a chance to see evidence of that potential early in my analytical career.

I give an account here of my first five weeks of seeing a child "patient," aged six and a half. I shall call her Joy. Some alterations of personal detail have been made to preserve the anonymity of the family, but I have not concealed my sense of bewilderment and naivete. What seems to me so extraordinary about this sequence is how Joy managed to communicate her own sense of what she most needed. Of course it also shows the importance of a proper training in child psychotherapy. However, I trust that the reader will be able to share something of the experience of feeling my way until I discovered more clearly what this child needed of me.

I have included all the details that I have of Joy's play so that readers can assess for themselves what may have influenced this clinical sequence. I have also given my reflections, as they were during a session or immediately afterwards when I wrote up my notes. Sometimes I have added retrospective thoughts, in parentheses or as "comment," but for the most part I leave readers to form their own ideas about what could, or should, have been interpreted. I have therefore not changed or added to my original notes as I believe that it may be more interesting to be able to follow my struggles to understand and to manage what was happening.

The reader will be able to see from this account how Joy persistently prompted me until I made the moves which gave her what she needed. Thus, the reading lessons that her parents wanted her to have gave way to therapy, which she needed; the drawing-room provided for the reading gave place to a playroom; the need for a sufficient privacy from the mother's anxious intrusion was regularly signalled until I acted upon it; the freedom to make mess, as part of the therapy, was increasingly indicated until this was provided. Much more was to follow. This child really did lead the way whilst I had to pluck up my courage to follow.

Referral

I was in my second year as a student on an adult psychotherapy training course when I was asked to see Joy. She was referred to me by her mother's analyst, who recommended that I could be used as a "reading teacher," and that I might also "keep an eye on the psychotherapeutic needs" of the child.

I arranged for supervision whilst I was seeing Joy, but I started out with a strong reluctance to accept any interpretive role with her. This was partly because I had not been trained to work with a child in this way but was further fuelled by my recent reading of Klein's account of her work with "Richard" (Klein 1961).

I had formed an opinion from my reading of "Richard" that Klein had been providing that child with a symbolic language through which he could eventually communicate deep anxiety, or unconscious fantasy, with a possibility that this could be understood by the person who had been teaching him this language. But my reservations about working in that way were: that it assumed an extraordinary degree of certainty about a child's inner world which I did not have, and I was not sure whether compliant agreement with that certainty could really be distinguished from more autonomous communications that might not be in agreement with it. I also wondered whether Joy would be able to find her own language for communicating to me. I was therefore determined not to preempt her thinking with any interpretations that might assume that I knew more of her unconscious than I could be fairly sure of. So I waited for Joy to show me what she needed. I was, however, slow to respond to her increasingly clear demands for a change of setting and for unambiguous therapeutic work because of my own reluctance to be drawn into that.

Fortunately, Joy was not content with anything less than she needed, and from our first meeting she gave me repeated cues to understand that her inability to read was a symptomatic condition: she needed someone to recognize that she was having difficulties about her position in the family as the only girl. Later it also became clear that she did not have the words for her sexual curiosity and anxiety, but she remained healthily determined that I should not fob her off with merely euphemistic acknowledgements of what she was trying to say through her play. She needed to have interpretations spelled out quite directly and, when I was eventually able to help her discover the hidden positives of her female body, she immediately rewarded me by showing how much she had been learning from my attempts to teach her to read.

Family Background

Joy was six and a half when I first saw her. She had two brothers—I will call them Richard (aged nine) and Tom (aged two). The referrer had told me that Joy's mother had difficulty accepting her because she was a girl. Soon after she was born, Joy was handed over to a nanny and there had been minimal physical contact between Joy and her mother since then. I was also told that Joy was overindulged—that she had been allowed to have and to do much as she pleased. By contrast there was a more openly affectionate relationship between the mother and Joy's brothers, and it was particularly striking how much more physical care Tom was receiving from his mother, who took care of him herself, whilst Joy had been in the care of a series of nannies.

Meeting the Parents

I naturally met the parents before I saw Joy. I saw them in their home and they gave me details of her schooling. The father also told me that he saw Joy as "a very sexual child," and that she was quite seductive towards him. He and Joy had recently begun to spend weekends together at their seaside cottage, where she loved to run up and down the beach playing with him. He explained that he made her special in this way to make up for having been away so much in the past. (His job had frequently taken him abroad.) He said that he rather hoped that Joy would "fall in love" with me and so learn to read—for me.

The parents said that their poodle, Polo, was very important to Joy, and they had told her that Polo might have puppies in the spring as they had recently taken her to spend a few days with a "boyfriend poodle."

It was agreed at this meeting that I would see Joy every weekday morning, for the first week until Christmas, and less frequently thereafter.

WORKING WITH JOY

First Meeting with Joy (a Tuesday)

I could see Joy only at her home. When I arrived for the first time, her mother showed me into the room that she had allocated for "the reading lessons." This was the family drawing-room where, it was suggested, I would be "least disturbed by other noises and goings-on in the house." Unfortunately, the room was huge and (for the purposes of any play-therapy) it felt oppressively clean, tidy, and respectable. But because of my ambiguous brief for seeing Joy, I did not feel able to ask for alternative arrangements at this point.

The mother asserted her control from the beginning by coming in with a tray of coffee and biscuits, which she put on a table beside the chair she had designated as mine. Before leaving me alone with Joy, the mother asked me what Joy should call me: "Patrick" or "Mr. Casement"? I suggested that Joy could decide this for herself after she had got to know me.

I had brought with me a medium-sized, flabby, and well-used "holdall." In this there were some felt pens in lots of colors, a scribbling pad, some colored sticky paper and scissors, some plasticine (clay) in various colors, and some remedial reading material.

I asked Joy if she knew why I was there and she replied "to teach me to read." I asked her if she wanted to be able to read. "Part of me does and part of me doesn't," she replied. I asked about the part that *did* want to read: "I would like to be able to read like Anne," a friend who had moved up to the next form that term when Joy had been left behind. (I realized later that I had not asked about the part of her that did *not* want to read.)

I told Joy that we would be doing some reading games eventually, but first I would like her to play—and I let her explore the contents of my holdall. Joy chose to play with the plasticine. She wanted to make Polo (the family poodle) and chose brown "because that is Polo's color." She made a large fat sausage from which she pinched legs, head, and tail, making quite a skilled model of a dog. I said "Polo is rather fat isn't she?" and Joy replied "Well she is going to be fat because she's going to have puppies." I asked how she knew this. "Of course she is because she went away to stay with Gonzo; he's a boy poodle, and Mummy and Daddy say that she's going to have puppies."

Joy made a model of her brother Richard out of red plasticine. "We'll make him big because he's ever so big—almost as big as you." I asked her how we could tell that he was a boy. (I wanted to give her permission to be more explicit about sexual differences, because of the apparent discrimination against her by her mother.) She replied: "Of course you know." When I asked her to show me, she took more red plasticine and made a long thin sausage. She looked at me mischievously and pressed it flat saying that's his school cap. She pinched this and drew out a long peak. I commented on what a large peak he had and she replied "Well, that's to keep the sun out of his eyes." She made another thin sausage, hesitated where to put it, squashed it and made it into his "satchel." She made a very thin length of plasticine, again hesitated up and down the body, and then quickly put it on to the satchel. She told me "that's his big pencil." Finally she made a tiny lump of plasticine and, after more hesitation and knowing looks, made a quick decision: "That's his ink pot," and she stuck this on to his satchel too. Richard was made to sit astride Polo but he kept falling off.

Reflection

In this material we can see several issues already emerging. Joy knew about pregnancy. She also knew about sexual differences, having been given a lead from me to be able to acknowledge this, but she was afraid of being explicit. The penis symbols were all eventually disguised—as a peak cap, a satchel, a pencil and an ink pot. There was also some reference to being able to see more clearly, helped by the peaked cap "to keep the sun out of his eyes." (This was the first of many references to eyes and seeing.)

There may have been an early indication of transference in Joy speaking of Richard as "ever so big—almost as big as you."

Joy then began drawing. She drew her mother first, adding Polo beside her. Then she dotted the picture saying "It's raining." She drew her father and added: "He must have an umbrella—we'll give him one." She began to draw an umbrella but changed this into "his brief-case." "He doesn't need an umbrella," she said, "because the sun is shining." She drew a black radiant sun. Then she drew Richard and Tom.

While Joy was still drawing she looked up to me and said very confidentially: "I'm going to tell you a secret. You are not to tell anyone." I asked if this meant that she didn't want her mother to know. "*No-one* must know," she said with great emphasis. (*Pause.*) "I have a secret telephone under the chair. I ring up Anne on this whenever I want to, without anyone knowing." This was the end of the session.

Reflection

I felt that I could see something of Joy's ambivalence towards each of her parents in her drawing of them. In relation to her mother she seemed to wish to be allowed to be special to her with Polo, the only other female in the family, drawn close to the mother. (Joy had added rain to the picture, and later I learned that she had been persistently enuretic since her mother's pregnancy with Tom had begun to show. She had been dry before then but wet every night since.) I was not sure about her representation of the father, with a black sun shining down on him. In relation to me, I felt that she sounded conspiratorial in telling me her secret—something that must be kept just between her and me. But we may also be seeing an unconscious prompt for me to establish boundaries around her contact with me. With her mother bringing in coffee at the beginning, and hanging around to see me before I left, these boundaries did not yet properly exist.

At the end of the session I thanked the mother for bringing me coffee but added that I would prefer not to have this in future "because it rather gets in the way."

Session 2 (Wednesday)

During this session Joy drew Polo again but made her very thin. I commented "You've made her thin today." Joy said "She's had her puppies" and drew a red puppy and red rain which fell on both mother and puppy. She added another puppy in blue, dotted the red puppy with blue and added blue rain which drizzled down on the blue puppy.

Reflection
I felt that Joy was representing a wish to be alone with her mother (Polo with one baby, both mother and puppy in red). After she had added another puppy in blue she went back to dot the red puppy with blue, perhaps expressing the wish to have some of the blue color in herself to make her more like her brother. I wondered about enuresis around the birth of Tom, but I didn't yet know the details of this. I did not interpret any of this to Joy.

Joy drew a gorilla. She said: "We'll put him on another page because he has big thumbs." She drew the thumbs. She drew squiggles to make a tree, drew a banana at the top, put a banana in the gorilla's hand and said: "I like to take bananas when Mummy's not looking." She drew a hand reaching into the picture from below. I asked her to show me that the gorilla was a man. She covered him over by drawing trousers on him.

Reflection
I felt that Joy was indicating jealousy towards her brothers, and perhaps her father, because they were allowed to have what she would like to have. She had to steal a banana whereas the man gorilla had a banana all to himself. The phallic symbolism of the big thumbs, and the banana, seemed obvious. Again, I made no comment.

I had the impression that Joy was refusing to look at the more visible maleness of her brothers because of the disturbing preference given to them in the family, and because she had not yet discovered a positive view of herself as female. So I invited Joy to show me the maleness of the gorilla, in order to let her know that it was all right for her to acknowledge this more directly. But she couldn't yet dispense with her need to retreat from more direct references to the distinction between the sexes, and she used plenty of other symbols of her own.

Session 3 (Thursday)

During this session Joy remarked: "You must get rid of that case and get a new one. That one is all dirty." It seemed that she didn't like the thought that I had taken it with me to see other children. She wanted me to be "new" with her. The case, however, remained unchanged and she eventually accepted it.

Joy began immediately with drawing. She drew a mound and drew two lines across it, calling it a cave. Beside this she drew a square with wheels. I asked her if this might be a car. "No." She drew more wheels and made it into a crane, drawing a large extension up into the sky. She blobbed in the end of this, drew a line coming out of the blob, thought about it and drew another line. From this she dangled a man. "That's you," she said. She filled in the bottom of the cave with little dots and asked me "What are those?" I said: "You tell me." "They are treasures and you have to go down into the cave to fetch them out, and here [drawing more] is a rope ladder to help you down, and here [drawing] is Polo standing over the treasures to keep them safe for you, and here to the right [drawing] is a passage—you can escape out of that if you need to." She drew Gonzo (Polo's mate) standing in this passage "to help Polo keep everything safe." She drew a figure half-way up the crane: "That is Richard who is watching to see that everything is all right." She drew a large support to keep up the end of the crane. She looked at the picture and was clearly pleased with it.

While drawing this Joy had told me about the gardener, who had recently made a big bonfire and how she had to run away because of all the smoke. Later, whilst she was still drawing, I happened to rub one of my eyes. She stopped drawing and said very earnestly: "I should have told you—you mustn't rub an itch, because although at first it feels nice it soon begins to hurt." I noticed the allusion to masturbatory experience but chose not to comment.

My first remark to Joy about her drawing was: "It seems to be rather like Polo and Gonzo making babies, because the man has to go in here, where the treasures are, and later the baby comes out where the man had gone in." Joy said: "No, Polo and Gonzo are here; and you are not one of the animal family." I said: "Well, perhaps it is like you having secrets which have to be guarded carefully, and you won't let anyone except me in to know about them." Joy was quite happy with this second comment, but she still wanted to maintain that a drawing is only a drawing. (I had made these comments so that she knew she was allowed to speak about sexual matters, which I could tell—from what I knew about her and from her play—were evidently preoccupying her.)

Reading: After this drawing, any attempts by me to get Joy to concentrate on reading were quite fruitless.

Session 4 (Friday before Christmas)

When Joy began drawing she started with a top hat out of which she made it "rain upwards." She said: "I've drawn that upside down so you won't know what it is." She made this into a clown. "But he is really a spy dressed up as a clown, disguised so nobody will recognize him." I asked her what he was trying to find out: secrets? "Yes, secrets." She continued to draw. She made the spy look very unhappy—adding tears to his eyes. At the top of his head she drew a circle and said "In here he has a little man with a gun, and [still drawing] down here [she drew another circle in his tummy] he has another man with a gun." "These are his friends," she said, "but here comes a flying ball—a ball with teeth." She drew the teeth in red. She then covered them over: "So no-one will see that it has teeth" and turned the teeth into a broad smile. She further disguised the ball by drawing petals around it, saying: "It now looks like a flower . . . but here it has a gun" (which she added to one of the petals). She took up the blue felt-pen and drew in the teeth again, and made the eyes blue too.

I asked Joy who were the "goodies" and who the "baddies" in her picture. She immediately took this up, saying that the little man inside the spy was "a goodie" and "the flying ball with teeth comes from the baddies." She added: "I'll be like that and I will have a go at Richard . . . but I haven't got a gun. I'll get a Dalek suit for Christmas, and then I'll have a gun and I'll fight Richard."

Reflection

I saw in this sequence a recurring conflict around Joy showing her aggression and a defensive need to hide it. I also thought that there was a disguised allusion to enuresis in her making it "rain upwards," drawing rain upside down so that I would not know about it. But, at the same time, she told me that this was what she was doing—to make sure that I did know. The theme of disguise continued with the spy disguised as a clown, and the flying ball with hidden teeth. The petals offered further disguise but there was still a gun which was added to one of the petals—a gun which Richard had, and Joy would like to have.

Monday. *Christmas Holiday*

Session 5 *(Tuesday after Christmas)*

Joy was difficult and very restless. She wouldn't concentrate so no effective reading work was done. She pulled the table cloth off "to make everything go on the floor" so I had to remove it. Her only interest was in drawing.

She began with a ground-level line. She drew a little man in a cave and then obliterated him. She drew a dog, crossed it out and turned it into "an animal with a snaky tail." She drew what looked like a ladder: "That is a well, and in the well there is an octopus." She drew a "Mummy figure" underneath, a "Daddy figure" to the right, and "a boy" to the left. She turned the boy into a girl and drew a hat on his/her head. She drew another black octopus at the top right and a red octopus on the left. She ended by drawing tufts of grass at the bottom. "This is hair-grass," she said. I made no comment except to say: "The octopus in the well looks very sad." She agreed with this. She decided to give him a clown's nose so she drew a cross on the nose. She added a final touch by making the man hold a gun which he was shooting.

Reflection

This was the first session after the break and Joy may still have been overexcited from Christmas. Equally she may have been angry with me for being away. I felt that she might have been telling me that she had felt obliterated by my absence, giving my attention to other people rather than to her, and I noticed that she had obliterated the "little man" who was by the entrance to the cave. I thought I had been made small in her mind so that she would not miss me.

I felt that the "sad" octopus might well be herself. By contrast the parent figures were together, outside the well containing the sad octopus, and they had a boy with them (Tom?). She turned this boy into a girl—perhaps placing herself where the boy was.

Session 6 *(Wednesday)*

Joy was exceedingly difficult. She pushed things off the table and then put her feet on it. She wouldn't even look at the reading material I tried to assemble, and at times she was so frustrating that I felt drawn into becoming a "punitive parent." This was clearly a mistake but it also indicated what she was doing to me.

Once I had decided that it was useless to pursue Joy further with the reading material, she began to draw and she became very excited as she did this. In one drawing there were two little men which she called "Chinese mice because they have long tails." She drew a bird and an aeroplane "with a bag underneath which it puts round the bird to keep it safe." And there was another dangling man, hanging from a parachute.

Before the end of this session Joy drew a second picture. "This is Polo. She is all dressed up for a fancy-dress ball. Mummy and Daddy are going to a ball in fancy-dress. We'll give Polo antlers then no one will recognize her: she will be all disguised. And here are her puppies, and they are disguised too." I said: "It looks rather like your Mummy with Richard and Joy—and Tom on her back like a baby that has to be carried." Joy denied this, saying "Tom doesn't need to be carried now. He can walk." She didn't go so far as to deny altogether that this could represent her mother and the three children, but on the whole she still insisted that a picture was "only a picture" and no more.

Reflection

This session began with an even stronger protest against reading and a wish instead to do drawing. There were further examples of her using disguise.

Session 7 (Thursday)

I was determined not to give in to Joy's attempts to make me angry, but to wait until she decided to join me. She again began by pushing away all reading materials. She wouldn't look at anything I put out for her. She walked round the room ignoring me. But when I continued quietly to put letters out on my own Joy began to be curious. In this way we managed to make a few words that she was prepared to read.

Joy drew her friend Anne, saying that she now thought Anne was silly. She didn't think she wanted to be her friend any more. She put "A" for her name. She said: "This is you." I said: "But isn't this a girl?" "Yes," she replied, "but it's still you!" She drew the octopus motif on the skirt, drew a face in the tummy, covered it over with red, drew a circle in the tummy then crossed it out. We looked at the drawing together and I said that it seemed to be a rather angry drawing. She replied with emphasis, "Now you are right there!"

As I was leaving the room the mother came to see how we had been getting on. Unfortunately, I allowed myself to be persuaded into showing her what progress we had made and I asked Joy to read out our list of words. She did this quickly and confidently, getting the first half right without a pause. When she came to the word "POT" she hesitated and guessed the rest. She had reverted to her old method of "reading" by guessing.

Reflection

Joy had begun to show curiosity when I did something on my own rather than thrusting it at her. Her reference to Anne may have been to let me know of her feelings about me. Anne was silly and she didn't want to be Anne's friend any more. (Anne had been associated earlier with reading and wanting to read.) In case I was too silly to get the point Joy made this very explicit by telling me that Anne was me. Joy elaborated on this by using the octopus motif (which she frequently used to represent her mother), and put a baby in the tummy with an "O" (presumably Oggie—her name for Tom when he had first been born). She had then crossed out the "O." I wondered if Joy was beginning to experience me as the mother who didn't spend enough time with her: and what other children or babies did I have that took me away from her when I was not seeing her? She didn't want me to have other babies and crossed out the Oggie baby in her drawing.

Session 8 (Friday)

We started with more three-letter games, as on the previous day, but Joy would not read any of the words that I made. She preferred to continue guessing. She was largely obstructive and refusing to be cooperative.

When she began drawing Joy again drew an octopus. She "disguised" this by putting trousers round all the legs. She added clown's eyes, a clown's hat and another hat. She drew "a fish, with teeth, that comes and bites off one of the legs." Still drawing, she said: "Now here is a rat with a tail and big teeth. And here is a man with one leg bitten right off. The teeth are red. And here is a hat for the man who has lost his leg, and the fish has a hat. And here is a crab."

I commented: "You've drawn a lot of teeth today. Does that mean that you want to bite people because you are angry?" She replied, "No." I continued: "Well, I have noticed that you do draw teeth when you've been angry with me over the reading." She seemed to accept this but made no actual reply.

Reflection

I had not yet interpreted to Joy the mother transference as I had regarded that kind of interpretation as beyond my "brief" with her. But she was not deterred. She went straight back to the octopus. She disguised this with trousers. (I was later told by the mother's analyst that the mother "liked to add to her body image sometimes with hats, sometimes with trousers, and with her phallic behavior.")

Joy used clown's eyes as a specific symbol of her own. It could be used to represent me as someone stupid, or to indicate eyes that didn't see, or both. At the time, however, I was still not letting her know if I was seeing what she had been telling me or not. The clown had two hats. I wondered if Joy saw me as "wearing two hats," one when I was alone with her and another when I was with her mother—as at the end of the previous day's session. This could add to any tendency she may have had to see me as having a split loyalty or as being there really to do mother's bidding.

In her drawing there was a man who had a leg bitten off, and there were also several biting creatures. There was plenty here to suggest castration anxiety but I did not take this up. Instead I focused on the biting. In her response to my comment here Joy showed that I was not getting to the point. I was avoiding the more specific elements in the material. I had also missed the possible allusions to the coming weekend, the days when I would be wearing yet another hat—in my life away from her.

Session 9 (Monday)

A frustrating day. Not much reading got done and her play was listless. I wondered if this could have been her response to the weekend.

Session 10 (Tuesday)

I brought with me (for the first time) a magnetic blackboard with letters. Joy played happily with this but unfortunately her mother came to see me on her way out. I was feeling a bit conscious of having submitted my first account to her and once again fell into giving her some idea of Joy's progress. I told her that we had made about 20 words today. "Oh good," she replied, "so Joy will soon be able to start reading the book we have that has only 36 words."

Reflection

I realized that I would have to resist any premature introduction of reading books into our sessions. Furthermore, I would have to avoid slipping into giving indications of Joy's progress, as this only fed into the mother's anxiety and impatience for tangible evidence of progress. The mother's constant access to me, as I came and went, was also becoming a severe disadvantage.

Session 11 (Wednesday)

Trying to read with Joy was futile. She wanted to put two random letters together and give them names. She resisted all my attempts to get her to make words with me or to read words. This may well have been a reaction to the further contact with her mother the day before.

When Joy began drawing she chose, for the first time, to copy. She copied a painting from the front page of a magazine on a coffee table in the room. The picture was of a "visitation" scene of some sort, a man approaching a woman sitting under a canopy. Joy made the woman a queen who looked as if she was sitting up in bed. The canopy was used as another version of the octopus motif. There was a king approaching on a horse, sword in hand. Joy added "a Dalek" standing behind the queen. Over the king she put "an aeroplane with a nose," and above that an octopus with a clown's hat. She made lightning attack the canopy over the queen, and the octopus fired from one of its legs. Towards the canopy, and behind the king, there was "a hidden baddie" who was "firing and making it lightning." At the top she drew the sun with a little man in it.

I made no comment except to say that there seemed to be a lot of fighting in the picture. Joy seemed happy drawing this picture, and I think she liked my comment. I added that she seemed to like drawing octopuses. She replied: "But you have to be very careful with them as they can catch you and can eat you all up, so that you would then be inside the octopus."

Reflection

We continued to have the octopus motif, here placed clearly in relation to the mother. There were several implied attacks against the dangerous octopus-mother, the "Dalek" standing behind the queen and the "hidden baddie" behind the king. I thought that Joy would like to be on her father's side (the king's), so that she could feel safe there and be able to be "firing and making it lightning." I wondered who the little man in the sun might be. Could this represent me—seen today as little?

Session 12 (Thursday)

We began with the blackboard which still had the alphabet laid out on it. While I was laying out the vowels, and two rows of lower-case letters that could be used with them, Joy made a fresh exploration into my holdall. There she found a box of magnetic capital letters. She was delighted with her find and thought her letters were much better than mine. She immediately put out her alphabet and laid out three columns of random letters, like in the spelling game I had been arranging. This was to be *her* game and *she* would make the rules! "You have to close your eyes," she said, "to pick your first letter. Then you open your eyes and you pick two more letters and make up a word. We take turns.... I'll start."

Joy first picked "F" and "H," which she put together. I took this opportunity to show her that we would have to use one of the five vowel letters I had put out too. Even in her game we could not make words without using vowels. I showed her a sequence I had put out for her—PA, PE, PI, PO, PU—following each with a "t" to complete the words. Joy seemed interested when she discovered that some letters (vowels) are special in this way. We began playing "her" game, with vowels accepted into it from "my" game. The first word she made was her "favorite word"—NIT. She put this as far away as she could on the board "so we can't cheat by looking at words we have already made." The next word she broke up after she had made it, and put it in another corner of the blackboard saying "I don't like it any more." I asked if she always pushed things away that she didn't like. She didn't reply.

After this Joy decided that we would write down the words we had made. She took the scribbling pad and roughly ruled a page with a line down the middle. She had a red pen for herself and chose blue for me (the color that she had used for "ruling" the lines). She wanted to make a word with AG. I helped her with "H" and she wrote down HAG on her side. I changed the "A" to "U" so she wrote down HUG on my side. She decided it would be better if I chose next. I made the word FUN. She wrote this down on her side as well as mine. She made MEN and again wrote this down on both sides. By now it was the end of the session.

Reflection

For a second time we had been too engrossed to do any drawing. I felt the session had included an important moment because Joy had taken over the spelling game and made it her own. Elements of her controlling me were certainly present too, but she was prepared to accept part of my "rules" into her game so that vowels were included and real words could be made instead of nonsense combinations. There was a new sense of sharing.

Session 13 (Friday)

When I arrived, Joy was playing with a ball which she had taken from the Christmas tree. This was made from malleable tin foil. She had pushed some dents into this and she showed me proudly how she could make the dents disappear "by pushing at the corners—on the points," so that she could mend it as well as push it out of shape. She showed me one side of the ball where she had made a lot of holes with a pin. I shook the ball, when she handed it to me, and noticed that there was something rattling inside. I suggested that there was a pin that may have got inside. Joy strongly denied this, insisting that there was nothing at all inside. "I'll show you," she said. She tried to push a hole in the ball with a pen but it wouldn't go through. She went to look for scissors and said that she would cut it open to show me. I asked her whether she would get into trouble if she cut up the ball. She was sure that nobody would mind, "and anyway there are plenty more balls on the tree," she added. She made a hole with the point of the scissors. "That is for you," she said. "For me to get inside?" I asked. "Yes, to find out what is in there." She made the hole larger. We didn't find anything because whatever it was had fallen on to the floor. She then made it into "a purse." "We can put things into it," she said. I asked "What shall we put inside?" She continued: "Money of course, but we haven't got any money so we'll have to make some things to put inside." She carried on cutting. "We can make the purse smaller." By this time it resembled a dish and I commented that the purse was now quite open. "But we can still shut it up," she replied, "I'll show you." She folded it over but it kept springing open again. She then tied it shut "so that the things inside won't get out." I asked her if these were secrets. "Yes," she said. "And, so that burglars like you won't get in, you are not allowed to know the secrets." I replied: "But you can tell me your secrets because you know I won't tell them to anyone else." (With more experience

I would have avoided the use of reassurance here and would have explored her anxiety that she could not yet trust me with her secrets. I should also have recognized that she might experience this as seductive.)

Joy put the purse into her "pocket." To do this she had to undo the zip of her skirt. She was ignoring the pocket which I could see on the other side of her skirt as she searched for an imaginary pocket. Joy was trying to hide the "purse" in her pretend pocket but it wouldn't stay. I suggested that she might use the pocket on the other side (where I could see it). "No, that pocket has a leak in it, and this pocket has a leak in it too." She pushed her hand through, to demonstrate this, so that it appeared between her legs—under her skirt. She added: "You put your hand in here and you'll see that it has a leak." I answered that I didn't need to do that as she had just shown me. This play ended there and Joy turned to other things.

Reflection

Joy began by playing at damaging the Christmas tree ball, then repairing it. Later she "destroyed" this and "created" something else—the purse. She was beginning to explore the question of what is inside things. She made a hole in the ball for me to see what was inside. She made a purse for her "secrets." When this wouldn't stay closed she made it smaller. If it was small enough burglars wouldn't be able to get in. I was not allowed to know the secrets today, but then she enacted a seductive invitation for me to look under her skirt at the pocket she has which leaks. (Might this have been her response to my invitation to tell me her secrets? And is she showing me here that she experienced that invitation as seductive? I think so.) What I felt unable to interpret was the richness of her symbolism—her search for the pocket that cannot be seen. Lacking the words to help I focused only on the visible, literal, pocket although she was clearly pressing me to acknowledge the inner "pocket" that was not being acknowledged by *anybody*—and not yet by me.

Reading: Joy was not interested in spelling games. But, for a time, she was prepared to play "her" game—making nonsense words. She decided, however, that she would spell POLO because she could do that. She told me that Polo had been away to see somebody who had told them she wouldn't be having babies after all. She was "half sorry but mostly glad" about this. I tried to get Joy interested in more spelling but she pushed away the words I was making with the magnetic letters. She walked round the room appearing uninterested, but she soon came to look over my shoulder to see what I was doing. She watched for a while. I was making a few words on my own. She then announced: "I can spell LOOK, because I know that." We did this on the board; also BOOK, COOK, and ROOK. I asked her to write down LOOK, which she had correctly spelled out aloud to me. She wrote KOOL. I removed LOOK from the board and suggested that she make it with the letters on the board. This time it was correct. She compared this with what she had written and crossed that out, obliterating it completely, and wrote it again correctly.

Reflection
Having introduced a curiosity about the shape of things, and the "inside" of things, Joy showed her curiosity with what I was doing. She looked over my shoulder to see and announced that she could spell "look." When she wrote this down she reversed it. Here I thought Joy was giving me an indication of her taboo on looking, and her need to reverse what she sees because of the implications for her of seeing things as they are. This may be particularly true in relation to herself and her brothers, who were different from her and were probably treated differently because of this.

Drawing. Joy described what she was doing as she drew: "I am going to draw the zoo." She wrote ZOO at the top. She drew a cage. Inside the cage she drew a seal. I said I didn't think seals were put in cages. Joy put in some water. "They have to be in a cage because, when people come to feed fish to them, if they are not safe inside a cage they might come and water at them—I mean snap at them." I said I wondered why she had said "water" just then and she replied that she had meant to say "Come out of the water and snap at them." I asked her if she was going to draw someone holding a fish to the seal. She almost shuddered and gave me an emphatic "NO." She told me that there was a notice NOT TO FEED THE ANIMALS. "We'll put it on a notice here," she said, and she wrote "NOT." She said: "That could be for all the things you're not allowed to do." She decided that it would read NOT TO FEED THE OSTRICHES. She began to draw an ostrich, made it into a seal and called it "A fat lady resting." After more thought about her "NOT" notice she said: "That notice now says DO NOT DISTURB." (I gathered later that her mother had been much given to resting and saying that she should not be disturbed, particularly during her pregnancy with Tom.) Joy scrubbed out NOT and drew a spider. She drew a man putting his hand in the cage. "We'll make him a clown, and here's his clown's hat, and there's his big nose—but it is an artificial nose."

As I was leaving, Joy said: "If Mummy asks about the ball I want you to say that you made me cut it open." She was clearly trying to manipulate me, but she may also have been testing me to see if I would stand up to this. I told her that I couldn't say that because she knew that it wasn't true. She seemed to accept this.

Reflection
The slip of the tongue ("water at") might have referred to Joy's continuing enuresis. There might also be a further allusion to her view of herself as "castrated" when she shuddered at the thought of someone feeding the snapping seal. In her elaboration around the "NOT" notice, it was interesting that she saw the prohibitions that she had been subjected to as summed up in the single order not to disturb (the fat lady—a pregnant mother). The "NOT" notice was replaced by a spider (another archaic symbol for the mother). She followed my earlier lead and drew a man putting his hand into the cage, but he is a clown (stupid?) and his nose was artificial. The "male" protrusions were either in danger of being bitten off or were artificial (the nose is not really as big as it seems). What might have been there at the very end of the session was a further prompt about Joy's need to be allowed a safe space to play where if necessary she can cut things up and "destroy" them without having to be anxious about her mother's reactions. I had not yet managed to tackle this problem.

Session 14 (Monday)

Joy came in carrying some artificial ferns, a long pencil, and some white cloth. With these she played quite contentedly, but after a pause she looked around for something else. She collected an ashtray from the window-seat which contained the ash of one cigarette and one stub-end. "This is more like it," she said with glee. She obviously enjoyed spilling the ash on to the cloth scraping it together, digging out the filter tip for more, pulling the ferns to bits and "planting" these in the ash. After a while she began bombing the ferns with the pencil, saying "stinky, smelly smelly bum; bumble bee; the pencil is a bumble bee." She was content with this for a bit, but added: "What we really need now is some water to mix with it." She wanted to "slip out" to get some straight away: "No one will see." I suggested that it might be rather difficult to use water in the drawing-room. "Well I'll use it afterwards, but I'll have to do it in secret afterwards so no one will see me. But if I could do it here I wouldn't have to hide it." I suggested that there were quite a lot of secret things which she would like not to have to hide, and which she could perhaps share with me. She agreed enthusiastically.

Reflection
Joy indicated quite openly her need for greater freedom to play with water and mess. Having been placed so firmly in the drawing-room by the mother, I had not yet found any way to free myself from the mother's control over Joy's "reading lessons." The arrangement had therefore remained a compromise between reading and therapy, but Joy could not have made a plainer plea for me to allow her to use her sessions as real play-therapy, without the restriction imposed by the parental setting. She added, sadly, that she would have to do it in secret afterwards, but she wouldn't have to hide this if it were allowed in her sessions.

Reading: Whilst Joy continued playing with the ashtray I began to put some words out on the blackboard. I tried to encourage her to come over and join me at the board, but without success.

I turned the board so that she could see it and asked her to read one of the words there. She turned away. I said: "Look at it and tell me what this word is. It's a word that you know." "I can't look because I haven't got any eyes," was her reply. I said that I thought it was because she didn't want to look that she said she hadn't got eyes.... "There are some things you don't want to see."

Reflection
Joy may have been telling me that I was the one who seemed to be blind. At that time I failed to see this and interpreted the blindness as hers, not mine!

As I left, I was again met by the mother who wanted to know how we were getting on. I took this opportunity to tell her that I appreciated her wish to see results, but I felt that Joy needed a time without being expected to perform for her parents.

Comment: Even though I had made a step towards establishing better boundaries for Joy's sessions I had still not asked for a more appropriate play-space for our sessions.

Session 15 (Tuesday)

I tried in vain to do reading with Joy but she blocked at every stage. Instead she made up a game with the magnetic letters, collecting small "o"s and "e"s. She arranged these with the letters on their sides (they were oblong in shape) "so that the 'o's will be smaller than the 'e's," and she told me that the letters were "going to school." She took a big "C" and two little "c"s, saying: "These are the teacher and her two friends who are helping her." She built a cage round these with straight letters. "The 'e's are the older children, because they are bigger," she explained. "I saw Anne yesterday," she said after a pause. I asked if Anne could read now. "Yes, easily." I asked if she is in the class of the "e"s now, with the bigger children. "Yes." (*Pause.*) "No, the 'e's are the smallest children now." I asked her if she wanted to be able to read like Anne. "No, I don't want to read at all." Joy pushed all the letters to the sides of the board and said: "There, I've *never* seen the board so clear as that!"

At the end of this session I asked Joy why she had wanted to play and not do any reading today. She replied: "I don't want to read. I want to play."

Reflection
I still felt under pressure to be the "reading teacher," and I may still have been wishing to protect myself from entering the unknown area of real play-therapy for which I felt singularly unprepared. Also, I thought that Joy had been giving me further indications of her unease about my contacts with her mother. In fact, in this session Joy seemed to be emphasizing her need for clearer boundaries, by building her wall with straight letters to keep me out, the cage around the big "C" (for Casement?) and the two little "c"s who were helping the teacher. The need for an adequate play-space was again evident when Joy pushed all the letters to the sides of the board, thus making it clearer than ever before.

Session 16 (Wednesday)[1]

We began by writing. After a while Joy announced that she had forgotten something, and asked to be allowed to go and fetch it. She went out and brought back a torch. "This is my gun," she announced. She began exploring behind the cushions of the settee, saying: "This is a secret passage." She climbed into this, burrowing and emerging. I responded to this reference to "secret passage" and said to her that it was rather like being born. She wasn't too sure about this, but she had so far always rejected such comments from me. (Joy had a rich capacity for fantasy and imagery in her own terms. Interpretations still seemed to be experienced by her as an intrusion into her private world.)

Joy continued playing for most of the session—still burrowing behind the cushions. She turned this into a game. "I want to see how many cushions I can knock over at one go." I didn't feel able to offer any interpretation of this, but as these were drawing room cushions they were clearly parent-related objects that were being knocked about. I felt even more uneasy about this play taking place in such an obviously "parental" space.

Joy tried fixing the lighted torch under her jumper. "Look, now no one will know where my torch is," she said. However, as it was still alight it could be seen through her jumper. I thought (to myself) that she was wanting to boast of an obvious penis-like protrusion that I couldn't fail to notice. But, as I didn't know what she called a penis (or if she had any word for it at all), I tried interpreting this more vaguely by saying "It makes you look like a boy." She wouldn't accept this. "What do you mean?" she asked. I replied lamely: "You know what I mean."

Reflection
I failed to follow Joy's cue for me to be more direct in speaking of sexual differences. We were not able to put these into words at this stage, because of my continuing reticence about making a specifically sexual interpretation to a child. I did not know whether I could handle whatever might follow from such direct interpretations. (Later events proved that the inhibition here was much more mine than hers.)

Joy probed the lighted torch into everything; into my ear, into my mouth, up her nose. "Look, I can make it red," she exclaimed. I hesitated to interpret. She told me that she was going to hide under her mother's bed with the torch "to find out what I can see." I asked her if her parents slept in the same bed or did they have separate beds. "The same bed. A big bed. You can see it if you want to." I asked her if she had ever slept in the same room as her mother and father. "No, but Mummy sometimes sleeps in my room—when I'm not well." I said that she probably wondered what her Mummy and Daddy did together in bed. "No I don't!" she replied with great emphasis. I suggested that she had denied this so strongly because she really wanted to know very much. She turned to the settee for a last bit of cushion-bashing. I said: "Well, I am going now. You can do that when I have gone. Joy didn't want me to go. She said "I haven't finished my bashing yet and I can't possibly do that when you have gone. *I can only do this when you are here.*" I said that there were probably a lot of things that she felt she could only do when she was with me. She agreed. She helped me to tidy everything up "so that it looks all right again," she said.

Reflection

Joy enacted with the torch her wish to look into everything. She needed me to help her understand what she sees (to throw some light on it). She could also have been using the torch to highlight what she is "saying" in her play, and to demonstrate that she needed me to put this into words for her (the torch into my ear and my mouth). She wanted to show me her parents' double-bed, having indicated that there were secrets there which she needed me to know. The plea for a play-room was present as ever, and I continued not to act upon it.

Session 17 (Thursday)

Joy wanted to begin by drawing. She drew a house. "That's your house," she said. She drew round windows with a cross over them. I said they looked like clown's eyes. I asked whether the house had clown's eyes so that you couldn't see *out* or couldn't see *in*. She said "So you can't see in." She obliterated the windows, saying "These are curtains." She drew a penis-shaped projection out of the side of the house. "Now, here we have a big sort of thing," she said. I asked her if she had a "thing" like that. She asked me what I meant, and once again I said "You know what I mean." (It was beginning to be almost impossible to stay with euphemisms to describe parts of the body. Names were becoming essential.) "No," she said, "I haven't got a thing like that." She drew animals on "the thing." She said, still drawing: "Here's a great big bird, an eagle—a Condor—with a great big beak and a long tongue, and it's going to come down and attack the animals here. We'll use some red because it is dangerous. Now the bird is coming to get some precious things that you have in your house. You know what?" "Treasures?" I asked. "Yes," she replied, "you keep them in your bedroom there. We'll draw the stairs." She drew the stairs in red. I asked her if these were in red because it might be dangerous to go up the stairs.

"No, it is not dangerous here because it is in our house . . . but it is dangerous where a bird wants to come in. I am going to make a special trap there so that the eagle bird will be caught and you will be safe." She drew "a cage thing." (Pause.) "Now there are other birds here, and they are dangerous too. They're baddies. But this bird is a good one who has come to look after you to keep you safe from the eagle bird .... And here's a cow, no, a bull." I asked her to show me that it was bull. She drew horns on its head. I asked what it had underneath that made it a bull. She said she had never looked. She continued, "Now the treasures are hidden in your room. I'll show you ....They are hidden behind a picture like this...." She described the picture as she drew it, saying "It's of a cow; no, a horse." (I wondered if she had chosen a horse because the sex differentiation is less obvious, and I had questioned her about the bull.) She went on, "And all round there are secret bomb-things, which will go off if anyone tries to get at the treasures. But they won't go off at you because I will give you the key, which will go in here, and you are the only one who is allowed in."

Joy drew the detail of the bomb gadgets. She said: "There are little bombs like these (red spots round the picture) which come out by mistake if you are not careful.... And the other big bombs are water-bombs." I asked which bombs Joy preferred. She replied: "The water-bombs."

Reflection

Joy pursued the previous day's theme. This time the bedroom secrets were put in my house where they would not be dangerous. The danger was identified as coming from the big eagle bird from which I would need to be protected. She took particular care in drawing the bomb-gadgets around the picture, behind which the secret treasures were hidden. I noted that only I was to have the key to reach these secrets safely. Joy was pressing home the point that her pictures hide (but also show) things, which could be dangerous with other people, but were safe for me to reach with the key. There still seemed to be an unconscious hope that I would interpret these bedroom secrets to her via her pictures.

Reading: I had made a sentence on the magnetic board: IT IS FUN FOR A NUN TO RUN IN THE SUN. As we talked about nuns, Joy said that she knew that they do not marry. She told me that they are not allowed boyfriends because "If one nun had a boyfriend, the others would want him too, and they might start fighting." Joy also knew that nuns do not have babies. I noted the implications of the play and the theme of competition for the same man (possibly alluding to Joy competing with her mother for my attention—and for father's) but I did not interpret.

Session 18 (Friday)

Joy played with coal, wanting to smear me with it. She wanted to fetch water to put with the coal so that she could make more mess. She asked me if I could get something so that she could draw on the blackboard. I agreed to get some chalks for next time.

Comment: It was difficult to recall the detail of this session, but the plea for a freer play-space was clearly repeated.

Monday (No Session)

Now Christmas was past, the arrangement was that I should see Joy four times week. This was the first week of the new arrangement.

Session 19 (Tuesday)

Joy started with the white chalks whilst I began writing a few words. Joy began crossing these out with the whole length of the chalk, which she scrubbed up and down making a lot of chalk dust. She went to fetch her mother's box of paper tissues, so that she could wipe the board. This produced more dust, which she started collecting in one corner of the board. She wanted "to make as much dust as possible....I will throw the dust into your eyes to make them itch so that I can watch you rubbing the itches in your eyes which I have made." She took a piece of coal, which she wrapped up with one of her mother's tissues, and said: "This is my baby, a coal-baby, and it is very useful.... We can rub out the board and we can rub all the white off." She experimented putting the coal into her mother's box of tissues, leaving quite a lot of coal dust inside the box. I felt it necessary to shake this out before I left. I was becoming increasingly distressed by Joy's clear need for a different room where she could more easily make mess as part of her play. I decided finally to discuss this with the mother as soon as an opportunity presented itself.

Reflection
The pressures to find a freer play-space had developed to an

unmistakable crescendo, and yet I was still avoiding action. But Joy persisted with her own need for something other than the nice polite "extra reading lessons" envisaged by her mother. With hindsight, I am struck by how strongly I was inhibited by my anxieties about seeing Joy without the constrictions for both of us represented by this parental setting. I had been protecting myself by not acting earlier.

Session 20 (Wednesday)

I didn't take the chalk with me for this session as it had been so distracting last time, and I was not sure how I could contain the use of the chalk without it spreading freely over the drawing-room. (I was now quite alarmed by Joy's determined messmaking, and yet again I had to witness her continued pleading for a more appropriate play-space.)

Joy began by taking more pieces of coal and rubbing the black into my hands. She asked me, just a little anxiously, whether the black would come off again. I reassured her that we could wash it off afterwards.

Attempts at reading were fruitless and I did not press further for this. During the session Joy told me that "coal-baby" was still all right—she had kept the "baby" behind the sofa in the drawing room since the day before. At the end she took me into her parents' bedroom, and through to their bathroom where she watched me washing my hands and "making everything all right again."

As I was leaving, I met Joy's mother in the passage. I told her about the need for a real play-room. She said that it would be quite all right for me to see Joy in the children's play-room downstairs, and if we wanted access to water we could use the cloakroom near the front door. (I wasn't all that happy with the cloakroom arrangement, even though it was separate from the adjoining lavatory.) The mother seemed keen to continue talking with me but I felt uneasy about this as I knew Joy always found it difficult to tolerate my contact with her mother. It could mean that her mother might take me away from her, just as her father and her two brothers seemed to have become mother's in some way. I expressed my concern about talking to her without Joy being there too. She took my point, a bit reluctantly I thought, and I left.

Reflection

Joy showed the need for continuity—with the coal-baby that had been hidden in the drawing-room since the day before. She also made it abundantly clear that we were going to need water as well as the freedom to make mess. At least, and at last, arrangements had now been made for us to use the play-room.

Thursday (No Session)

Joy's mother had tried to contact me, without success, to say that Joy had become ill suddenly during the night. As I had left before she telephoned I had come as usual. I was let in by the Nanny, who gave me a cup of tea. She explained that Joy had kept her mother up most of the night, having started running a temperature at 11:00 p.m. I wondered to myself if there could have been any connection between this and her feelings about me seeing her mother the day before. I also realized that it might reflect anxieties about the impending change from the comparative safety and parental control of the drawing-room to the play-room which, by comparison, seemed to present no controls at all.

Friday (No session)

I was telephoned at home to be told that Joy was still not well enough for me to see her. Then, because I no longer saw her on Mondays, and I could not change my arrangements to offer a make-up session, it was left that I would see her on Tuesday unless I heard otherwise.

Session 21 (Tuesday)

I was let in by the Nanny who told me that Joy was all right now.

This was our first introduction to the play-room and it was pretty chaotic. Joy was not prepared to attend to anything I said, or to anything remotely connected with reading. She pulled things out of the toy-box and played with these. She climbed around on the swing. She picked things up and hit me with them. She even climbed up on to the back of the chair and jumped on to me several times from behind. I tried to interpret to her what she was doing, saying that she was forcing me to control her. In the end I held her arms to prevent her being actually dangerous to me. When she shouted at me to let her go, I said: "I will let you go when you are ready to hold yourself." After testing me once or twice, to see if I meant this, I could feel that she had relaxed in my grip. Then I said: "I think that you are now ready to hold yourself, but if you are not

I will hold you again," and I gradually let go of her. She calmed down immediately.

Comment: This sequence came to be repeated several times during the time I saw Joy, and it always struck me that she would reward me with some particularly creative play, or work, when I had set limits to her otherwise uncontrolled behavior. I came to feel sure that this reflected the lack of limits in the home, to which the referring analyst had initially hinted.

When Joy settled down she turned her attention to the seat that she had chosen as hers. She told me straight away that I was not to look behind it, because she had "secrets hidden there." She launched into a discussion about mice, saying: "Mice are funny things, because they have big ears so that when one mouse is putting his nose into another mouse's ear you don't know whether he is feeding the other mouse or whether he is telling it secrets." At the end of the session Joy took from behind her chair one of her "secrets," which was something that she could chew. Having chewed this up she made an oblong shape, which she tried to push into one of my ears. I did not interpret this. She made a tiny little plasticine figure, which she said was me, and she put this inside a small plastic purse. I said she had made me into a baby and had put me into this purse, which was "like a baby bag." She accepted this without comment. At the very end of the session Joy picked up a toy car, which she tried to put into my mouth. Again I didn't interpret.

While Joy had been making her model in plasticine, I had made a plasticine figure of a man. I made him with a very obvious penis. (I was still trying to delay making a verbal reference to the differences between the sexes, which I felt to be preoccupying Joy.) She said to me, on seeing what I had made: "He shouldn't have three legs." I told her that she knew quite well really that it wasn't a third leg, but that it was what her brother Richard has and calls "a penis." (I did not know what word, if any, was used in the family for "penis" but clearly I could not delay any longer my moving beyond non-verbal and euphemistic references to it.) She looked puzzled and didn't seem to like the word. I began to lose courage so I offered her a baby-word, saying that if she didn't like the word "penis" perhaps she might prefer to call it a "winkle," adding that some people called it that instead. She laughed to herself, saying: "Winkle, twinkle, little star; how I wonder what you are!" and she pulled the penis off the figure. She later pulled various bits of plasticine apart and threw them about the room. She was making a great joke of it—laughing at the word "penis," at the penis itself, and at me.

Reflection

I thought that it was extraordinary how explicitly Joy had been illustrating her need for me to interpret her sexual curiosity and anxieties about it. She had put into my ear one of the chewed up secrets, which she had produced from behind her chair, as an acted-out version of what she had described earlier as going on with the mouse (his nose in another mouse's ear) which I had failed to take up at the time. It seemed that Joy was indicating that the absence of words for the vital questions and areas of anxiety was becoming an urgent matter for her as well as for me. She was almost forcing into my mouth the words for her secrets that she had so often pointed to.

At the end of the session I was feeling depressed by the amount of mess and "destruction" that seemed to have come out in the session. (I was also wondering whether it had really been all right to have been so direct with her.) But Joy then surprised me (as I was about to leave) by announcing: "Tomorrow we will do writing." She seemed to be saying "thank you" for this very different session.

Session 22 (Thursday)

Joy started with writing but this soon turned into play. She drew a large snake. Now, feeling somewhat encouraged by Joy's response to yesterday's session, I said quite directly that this was a penis and she replied with delight: "Yes, a great big dangerous penis." She drew two baby snakes beside the big one. I said perhaps these were Richard and Tom. She took the pen that she was using and began poking it into a hole she had made in some paper. I told her that she was pushing a penis into a baby-hole, because a part of her would like to have a penis like Richard and Tom. She accepted this and extended the idea to the wish to have a water-pistol. Richard used to have one and she loved shooting water at people and playing with his pistol. "I know what you would call it," she said, "you would call it a star." I told her that she had called it a "star" because the previous day I had suggested that she could call the penis a winkle, and she had then said "Winkle, twinkle, little star...." She continued to play around this theme. At one point she began pushing a pencil in and out of my hair, saying that she was washing my hair. I asked her what she was washing my hair with, was it with a water-pistol? "No, it is a penis .... A great big penis."

In the course of this play Joy made a plasticine "Daddy" and gave him a huge and unmistakable penis. She also made a "fat Mummy." She was happy with my comment that the Mummy was fat because the Daddy had given her a baby with his big penis. I added "One of your most precious secrets is that inside your own body you have what Mummies have, which one day (when you are grown up) will make it possible for you too to make a baby inside you." She smiled happily at me and announced: "Tomorrow we will read."

Reflection

I had at last begun to speak directly to Joy about the parts of the body, and she had responded with an equal directness. But, as if to check that she was really allowed to be direct, Joy half teased me by saying that she knew what I would call a penis: I would call it "a star." She may also have been reminding me what was echoing in herself "How I wonder what you are!"—referring to the penis. (There is of course an even more important question around here in Joy's wondering about her own sexual identity, particularly in the light of the preference given to boys in her family.) Joy then showed me that she is wondering about poking a penis into holes. I took this up and put it into words for her. She continued the session by playing at giving me a baby (washing my hair "with a great big penis") and she played at "Mummies and Daddies" with the plasticine.

Session 23 (Friday)

Joy seemed to be very much in control of the situation from the moment I arrived. There were some children playing outside the French window "having a tea party." Joy came in from the garden, closed the window, and made it quite clear to these other children that if they didn't go away she would draw the blinds down on them. She also waited until the Nanny had gone out of the room before settling down.

Joy wanted to start the session straight away with the blackboard. First she put out the capital letters. While she was sorting out the little letters, she hesitated over the difference between the little "h" and the little "n." I told her that the "h" had a tail but the "n" had had most of its tail cut off. She looked at me mischievously and said she knew what I meant: "The 'n' had had its penis cut off . . . cut off by a big snake." She added: "But not a man snake . . . a lady snake." Having finished with the letters, she asked me if I had remembered to bring some reading books.

We looked at the two books that I had and she chose the easier one. She read this without help from me except for the words "at" and "to." Apart from these words she read the whole book un-aided. (This was the first time that she had ever read anything except isolated words.) She had got within a few pages of the end when the time came for the end of the session. I told her that we could leave the rest of it until next time, but she asked if she could have extra time. I replied that she could have ten minutes more if her mother said she could, so she ran outside to ask. When she returned she finished the book in no time at all.

We still had some time left and Joy began playing with Richard's airgun. I told her that she was playing at having a penis. She accepted this and produced a box of beads. She began playing with these, putting them down the barrel of the airgun. I said that she was loading a penis with baby-seeds, and I added that I could use the airgun and the beads to show her how babies are made.

I took a teddy bear and "hid" this inside my holdall which I had continued to bring to each session. (This still contained all "her" things.) We put more "baby seeds" into the gun and we poked the gun into the bag. I said to her "We are now putting the baby seeds into the Mummy." She immediately added: "And then the Mummy becomes all fat and then the baby comes out from inside the Mummy." After a pause she said: "I think the baby is ready to come out now." I produced the teddy bear from inside the bag and gave it to her. She looked radiant.

After this I cleared up my things and Joy went into the kitchen to have her tea. However, as I was turning my car outside the house, she came out of the front door and made sure that she caught my eye to wave "good-bye."

Reflection
I felt that Joy and I had shared an important experience, which we would be able to build on in the future. I had at last begun to respond to her cues openly and directly, and there was a great sense of relief (for me as well as for her) from my having been able to put sexual issues into words. It seemed to follow that this "allowed" Joy to begin to attend to written words, to look at them, to recognize them, to say them aloud and in fact to reveal to me the extent to which she had already begun to learn how to read. In parallel with this I had let myself "read" what I had

written in my own notes, and I had let myself "see" and to begin to understand the implications of this for Joy.

What also seemed now to have become clear was that Joy had developed a resistance to looking. Although she could clearly see the sexual differences between herself and her brothers, nobody had helped her to understand these differences except in terms of some lack in herself. It had therefore become far more pressing for her to be helped to understand the hidden things about herself as a girl, for which she needed me to provide the words, than for her to be expected to understand those other words that her parents so much wanted her to be learning. Reading followed naturally after her own more urgent needs here were beginning to be attended to.

FOLLOW-UP

My detailed notes on this work with Joy ended with the last session given here, but the therapy went on. It was not the end of her problems but the beginning of a more direct way of dealing with them.

I continued to see Joy for another fifteen months. During this time her reading was handed back to the school and the parents, with whom it seemed more properly to belong, whilst I continued to offer a setting in which Joy could regress when she needed to. She moved up at school from "kindergarten" to "remove," but said that she liked seeing me "because with you I can be kindergarten when I feel that's what I want, and you don't mind that." She also began to discover that her capacity to read could bring attention just as her refusal to read had previously.

A lot of movement occurred in Joy's therapy around the birth of a daughter in my family. I eventually decided to mention this impending event to her because I had always been reliably there for her sessions, but now I might have to miss seeing her on the day of the birth. So I told Joy that my wife was expecting a baby and that it would be born fairly soon. However, I promised that I would telephone if I could not be there for her on the day.

Joy was able to work through her anxiety about this information during the remainder of the pregnancy and she was in the end able to accept, as a good event, the arrival of this baby as it did not take me away from her (as had happened with her mother after Tom's birth). In her fantasy, the baby became "her" baby and in her play she explored having the baby inside her, giving birth, feeding and looking after it. This helped to reinforce a positive value in her being a girl, and she began to enjoy the fact that women can do important things that men can't do. She was also pleased that I was so clearly delighted at having a daughter.

As Joy began to discover her growing ability in reading, my role of "reading teacher" became redundant. Her investment in my therapeutic role, however, remained.

The most crucial need that Joy continued to present was for help with her view of herself as a girl, not only different from her two brothers and her father but also so glaringly different in her mother's attitude to her. And it had been a female snake, not a male snake, that she spoke of as cutting off a penis (see session 23). Having felt so much less valued than her brothers, as though something might be missing in her, we can readily appreciate Joy's excitement and delight upon discovering that her femininity contained hidden mysteries ("secrets") which could give her a positive female identity. She had needed a relationship in which her sexuality could be both acknowledged and contained, and I believe that it helped that she was seeing a male therapist.

Joy's bed-wetting also showed a great improvement and finally disappeared altogether. She had decided to take over the management of this, with the help of an alarm clock (her own idea), and began getting herself up in the night. As with her reading, she discovered a pride in her own achievements.

DISCUSSION

I feel that there is much to be learned from this case. If Joy had been referred to a qualified therapist, she would presumably have been seen in a consulting-room away from her home; the mother would have been much less able to impose her presence upon the therapeutic relationship; there would have been facilities immediately to hand for Joy to use, including water and sand or other means of making mess; there would have been a play-space that allowed for greater freedom than the parents' drawing-room did; and the therapist would have been trained to recognize, and to act more promptly upon, the need for more direct interpretation. The therapy would, therefore, have started better and would have proceeded along expected classical lines.

Instead, we have an opportunity here to witness a child repeatedly giving active cues for me to respond to her most pressing needs. And, by following these leads (as I gradually developed the courage to respond to them), I eventually began to grapple with those key issues.

The naivete of this untrained approach highlights what Joy needed from a therapeutic relationship. Persistently, and with increasing clarity, the process of her unconscious search showed me where she needed to go. I had to learn to follow.

❖14❖

Countertransference and Interpretation[1]

What the analyst feels in the session may convey important diagnostic clues for understanding elusive communications from the patient. Ways have then to be found to make use of such clues. A detailed clinical example is given to illustrate some of the problems of interpreting from the countertransference and the therapeutic benefits that can emerge.

In this chapter I present a case that will illustrate more fully some of the concepts outlined in Chapter 11, in particular those of role responsiveness and projective identification as forms of unconscious communication. I shall give a detailed account of my work with a patient with whom these issues turned out to be crucial; and I will share with the reader some of my internal supervision, as I tried to distinguish what belonged to me (in what I was feeling) from what my responses to the patient might be indicating about her.

It is, of course, essential that we do not interpret just on the basis of what we are feeling. This is all the more important because some patients will actually welcome it, when it gratifies their passivity and their wish to be drawn into a state of merging with an analyst who appears to be all-knowing. Other patients, however, will experience it as omnipotent, intrusive, and persecutory.

A further problem with this patient was that of finding ways in which I could validly draw upon what I was feeling, without having her experience my interpretations as a repetition of her traumatic experiences. To that end I relied upon two safeguards in particular. First, I knew that I had to take note of my own warning to others:

Any . . . interpretation that is based upon interactive communication needs to be linked to some identifiable cues from the patient, that he or she can recognize when made aware of them. When we cannot identify these cues, this usually indicates that there are not yet sufficient grounds for an interpretation if it is arrived at solely through the therapist's responses to the patient. (page 86, this volume)

Second, I made regular use of trial identification with the patient before attempting to interpret. (I examine the issue of trial identification and interpretation in more detail in Chapter 19.)[2]

CLINICAL EXAMPLE

The patient (Miss A.) was thirty-five when she came to me for help with a severe agitated depression that had a very long history. At the time of the first sequence that I shall describe she had not yet committed herself to analysis. I was then seeing her twice a week. By the time of the second sequence she had been in five-times-a-week analysis for about a year. The analysis continued for three years after that.

Miss A. came to England in her early thirties, having lived her life until then in Scotland; the second child of rigid Presbyterian parents, she has an older brother and two younger sisters.

At the age of seventeen Miss A. was seriously injured after being knocked off her bicycle by a lorry. She was thought to have sustained some brain damage but the extent of this had never been clear. For most of the next ten years she had been in hospital.

About six months after the accident Miss A. had begun to develop agitated movement of her arms and legs. This soon became so severe that she could no longer walk. The cause of this agitation was assumed to be the supposed brain damage. Very soon she became confined to a wheel-chair, and within months she had also become doubly incontinent. Because of this her hospital management was relegated to a geriatric ward. There, still a teenager, she was shut away with elderly deteriorating patients; and there she remained until she was discharged ten years later.

While she was in hospital Miss A. had been treated by a psychiatrist who had persistently used a treatment method that he called "catharsis." (Although not psychoanalytically trained he had apparently called himself a psychoanalyst, and this made for considerable problems in the patient's transference to me when I later took her into analysis.) That cathartic treatment involved urging the patient to recall details of the accident using suggestion, hypnosis, and various "truth" drugs. After some of these sessions the attendant nurse was called to witness that Miss A. had shown "unmistakable pelvic movements" whilst unconscious. This was meant to prove the sexual origin of her conversion symptoms.

Ten years later, the agitation in the patient's legs was sufficiently controlled for her to recover her ability to walk. This recovery resulted from an experimentally intense course of ECT. She did not, however, lose the agitated movements of her arms, which meant that she still had to control the shaking of one hand by holding it in the other. This had been her condition until she came to me.

For much of the first year of my seeing Miss A., she would come to each session in a ritualistic way. The ritual included defecating before many of her sessions, and quite often again afterwards; and in each session, as if by contrast, she talked in a lifeless and boring way of the daily details of her many years in hospital.

My capacity for sustaining a spontaneous interest in this monotonous outpouring began to be sorely tried. I would find myself switching off, sometimes almost entirely. How then was I to go on seeing this patient who was beginning to bore me out of my mind? This became a crucial issue, requiring active and thorough self-examination.

I struggled with my unruly feelings towards this patient in every way I knew. Was this just personal countertransference? Did Miss A. represent some other relationship for me, from which I might be retreating into boredom as a defense? But I could not recognize anything that really confirmed this. Or was it simply that I did not like the patient? Had Winnicott been pointing to something like this in his paper "Hate in the Countertransference" (Winnicott 1958: Chapter 15)? Perhaps I just couldn't stand her! And yet I felt a real concern for her—basically I liked her. I therefore did not think that I had yet understood this response that was troubling me.

Gradually, however, I began to notice a striking similarity between how I was feeling towards this patient and how she described her father being with her. He had visited her in hospital, regularly twice a week, but he had merely listened to her complaints about the treatment of her. He never did anything to have this changed. It was as if he either did not care, or perhaps he could not cope with seeing his daughter in a geriatric ward—unable to walk and doubly incontinent. Perhaps he just switched off from the appalling facts of her life. (The mother was even more absent, having felt unable to see her daughter in hospital.)

I wondered how Miss A. might have related to this switched-off father. Perhaps she had retreated into a hopeless nonrelating, telling the details of day-to-day life in the hospital as a substitute for real relating. I then began to feel convinced that this was what she was doing with me. She was relating events to me; she was not really relating to me with anything of herself. She was also not expecting me to be emotionally engaged by her, or interested in her. In effect, therefore, I had virtually become an embodiment of the switched-off father. I now saw this as a clear example of unconscious role-responsiveness, the patient's contribution to this being her *nonrelating* to me in her sessions.

My next problem was to know how to use this insight interpretively. By monitoring each possible interpretation, through trial-identifying with the patient, I discounted the idea of making any direct reference to my feeling bored. It was easy to see that Miss A. would immediately have become defensive, feeling criticized, if I made any reference to this before I had found a clear context within which we might be able to look at this phenomenon together.

However, I soon realized that I could approach this from another angle. I could explore with her the way in which she was relating to me. It was then quite easy for me to say to her: "I am feeling puzzled about something.... I have noticed, for some time now, that you frequently speak to me as if you are not expecting me to be interested in what you are saying."

The patient remained silent. After a pause, I continued: "It has occurred to me that you may be relating here as you did to your father—at the time when he used to visit you in hospital. You became used to him not doing anything about what was happening to you. I think that you are also expecting me not to do anything with what you are telling *me*." The patient then came out of her silence and remarked upon other similarities between her father at that time and how she was experiencing me now. For instance, she also noticed that I was seeing her for an hour twice a week—just as her father had at visiting time.

After this confrontation the patient began to relate to me more as a person, and there were occasional glimpses of some kind of emotional relationship to me beginning to develop. I stopped feeling bored, and the patient became more committed to analytic treatment. Soon afterwards she asked me to take her into analysis; and, when I could, I began to see her five times a week.

During the first year of full analysis the patient continued to use her sessions to pour out details of her resentment to all those who had failed to help her in the past; and I was silently wondering how I too might be failing her in the present. Sometimes I would try to explore this with her but with little result. For much of the time the patient would revert to using me as a passive container for all that she was trying to get rid of in herself.

I was also aware of the patient's continued use of the toilet, before and after her sessions, which prompted me to think that she was using this to reenact what she had been doing in her sessions with me. Perhaps I was still a "toilet-analyst" into whom she was seeking to evacuate all that she wished to be relieved of.

However, the way in which I next found myself being disturbed by this patient took a more difficult and worrying form. I found myself quite regularly becoming aware of a slight sexual arousal in myself during her sessions; and this happened only with this particular patient. What was this about? I had to wonder whether I was in some way experiencing the patient transferentially, and responding to her as a sexual object: had my earlier boredom been a defense against this sexual arousal?

I was unable to find any confirmation of this. I could not sense within myself any sexual interest in this patient; nor did she remind me of anyone from whom I might be transferring a sexual significance to her. Nor was I convinced by an alternative supposition, that this sexual arousal was an avoidance of my previous boredom.

I began to wonder whether I was picking up some unconscious communication from the patient. Could my response to her be evidence of some projective identification? But, even if this were so, there was no obvious link between what she was saying and what I found myself feeling. What she was talking about was never in the slightest way related to sexual matters. Could it be that I was feeling what the patient was not allowing herself to feel?

I reviewed what I knew about the patient in this light. Then certain details of her history began to come back to me, and they could now be seen in a new way. For instance, I had heard so many details about her accident, and its aftermath, I had almost forgotten that the patient had not remained continuously in hospital from the time of the accident. She had actually recovered enough to return to work after only three months; and she had been back at work for a further three months before the agitated movements had led to her being readmitted to hospital. I then began to recall what precipitated her return to hospital. This had been an experience on holiday. She had met a man who had started petting her and then kissing her. She had never been kissed before; she was therefore very surprised when the man put his tongue into her mouth. She was disgusted by this and withdrew, feeling shocked.

When the patient got home from holiday she told her mother about this, wanting to know whether it was how people usually kiss—or was there something the matter with this man? Her mother had not helped with her anxiety or her curiosity. She had simply said "May God forgive you" (as if she herself could not) and had walked away from her daughter in disgust.

The patient had felt very let down by this dismissive response. She remembered feeling upset that her mother did not seem to see there was something about the experience which she needed to talk about. That same day she had found herself shaking all over. By the next day her shaking had become so bad that her parents had taken her to the hospital for investigation. Within the next two days she had become incapacitated to the point of no longer being able to stand or to walk. Her withdrawal from the world of sexuality became virtually complete when she subsequently found herself in a wheelchair, and later admitted to a geriatric ward.

A lot of things now began to make a new kind of sense. The patient had regressed from genital sexuality to anality; and she had been using the toilet for the evacuation of her anal excitement, as something still to be got rid of as disgusting. I now began to sense that she had also begun to use her relationship with me to get rid of her still disowned genital arousal—into me.

The technical problem was, once again, to see how to interpret from this unconscious level of communication. If I were to interpret too directly from my own feelings I would be behaving seductively. In effect I would be allowing myself to enact towards the patient a near-repetition of how the man on holiday had behaved towards her. Trial identification with the patient was essential here to clarify the technical issue of how *not* to interpret.

It now began to dawn on me that I had been missing an obvious clue. The patient was telling me about everything *except* about what she was feeling. And, in particular, she always spoke of herself as if she were entirely asexual.

I thus felt able to say to the patient: "One thing stands out, in what you have been telling me since you first came to me. You never speak of yourself as having any sexual awareness: at least, I have heard of only one exception to this—the kissing on holiday." Miss A. replied: "I never have any sexual feelings. I am probably afraid of them. In fact, it might be more true to say that I am terrified of feeling sexual, and I can't think why."

The patient told me more about the sequence which led up to

her return to hospital. The kissing incident, mentioned by her in passing at her initial consultation, was clearly central. For some reason the patient had become terrified. It was not just that she had felt disgusted by having a man's tongue in her mouth. There was something about her own feelings that had upset her.

The patient now began to realize that she had been excited by this sexual attention from a man, but she had feared that something terrible might follow from it. She at first thought that this might have been due to a fear of becoming pregnant. I therefore explored with her the effects of childhood fantasies, such as that of oral impregnation, as they might relate to this experience of sexual contact with a man. But something continued to be missing. Why should the patient have been so terrified?

At some stage the patient was telling me again how extremely upset she had been about the kissing incident on holiday. She added that she "could have died with shame" when her mother called upon God to forgive her. I found myself silently wondering about this casual remark. This phrase is a common one, but the patient may have been using the issue of shame to cover something else. The patient was linking her experience of feeling sexually aroused with the thought that she "could have died."

I returned to what I knew about the patient. In reality, she had very nearly died when she had been knocked off her bicycle. There was also another detail she had repeatedly included in her narrative of that event. She had always linked the accident with the fact that it happened on the very first occasion when she had ridden a bicycle with drop handlebars. She had asked her brother to turn the handles of her bicycle upside down to make it more like his.

We had previously explored this in terms of her wish to be like her brother. She had also tried to explain the accident in terms of her not having seen the lorry in time to swerve. She thought this had been because she was not used to having her head down rather than sitting more nearly upright as before.

I then started thinking again about my puzzling experience of sexual arousal, which I now felt sure was unconsciously being stirred in me through the patient's powerful disowning of this in herself. Had I been missing an element of sexual arousal in the patient at the time of the accident?

By this time I had been able to show the patient how she had been trying to eliminate from her life anything even remotely connected to her own sexual feelings: her not speaking of anything sexual in her sessions, the absence of any sexual interest throughout her life since the accident, and the use of the toilet as a way of trying to eliminate (outside of the consulting-room) any excitement that might be stirring in her.

Once again, using trial identification, I monitored what I thought of saying. If I were to be too direct with my hunch about her disowned sexuality, I would be putting ideas into her head and she could feel intruded upon. If I approached this too obliquely she could experience me as afraid of her sexuality.

I therefore said to her that we may have been missing something important about the accident. She had discovered that she felt terrified of feeling sexual, and she had responded to the kiss as to something terrifying. Could it be that she had come to see sexual feelings as in some way linked to her experience of a near-death?

What then gradually emerged, from this fresh wondering about the accident, was a recovery by the patient of a severely repressed memory. She recalled having discovered a quite new sensation from riding her cycle with the handlebars dropped. This position had brought her clitoris into contact with the saddle of her cycle. It then became apparent that, at the moment of her accident, she had been carried away by the discovery of a masturbatory excitement in this altered way of cycling. She had therefore experienced the accident as a terrifying result of having allowed herself to experience sexual stimulation. This had also established an unconscious link between sexuality and punishment, with near-death as a dreadful embodiment of that punishment.

The kiss now made sense in an entirely new way. The patient had not immediately associated this reexperiencing of sexual arousal with that earlier (but still repressed) experience. But, when her mother had responded punitively with her dismissive and critical remark, the unconscious link between sexual arousal and near-death was once again imminent. Her agitation since then had continued to express this associative link whilst also defending her from the risk of any further sexual encounter.

The patient was now able to tolerate having the "unmentionable" mentioned in her sessions. Much working through of this new insight was necessary and, of course, had to be worked through also in the transference.

One day, several months later, the patient reported that she had noticed something quite new. She no longer had to hold one hand in the other to stop it shaking. In fact the agitated movements had almost entirely stopped. This was after twenty years of constant agitation.

DISCUSSION

As well as the physical trauma that led to this patient being admitted to hospital, she had been further traumatized by her treatment there. As described by Miss A., this treatment appears to have been very invasive and was experienced as psychological rape. It was therefore not surprising that Miss A. had retreated behind her symptoms and her narrative, defending herself from any further closeness to a man.

By means of my unconscious role-responsiveness, during the early months of her treatment with me, I was able to get in touch with her fear of relating. Only then could Miss A. begin to engage with me in the analytic process.

The significance of what later emerged, when I sensed that Miss A. was ridding herself of her sexuality, can be better understood if we bear in mind that earlier treatment. From the patient's point of view, her psychiatrist had been seen as trying to force something sexual upon her—and even more persistently than the man who had kissed her. It was clear to me that this patient could not have tolerated any further interpretation of her repressed sexuality until she was ready for this. I therefore decided to wait.

I had little idea of how I would know when this patient was ready for sexual interpretation. Perhaps she would begin to have dreams with recognizable sexual content; or, maybe, she would begin to introduce her own more direct allusions to sexuality into her sessions. Neither of these things happened. Instead, however, I began to realize that the patient's disowned sexuality was beginning to be actively present in the session—*but not in her.* I was therefore able to arrive at the possibility of interpreting this to Miss A. with a timing that was specific to where she was in relation to her sexuality. This was now dynamically evident within the analytic relationship, whereas in the earlier treatment it had still been fiercely repressed.

I hope I have been able to illustrate the value of interpretations that arise from monitoring what the analyst is feeling in the presence of the patient. In addition, I have wanted to outline some of the silent dialogue within the analyst that constitutes internal supervision. We can often avoid giving premature interpretation by examining, from the patient's point of view, what we might say—before speaking.

Monitoring what I was feeling in the presence of this patient helped to alert me to what I might otherwise have missed. Later, by using trial identification with the patient, I became able to find ways of exploring the patient's contribution to what I was feeling, without traumatizing her by saying more directly how I got to my understanding. I believe that it was through working in this way that progress was achieved in this analysis that might otherwise have remained impossible. And when, eventually, I did formulate interpretations that were based upon my countertransference these were more than just an application of theory. In each case the impact on the patient was that of real discovery.[3]

✤ 15 ✤

The Experience of Trauma in the Transference[1]

It often happens that past trauma comes to be reexperienced within the analytic relationship. But for this to be effectively worked through, the patient needs to be able to recover an awareness of the difference between the objective present and the past that is spilling into the present. Sometimes the transference experience can be so like the past as to become in itself traumatic. Illustrations are given to highlight the implications for the patient of either too much incidental similarity in the transference relationship, or deliberate difference, as presented by the analyst.

SOME TERMS DEFINED

In *The Language of Psychoanalysis*, Laplanche and Pontalis describe *psychical trauma* as: "An event in the subject's life defined by its intensity, by the subject's incapacity to respond adequately to it, and by the upheaval and long-lasting effects that it brings about in the psychical organization" (1973: 465). However, not every experience of trauma is a specific event: it can be cumulative (Khan 1974: Chapter 3). *Silent trauma* (Hoffer 1952) refers to the effects of cumulative stress, whether in childhood or in the course of analytic therapy. This is often difficult to deal with as the causes are less clear than with more specific trauma.

In this chapter I also wish to emphasize the double nature of *transference*, and the overlap in this between past and present (see

Chapters 6–8). Klauber also says something similar: "The trans-ference illusion is not simply a false perception or a false belief, but the manifestation of the similarity of the subjective experience aroused by an event in the past and in the present" (Klauber et al. 1987: 7).

The patient's experience of the analytic relationship is certainly not all transference. There are often elements of objective reality that function as triggers for transference (Gill 1982; Langs 1978). This is part of what I understand Klauber to be referring to when he speaks of the need for "horizontal analysis" (of what is happen-ing in the here and now) alongside "vertical analysis" (the histori-cal approach to transference). And he says of this horizontal dimension in the analytic relationship: "What had been ex-perienced in the past was also being enacted in a relationship between two persons in the present" (Klauber et al. 1987: 26). This enactment in some measure involves the analyst as well as the patient.

Central to my argument in this chapter is the concept of *signal anxiety*. In defining this, Laplanche and Pontalis write: "The signal of anxiety is a reproduction in attenuated form of the anxiety-reaction originally experienced in a traumatic situation: it makes it possible for defensive operations to be set in motion" (1973: 422). Related to this, I believe it is also helpful, when considering the reexperiencing of trauma, to think in terms of *unconscious sets* (Matte Blanco 1975). This gives us a logic in terms of which we can understand how the mind unconsciously regis-ters particular elements of traumatic experience as belonging together—because they have previously been specifically experi-enced together. They thus come to be established as linked, timelessly and without exception. Matte Blanco also shows us that (to the unconscious) *the part can represent the whole* and that *past, present, and future are all the same.*[2] The result is that anything associated with a trauma can come to represent the trauma as a whole and may trigger signal anxiety, alerting the unconscious mind as if that trauma were about to be repeated. And if several things associated with a trauma again happen to occur together, there is a heightened sense of that trauma again being about to happen.

In order to embody these concepts, I shall give two clinical vignettes. In the first example we can see signal anxiety occurring in response to a set of associations that may still have been con-scious.

UNCONSCIOUS SETS IN THE MAKING

Example 15.1
A baby girl of one year was taken by her mother for inoculation, prior to going abroad. Before injecting the baby's thigh, the doctor asked the mother to pull up her baby's dress. Up to this point nothing unfamiliar was happening, except perhaps for the presence of this comparative stranger—the family doctor. However, after being shocked by the sudden pain of the injection, it was some months before this child was able to recover from the experience. It seemed to be for ever imminent. Most specifically, she demonstrated clear signal anxiety whenever her mother tried to change her clothes.

Any attempts by the mother to pull up the child's dress were reacted to by screaming. A similar response was evident upon removing other garments; the nearer to the lower half of her body the more intense was the reaction. Other people were trusted with more undressing of the child than the mother, but nobody was allowed to pull up her dress.

We can see in this example how various associations relating to the danger situation had been established around the original trauma. The most specific were the following: *the mother holding her baby on her lap* and *pulling up the dress.* Lesser associations could be identified too: *clothes near to the thigh* and *people like the mother.* It was noticeable that the father was trusted more than the mother, when the child was on his lap instead of hers. But when the child was on someone else's lap, the father became a source of anxiety if he then held out hands to help with any undressing.

Therefore, it would seem, there were different levels of association operating: a lap-person who was a woman being feared more than a lap-person who was a man, particularly if associated with trying to remove clothing. Also, a man holding out hands to help, if associated with trying to remove clothing, was feared more than a woman holding out hands to help.

In this example we can see that the trauma came to be associated with a set of principal elements: *being on a woman's lap; clothes being removed or lifted; a man holding out hands to do something.*

The mother, intuitively recognizing the associations to which her child was responding, found a way of dealing with this problem. She created differences by putting the child into a bath rather than try to undress her on her lap. She was then able to remove clothes that were wet rather than dry. Wet clothes had not been any part of the original trauma, so this difference enabled the child to accept a new way of being undressed even though *removing clothes* was still part of what the mother was doing. She was, therefore, not completely avoiding the feared experience but finding a way of facing it—as much of it as the child was yet able to tolerate. Gradually, the associative links became weaker and dry clothes could be removed too: first, if removed when sitting in an empty bath, and eventually whilst sitting on mother's lap.

UNCONSCIOUS SETS IN THE TRANSFERENCE

In my second example we can see evidence of signal anxiety in response to a set of associations that was more clearly unconscious.

Example 15.2
A male patient aged twenty-five sometimes experienced acute anxiety between sessions and over weekends. He sometimes had the fantasy that I had become ill or had died. If the telephone rang at such a time as this, he became afraid to answer it—as if this were bringing confirmation of his fantasy. What was happening in the transference?

It emerged that in his early teens this patient had begun to face his father with difficult feelings he had never previously shown so directly to him. During these confrontations he had begun to communicate much that had earlier seemed entirely taboo. For example, he had expressed extreme resentment at the emotional distance that had existed between them for all the remembered years prior to this, and anger at his father for preferring his younger sister.

In the course of several weeks with his father there were crucial changes taking place in their relationship. Most particularly, *the son was expressing difficult feelings* and *he was being listened to.* Previously he had imagined that he could never dare to confront his father in this way: "It would have killed him."

The son was now discovering, to his surprise, that it was actually safe to be this direct with his father. What was more, he discovered that he could also love his father as well as hate him. Then, one day when the patient was at school, the news was *telephoned* through to say that his father had suffered a pulmonary embolism and had died.

What had been happening in the transference could be better understood once we had identified some of the unconscious links to a past set of experiences. There were several similarities between the time before the father's death and what was happening in the patient's analysis: he was talking with a man whom he sometimes experienced as his father; in the transference he was confronting the analyst with his anger and his criticism; he was being listened to. These experiences were then followed by an absence—the analyst not being there. Because there had been a similar set of experiences associated with the father's death, absence at a critical time had come to be unconsciously equated with death. The telephone was therefore being feared as the means by which news of this death would reach the patient.

In the transference illusion, I had become (between sessions) the dead father. The patient's distress at his father's death, being reexperienced in these ways, could then be brought to sessions where I (who had not died) could help the patient with his feelings about my "death" (his father's death) during these times of absence. His mother, too distressed herself at the time, had not been able to help him in this way. For years, therefore, the patient had felt that only his father would have been able to understand how impossible his death had been for the patient to bear. But his father, being dead, could not be there to help him. So, it seemed as if no one would ever be able to understand, or to help him with, the effects of his father's death upon him and the timing of it.

DOUBLENESS IN THE TRANSFERENCE

We can see in this example a theme which runs throughout this chapter—that of the double nature of the transference. Clinical findings show that a patient needs to discover enough that is different in the analytic relationship to represent security, for it then to be possible for the patient to tolerate the reexperiencing of trauma in the transference. Elements of similarity in the analytic situation can then be used to represent traumatic experience as it was. Both dimensions are necessary, the similarity as well as the difference, for the analytic experience to be therapeutic.

Therefore, if the analyst is obtrusively different (from whichever key person in the patient's life), the patient is deflected from using the analyst in the transference to represent that particular object of intense or difficult feelings. But if there is too much similarity, the analytic experience threatens to be too nearly a repetition of earlier experiences, which could preclude recognizing the transference as transference. The analysis may then break down, the patient either leaving treatment for safety—or seeking refuge in renewed defenses against this further trauma now being reenacted in the analysis. Some similarity is necessary to sustain the transference-illusion (and this will always be found and used by the patient unless there are maneuvers by the therapist to prevent it) but sufficient difference is also necessary if the experience is not to become traumatic in itself.

I shall now give examples of both kinds of failure in analytic work with patients.

Example 15.3
A therapist in supervision with me confessed to feeling irritable with a patient who kept on complaining about her mother: she felt very identified with the mother of this complaining child. In her countertransference response to this patient she was becoming alienated from her patient's experience, due to a failure in empathy. The patient, therefore, could not get beyond feeling stuck in her therapy with a therapist who was being perceived as "just like" her irritable mother.

The problem relationship being complained of here was being brought directly into the therapy: it was not merely being talked about. However, until this was understood, the patient's transference experience had remained too real to be analyzed. The patient was once again in the presence of a mother-person who was failing to recognize the extent to which she had been shutting off from the patient's feelings. The traumatic degree of similarity between the therapist and the mother had continued to block this therapy.

The patient may, however, have been prompting her therapist (as with her mother) to recognize that she had a resistance to being truly in touch with what the patient was feeling. Therefore, the therapist had to restore a sufficient sense of difference between herself as therapist and herself as the transference-mother before the patient's experience of the transference could be analyzed. Antipathy had to give way to empathy. With this recovery the therapy could proceed more freely.

In the next example the therapist (at least manifestly) had seemed to be different from the patient's parents.

Example 15.4
A male patient came into analysis because he had come to realize that there was something he had never been able to deal with during his previous therapy: he still had difficulty with anger—his own and other people's. In his analysis it appeared that this patient's previous therapist had always been too nice to him for it to be possible to be angry with her. He reported the following interchange, which took place when he discussed the possibility of his going back into therapy with her. The patient had said: "I could never be *angry* with you." To this the therapist had

apparently replied: "Was there really so much to be angry about?" The patient now realized that his anger had regularly been deflected during that therapy, the therapist thus preventing him from using her analytically in any negative transference. The patient felt that his anger had been treated as unjustified—much as it had been by his parents. It had not been accepted as belonging to the transference.

In the subsequent analysis, it was possible to work through the anger because the analyst was able to tolerate being used by the patient to represent the mother or father, towards whom he still felt very angry, with the analyst surviving the experience of being battered with much that had remained unresolved from the patient's childhood: it was crucial that he could cope with direct expressions of anger. There was evidence to suggest that the previous therapist had been attempting to be a better parent, in trying to be someone who deserved gratitude rather than anger. Because of this, the therapist had unwittingly become traumatically like the patient's actual parents, who had likewise behaved as if there could be no valid occasion for this child to be angry with them. Analysis of the negative transference had therefore not been possible for this patient with that therapist.

From the viewpoint of the therapist, these two examples may seem to be quite different. But, when viewed from the perspective of a patient's unconscious perception, they are actually very similar.

The therapist in Example 15.3 had become too much like the patient's mother; but she was aware of being discomforted by the irritation that her patient was regularly evoking in her, and she was seeking help in supervision with this difficulty. The therapist in Example 15.4 seems to have made efforts to be actively different from the patient's parents, and the patient was consciously grateful to her until he recognized the unresolved problems with anger.

The point that I am trying to illustrate in Example 15.4 is that any attempt at "being the better parent" has the effect of deflecting, even seducing, a patient from using the analyst or therapist in a negative transference.

THE "AS IF" RELATIONSHIP

These two examples illustrate how important it is to preserve the "as if" quality of the analytic relationship. It is this illusion that allows a patient to reexperience in the transference whatever aspects of earlier relationships are being brought into the analysis, *as if* the analyst really were the original person to whom the patient is currently feeling related. Therefore, when trauma is being brought into the transference, it is the illusion of realness that accounts for the transference experience being so immediate. Paradoxically, if this is not to become traumatic too, there needs to be an adequate sense of safety in the analytic "holding" for it to be tolerable for the patient also to reexperience extremes of unsafety in the transference. Only thus can a patient find a viable security amidst the transference illusion of trauma reexperienced, without which there will not be room for the patient to "play" with that experience: an important part of working-through.

Of course, if a traumatic similarity is too pronounced, whether manifest or latent, there may be no analytic space within which to analyze this as transference. From the patient's viewpoint it is then no longer experienced as transference but as real repetition. This cannot be analyzed. It must first be remedied (if it can be) so that the potential space (Winnicott 1971: 100–10) of the analytic relationship is reestablished. Only thus can a patient "create" such transference as can at that moment be tolerated

If, however, a therapist insists on being experienced as different from the original object(s) (Example 15.4) there can be no analyzable transference in that area of relating. At best there can only be "charismatic cure," which evokes change by seduction. And, when that difference is based upon defensive behavior by the therapist, the repetition becomes more insidious—because it is concealed. It may then continue to be beyond the conscious awareness of either party, and so remain not dealt with.

SILENT TRAUMA

What we can also learn from the examples just given is that there are times when the analytic experience itself develops into trauma. This can happen when the patient senses something wrong in the analytic relationship that is not being dealt with, as in Example 15.3 where the therapist had been unempathic because of feeling ir-ritable; or when there is something more radically wrong that cannot readily be dealt with, as in Example 15.4 when the therapist was unable to accept her patient's angry feelings. In each of these cases, whilst the therapist's own behavior remained unattended to, the analytic process was being deflected or hindered. Patients do not always regard this kind of failure as traumatic, but the effects upon the analytic work can be longlasting. To this extent, there-

regard this as silent trauma, fitting the definition of trauma with which we started.

There are other cases where the patient becomes more obviously traumatized by the experience of therapy or analysis, but for reasons that are often not at all clear. In these cases, the childhood may not have been clearly traumatic, except perhaps cumulatively over a long period of time. The behavior of the analyst, likewise, may not be significantly traumatic in any of the ways so far described; and yet the patient becomes unable to work in the analysis.

I believe that this hold-up in an analysis can sometimes be provoked by aspects of the analytic setting, or by the analyst's way of working. For instance, if any particular style of analysis is rigidly adhered to, it may take much longer for the analyst to recognize when problems arising in an analysis are due to the patient's response to the analyst's way of working. Analysts, therefore, have to be careful that they do not hold too strongly to their own clinical style as there is a risk that they might rationalize as *technique* their own character traits, such as rigidity or having to be right; some patients may then find problems in their analysis which the analyst cannot see as directly related to him/herself. Thus, a patient's behavior may be due to desperation about a communication failure in the analysis, but it can be mistaken for resistance. It then becomes much harder for the patient to offer corrective cues (see Part One; Langs 1978). That is why it is important to have a technique that allows room for unconscious prompting by the patient. The possibility of movement in the analysis can then be restored.

I wish now to give two examples where patients were temporarily stuck in their analyses with me. In each case the problem turned out to be due to traumatic similarities between my way of working and the way that each patient had experienced a parent. Renewed progress became possible only when the reasons for stalemate had been recognized and dealt with. This required some flexibility in technique.

The first clinical sequence is from work with a patient early in my analytic career.

Example 15.5
A female patient, Mrs. G. as I shall call her, often used to complain about her parents, who had separated and divorced by the time she was seven:

she was an only child. She described her mother as someone who was distant and unresponsive, who thought she always knew best, and who frequently saw faults in others but never in herself. Her mother could not tolerate criticism, and if Mrs. G. ever made perceptive comments about her she would be accused of being out of her mind: "You must be crazy even to think such things of your own mother" would be a typical response. Her father was mostly absent from her life.

In her analysis Mrs. G. became very stuck. She would often lie silent and paralyzed. Interpretations, even if accepted, did not help. Instead, she came to feel persecuted by any attempt of mine to interpret; she experienced this as my trying to "see into her." She once remarked: "My mother used to say that she knew what I was thinking, and it often felt as if she did."

The patient increasingly came to see the analytic relationship as traumatically similar to her experience of her parents. For instance, her mother (like a caricature analyst) used not to answer personal questions; instead, she would often parry with other questions, or she would query the patient's motives in asking such questions of her. The father, by contrast, remained a shadowy presence in the background. Mrs. G. thus came to see me as just like these parents. This was very difficult to treat simply as transference as these parents had, in some respects, behaved much as I then used to think analytic technique required of me to behave.

For this patient, therefore, the analytic setting and the usual techniques of analysis had in *themselves* become a traumatic repetition of her childhood relationships. As a result she became unable to recognize the transference dimension within this context of sameness. She had to discover a sufficient difference between me and her parents before she could resume working analytically with me.

I shall not describe in any detail the prolonged period of analysis during which this problem was being worked out. In essence, I had to discover ways of being more flexible with the patient. For instance, when Mrs. G. asked me a personal question she used to defend herself from any rebuff by saying: "Of course, I know you won't answer that." Sometimes, to her surprise, I chose to give her a straight answer. Also, when she had accurately read what I was thinking or feeling, I would sometimes affirm her impression rather than fend it off.

In ways like these Mrs. G. was able to elicit responses from me that she had not been able to get from her parents, and which she likewise did not expect from an analyst. Naturally, I had to watch carefully for repercussions from such self-revelations, but the gains in the analysis clearly outweighed the occasional difficulties that arose from this openness.

Mrs. G. eventually became able to discover for herself the paradox of transference, becoming able to explore the recurring sense of sameness within a growing awareness of difference in the analytic relationship. Gradually she recovered from the paralyzing conviction that I was really just the same as her parents. She could then use me more freely in the transference *to represent* the relationship difficulties that she had had with each of her parents, which continued to be the paramount focus of the analytic work. This had not been deflected by the evidence of difference: it was this difference, in the end, that had made it possible to analyze the patient's transference experience.

In the following clinical sequence, I can illustrate something more of this discovery of difference.

Example 15.6
As an infant, Mr. H. had often been left to choke upon his own crying. He used then to experience his mother as having abandoned him. A phantasy[3] was subsequently developed whereby this abandonment had been seen as related to the intensity of his need for his mother's attention. The more intensely he needed this—the more sure he became that he would be abandoned.

Silences in the analysis were frequently experienced as abandonment or retaliation. This did not mean that I therefore felt this patient should be protected from all silences; but it was clear I should monitor the degree of anxiety that he could tolerate—and space my silences accordingly.

A technical problem here was that Mr. H. also expected me to be unable to tolerate the intensity of his anxiety and his anger. Therefore, if I responded too quickly to a silence I was seen as afraid of his violent reaction to my silences. Gradually, I came to realize that the transference experience sometimes became so total for Mr. H. that the therapeutic alliance was in jeopardy or seemed to be entirely absent.

Eventually, Mr. H. pointed me towards a way of beginning to deal with this problem. He began to complain that the lights in my room made his eyes ache. Would I please turn off the light in front of him during his sessions? I then recalled a discussion, with Dr. Martin James, of his paper "Premature Ego Development" (James 1960). In this discussion, Martin James had made the following statement: "All analysis has to be conducted within the omnipotence of the patient, which has to be challenged sensitively and very very cautiously." He later illustrated this by giving an example of a patient who needed him "to provide the basic sameness of the initial mothering, within the analytic situation, before the patient could tolerate change and thus begin to grow."

The impression I had of my patient's mother was that she had become prematurely unavailable to him. I, therefore, did not think there had been an adequate preparation for this sudden distance. There had been no "progressive failure to adapt" (Winnicott 1965: 87). Maybe, then, Mr. H. needed me to provide symbolic evidence of my basic sameness, as a thread of continuity by which he could hold on to me (as someone still controlled by him), whilst he was experiencing intensely violent feelings towards me, as towards the mother who had remained unresponsive to him even when he had been most needy.

For about six months I regularly turned off the offending light. In doing this I was responding to what I regarded as a need that should be met. I was not simply trying to placate the patient; rather, my flexibility here signified a difference from his parents that freed him sufficiently to rage at me in the transference—for instance, over my silences or my failures to understand. Inevitably, I sometimes forgot to turn off the light. I had then to pay for that too, and in no uncertain terms, the patient using that tangible failure to rage at me, as against failures in the early holding environment, in ways so well described by Winnicott (1958: 281; 1965: 258).

As we worked through what was required in this phase of the analysis, Mr. H. became able to relinquish his token of control. When he was ready, *he* told *me* one day that he could cope with the light being left on. This meant he could begin to use me as someone able to survive his rages. My separateness from him could then be more clearly established, and he became able to explore further his murderous attacks upon me in dreams and in his waking thoughts.

THE CORRECTIVE EMOTIONAL EXPERIENCE[4]

It is a seductive idea that what our patients might be needing, for recovery from past bad experience, is an analyst willing to provide opportunities for good experiences as a substitute for those that had been lacking in childhood. But things are not so easily changed in the internal world of the patient.

The analytic "good object" is not someone better than the

original object: it is someone who survives being treated as a "bad object." By surviving I mean neither collapsing under that experience nor retaliating because of it (see Winnicott 1971: 91).

Example 15.7
In Chapter 7 (this volume) I describe a patient, Mrs. B., who reached a point where she felt she could not possibly go on with her analysis unless I would let her hold my hand if the reliving of an early trauma became too unbearable. I will not go over the clinical sequence in full here; but, as the case illustrates my present argument most clearly, I shall draw out a few of its significant features and discuss it in a slightly different way.

At the age of eleven months Mrs. B. had been badly burned, and six months later her scars were operated on under a local anesthetic. In the course of her analysis, she began to experience me as the surgeon who had operated on her, and became utterly terrified of me. During that operation her mother, who was holding her hands, had fainted. In telling me that she might need to hold my hand, she was appealing to me to be available to her as a mother who would protect her from the transference experience of me as the surgeon.

Under pressure, and aware of the extremity of her early experience, I agreed that she might need this possibility. However, over the ensuing weekend I gave much thought to the implications for Mrs. B. if I offered myself to be a "better mother," and I realized that this could become a collusion with her wish to avoid the worst part of her experience by not facing it *as it was*.

The patient's subsequent use of me in the transference came to include the experience of not being physically held—after her mother had fainted. I then had to be able to face the impact of the patient's feelings from that time. And, eventually, Mrs. B. could find that I had survived in my own right; not by some manipulation of the clinical situation, nor by her continuing to protect me from what she experienced as the worst within herself. Only thus was I able to relieve her of the unconscious dread that nobody could ever bear to be in touch with her most intense feelings as they had been at the time of the original trauma.

As Winnicott says (1965: 258), this was something very different from the notion of cure by corrective emotional experience. A key distinction here is that the experience, unconsciously being looked for, was quite different from anything I could have prescribed for the patient. It was *she* who had found the analytic experience that was in the end most therapeutically effective. *It had not been provided for her*. What had been provided was a sufficient security in the analytic "holding" for her to bear to remember the early trauma of not having been held; and now, her remembering (by reexperiencing that trauma in the transference) could be in the presence of someone against whom she could safely rage—as at the mother who had become absent through fainting.

Much later in the analysis the patient reflected upon that time. She said of this: "What was so important was not just that you survived: *it was that you survived—but only just.*" It had therefore been vital to her that she had seen evidence of my being truly in touch with the intensity of her distress, for it had been that which had contributed to her mother's fainting. But it had also been essential that I had managed to find a way of staying with her most difficult feelings from that trauma—that I had not deflected these by trying to be the "better mother."

CONCLUSION

When we are treating a patient who has been traumatized, it is inevitable that the traumatic experience will eventually come to be represented in the transference—if we do not deflect this or prevent it. The reexperiencing of trauma then turns out to be a subtle blend of truth and illusion: it combines the realities both of the analytic situation and of the patient's internal world, where unconscious memories of trauma are still dynamically present. The resulting illusion, of the past and the present being powerfully experienced as the "same," is based upon an unconscious set of experiences that have remained timeless because in the unconscious there is no sense of time (Freud 1915: 187). A similar set of experiences in the present thus comes to represent the original trauma.

In learning to distinguish *the present* from *the past that spills into the present*, the patient has to find sufficient difference between the analytic relationship now and the situation as it had been at earlier times of trauma. This means that the analyst has to be careful not to be disturbingly similar to the patient's primary objects of the past; but it also turns out to be crucial that it is the patient who discovers the necessary difference—this should not be actively demonstrated by the analyst. Likewise, any similarity that may come to be used to represent trauma should also be found by the patient: in no way should this be consciously introduced by the analyst.

If the analytic process is not to be impeded or distorted, the analyst has to be careful not to influence or direct the patient. This means that he should not deliberately provide experience that is thought to be "good for the patient," as suggested by advocates of cure by emotional experience. But what *can* be provided is a security within the analytic relationship that allows the patient to feel understood, sensitively responded to, and analytically "held," by an analyst who can tolerate what is yet to come in the course of the analysis, without collapse or retaliation.

Therefore, when a patient is prompting the analyst to depart from classical technique, particularly if it is being rigidly adhered to, this need not always be seen as seductive or manipulative. The patient may be searching for a more viable balance between the similarities in the analytic relationship (that represent trauma) and a sufficient difference (that alone can provide the necessary security for the analysis to continue). It is the balance here that matters.

❖ 16 ❖

The Meeting of Needs in Psychoanalysis[1]

The process of change in psychoanalysis cannot be explained only in terms of the interpretive work of understanding unconscious content. The part played by the meeting of unmet needs is also taken into account–through the provision of a "second chance" to attend to the effects of trauma and to negotiate outstanding developmental tasks. The essential differences between this meeting of needs in psychoanalysis and any attempt at providing a "corrective emotional experience" are also considered.

INTRODUCTION

I have already indicated that in my view corrective emotional experience cannot be *provided* for a patient by the analyst or therapist. Here it is worth considering what patients *find* within the analytic encounter that can, of itself, be therapeutic. In particular I wish to draw attention to some of the many ways in which needs from childhood recur in the course of analysis or therapy. This representation of need by a patient is, I believe, unconsciously in the service of a continuing search for attention to needs that have remained unmet.

First, however, I wish to remind the reader of a distinction that I regard as diagnostically necessary in relation to the issue under discussion: between "libidinal demands," which cannot be gratified in any analytic psychotherapy without risking a serious disturbance of the analytic process, and "needs" which cannot be

273

frustrated without preventing growth. Winnicott (1965: Chapter 4) has called these latter "ego-needs"; in relation to later development, I have found it useful to think of them as "growth-needs" (see pp. 142–144; Winnicott 1965: 141).

Views on the concept of corrective emotional experience have been very polarized. The concept was originally proposed by Alexander (Alexander et al. 1946; Alexander 1954), and more recently by Moberly (1985). In the latter's view, corrective emotional experience represents essentially what is therapeutic in analysis. Many others, however, have been almost entirely dismissive of Alexander's concept, because the notion of an analyst actively choosing to play a role can now be seen to be antithetical to any truly analytic process. And this difference is most particularly evident when psychoanalysis is recognized as a process with its own dynamic and sense of direction—emerging from the unconscious of the patient.

At the time when Alexander was writing, however, it was pertinent for him to be drawing attention to the therapeutic value of the emotional experience of patients in analysis. For it was already becoming clear that patients do not benefit only from insight, nor was it the experience of transference, or of transference interpretation (as in Strachey 1934), that alone brought about lasting change. Beyond the experience of transference there is much else that affects the patient in the analytic relationship, for good or for ill. We still have much to learn about the effects upon patients of the analyst's presence and manner of interpreting.

It is my contention here that some key unmet needs of a patient may be met in the course of an analysis or psychotherapy. But I question any *deliberate* attempts at providing good experience for the patient. I believe that that can only deflect the analytic process: it does not enhance it.

CORRECTIVE EMOTIONAL EXPERIENCE

Taken out of context, the idea of the therapeutic factor in psychoanalysis being closely related to corrective emotional experience may seem attractive. We may also find Alexander's own description of his technique superficially quite appealing:

> the main *therapeutic* result of our work is the conclusion that, in order to be relieved of his neurotic ways of feeling and acting, the patient must undergo

new emotional experiences suited to undo the morbid effects of the emotional experiences of his earlier life. Other therapeutic factors—such as intellectual insight, abreaction, recollection of the past, etc. are all subordinated to this central therapeutic principle. (Alexander et al. 1946: 338)

He goes on to say that the therapist has a unique opportunity "to provide the patient with precisely that type of corrective experience which he needs for recovery." But we may feel rather cautious when he concludes: "It is a secondary question what technique is employed to bring it about" (Alexander et al. 1946: 338).

When we look more closely at this concept, and the technique advocated, we find that Alexander recommended the analyst should present the patient with deliberate provocations, selected on the basis of a "principle of contrast," the analyst consciously choosing to respond in ways that are opposite to the manner in which the parents had behaved (Alexander 1954). And he had previously given some examples to illustrate the kind of technique he has in mind:

If the therapist knows what kind of problem is emerging into consciousness, he will find it simple to elicit such reactions deliberately. He may, for example, praise a patient for therapeutic progress in order to bring out a latent guilt feeling about receiving the father's approval. Or he may express approval of a friend of the patient's in order to bring out latent jealousy. (Alexander et al. 1946: 83)

He does, however, admit that the response to such a provocation may be "of such intensity that it is difficult to control." And he goes on to say:

What is even more important, if the therapist has, in fact, deliberately provoked such a reaction, it may later be much more difficult to convince the patient that his reaction is really a repetition of an earlier pattern and not a quite natural reaction to the therapist's behavior. (Alexander et al. 1946: 83)

Alexander acknowledges here one of the problems with his proposed technique, but knowing the difficulty does not mean that an analysis of the transference can then be convincingly restored, especially when there has clearly been some manipulation of the patient by the analyst.

So, in thinking about a possible rehabilitation of the concept of corrective emotional experience, we have to remember that this term has a bad history. And it is questionable whether the concept can be altogether separated from its reputation.

SOME NEEDS OF CHILDHOOD MOST RELEVANT TO ANALYSIS

It is especially in relation to regression that analysts have to decide how to handle early emotional states, as these are represented within the analytic relationship. But it will be my thesis here that many of these early needs are met as a matter of course in the analyst's usual responses to a patient. They do not necessarily require any particular alteration of analytic technique so much as a sensitivity to the changing needs of the patient and an adequate responsiveness to them on the part of the analyst.

As background to a comparison between the needs of early life and needs expressed by patients, I wish to review some of the needs of infancy (and childhood) that are most likely to be represented at different stages of regression and progression in an analysis.

We know that an infant needs to be provided with warmth and security, in the presence of the mother and in her absence; needs to be securely held; needs to have the consistent care of a mother (or mother substitute) who has an empathic understanding of the infant's various indications of what is needed; needs to be fed but also to be given space in which to find the breast that feeds; needs a mother who can tolerate being "used" (in the preconcern phase of development) without the mother either collapsing or retaliating; needs a mother who can intuitively accept the infant's initially "omnipotent" control of her; needs a mother who can tolerate (at least) and even enjoy (without exploiting) the infant's capacity for an excited relationship to the breast—and (later) to her as a whole person; needs a mother who is at first able to be maximally available to her infant but who becomes progressively less available and less controlled by the infant's demands—as development makes possible a greater toleration of frustration; and, throughout, the infant needs to be able to discover his/her capacity to light up the mother's face—for here is to be found the fundamental basis of self-image and self-esteem.

As children grow, what they need of the mother (and father) continues to change. Manageable degrees of separation from the mother need to become an integral part of life. And, when triangular relationships are discovered, the feelings related to Oedipal development need also to be found to be manageable by the mother and father, and eventually by the child. Also, from the Oedipal phase onwards, children who are growing into an awareness of their sexuality need to feel that this can be affirmed by the parents, as valued and not to be exploited: they also need to discover that their sexuality can be accepted as healthy and manageable, and does not have to be ignored or treated as bad or dangerous. And at various stages, throughout childhood and particularly in adolescence, there needs to be the possibility of confrontation with a parent (or parents) able to survive the battering that can accompany a child's demonstration that it has an autonomous mind that is being tested in opposition to the parents' wishes (see Winnicott 1971: Chapter 11). Of course, there is much else that is needed in childhood but this sample will suffice for the purpose of the present discussion.

SOME PARALLELS IN THE ANALYTIC RELATIONSHIP

Omnipotent Control

Many patients need to be allowed to establish a provisional omnipotence over the analyst, in the early stages of an analysis, as a basis for primitive security; and this should be challenged only by degrees, and only as the patient becomes ready to relinquish this form of control over the analyst (see Example 15.6).

In practice what does this mean? If the analyst is going to be found by the patient as someone to be trusted, with the sometimes quite terrifying (because so intense) feelings that can accompany regression, the analyst needs to be able to maintain a delicate balance of being controlled by the patient without being rendered impotent. This balance will not be achieved if the analyst is too actively insistent upon preserving a separateness from the patient, nor will it be if the analyst remains either silently detached or too frequently intervening with interpretations. There has to be a time during which the patient can gradually "discover" the analyst in ways that belong to where the patient is in the emerging transference. Where, developmentally, the patient might be in this process is not always clear straight away.

Space

Patients, like infants and children of whatever age, need a sense of space which protects them from the experience of being impinged upon by the environment (or by the analyst). The analytic environment can then be discovered gradually as a patient becomes ready to find this and ready to be relating to it. (I return to this issue in

Chapter 20.) I therefore think it is presumptuous and intrusive when some analysts interpret *right from the start of an analysis* in terms of some assumed primitive transference. What is active so early in treatment is usually a more general transference to the *unknown* of the analyst or sometimes to the *known* of the analytic situation—particularly when there has been an earlier experience of therapy or analysis. It is only gradually, in my opinion, that more specific transferences begin to emerge.

In this respect, patients could be compared with a compass needle. Even a very faintly magnetized needle, if freely suspended, will eventually find its own magnetic North—thus revealing its potential for direction-seeking. But if some large object, with its own magnetic properties, is too near to the needle it will only point to that. Some analysts may disturb the emergence of more individual transferences by too quickly regarding themselves as the assumed focus of a patient's life and internal world.

The Need to be "Fed"

It is quite common for analysts to regard the analytic relationship as a feeding one, and for the patient's difficulties in feeding to become a focus for interpretation. The feeding here is symbolic and the "food" offered is in the form of interpretations. Very occasionally one hears of exceptions to this. For instance, Freud reports feeding one of his patients, the Rat Man (Freud 1909: 303), and sometimes one hears of an analyst giving food to an anorexic patient. But this is always a compromise which usually indicates some anxiety that what is being offered analytically may not be enough. And if the analyst takes over responsibility for some part of a patient's life this can be read by the patient as an implicit communication that the analyst may be prepared to take over other aspects of caregiving too. This can create considerable difficulties unless the analyst (like Winnicott) is prepared to meet the demands and expectations that are likely to be stimulated by such "acting in" by the analyst.[2]

It is also important that patients are left free to discover the analyst as "breast" or as "feeding mother" in their own time. In this respect the analyst needs to tolerate what Winnicott speaks of as the "period of hesitation" (Winnicott 1958: 53), allowing the patient to use the analyst as someone who is there to be found—a presence that is neither intrusively present nor traumatically absent to the patient. Thus the patient can begin to reach out, to find and to use the analyst in whatever way—with a timing that belongs to the patient's internal world and which corresponds to the patient's readiness to relate. If a mother presents her baby with the breast only when it suits her, regardless of the rhythm of the baby's needs, she may get a lifeless compliance. Similarly, if we ignore a patient's rhythm, the relationship to the analyst is in danger of being based upon compliance—the analyst being experienced as an impingement that threatens the patient's internal world and true self. What follows then can all too easily fall into further false-self relating. Often, this has been the patient's lifelong problem already. Therefore, when an analyst gets drawn into being too active, becoming a presence that impinges upon the patient, it is useful to review this interaction for the diagnostic clues that may be indicated. Sometimes, through the process of "unconscious role-responsiveness," the analyst may be being drawn into a reenactment of some central aspect of the patient's past experience. But this will not be recognized as such if the analyst's own style of working is already prone to be over-active and potentially impinging upon the patient.

The Need for Warmth and Security

A patient needs to feel securely held in an analysis, but the manner of this holding has to take into account the fact that the analyst is dealing with *the child within the adult*—not just a child—however regressed the patient may be.[3] So the analytic precept of abstinence continues to be crucially important here.

When, as we sometimes hear, an analyst rationalizes a physical holding of a patient, we cannot be sure how the patient will experience and interpret that holding. On the one hand, a literal holding will often, at some level, be experienced by the patient as sexual. On the other hand, it can become a collusive step by the analyst whereby the distinction between the symbolic and the concrete is confused. And, once this distinction has been lost, the analytic relationship may then become changed by the patient's hope that other gratifications may be granted, which sometimes are yearned for and fantasized. The patient may then be deprived of the analytic space which is so essential if there is to be a freedom to "play" with various aspects of relating without having to be anxious about these becoming realized between him/her and the analyst.

A patient feels secure through appropriate interpretation. Of this Winnicott wrote:

> A correct and well-timed interpretation in an analytic treatment gives a sense of being held physically that is more real (to the non-psychotic) than

> if a real holding or nursing had taken place. Understanding goes deeper
> and by understanding, shown by the use of language, the analyst holds
> physically in the past, that is, at the time of the need to be held, when love
> meant physical care and adaptation. (Winnicott 1988: 61–2)

This need of the child in the adult (for holding) has to be met, and
clinical experience repeatedly shows that, with very few exceptions,
it is more productive in the end for this need to be met analytically.
However, Winnicott's analysis of Margaret Little (see Note 2) might
be one of these exceptions.

Consistency and Firmness

Another way in which patients are able to discover a sense of being
secure is through the analyst being found to be consistent and
reliable. Here, too, deep needs from earliest infancy are met within
the analytic relationship. It is therefore of utmost importance to
the patient that the analyst keep to the arrangements made, with
as little change or interruption as possible, and for the analyst also
to work with the patient in ways that are consistent.

Paradoxically, a part of the consistency that a patient needs from
the analyst is that of *empathic responsiveness to changing needs*. This
may require the analyst sometimes to be adapting to the patient
rather than remaining rigidly the same. In this responsiveness the
analyst again parallels early mothering. For after a period of
omnipotent control of the analyst, a patient needs eventually to
find that a firmness is also available that can withstand testing—
even severe testing—and which can later be used for the purposes
of confrontation. The analyst can thus be found, after all, to be
separate from the patient.

Being Used by the Patient

When earlier differentiation has been disturbed, or has remained
incomplete, the patient has a second chance in an analysis to work
through the developmental tasks that belong to that process. But
this is only possible if the analyst's separateness can be gradually
discovered by the patient beyond the more regressed use of the
analyst during which he/she may have been experienced as merely
an extension of the patient.

This more primitive use of the analyst, as described by Winnicott
in his paper "The Use of an Object" (Winnicott 1971: Chapter 6),
is possible only when the analyst can tolerate the patient relating
in ways that belong to very early stages in life, in particular to the

stage that Winnicott (1958: 265) describes as "preruth" (ruthless = without concern). In this experience a patient unconsciously seeks to discover an object that can survive being "destroyed." But this typical sequence in analysis will be greatly disturbed, or even prevented, if the analyst is too quick to interpret this "destroying" of the analyst as sadistic—or as symptomatic of something in the patient to be eliminated—rather than to be lived with and worked through.

ASPECTS OF SELF-EXPERIENCE[4]

In the way of infants with mothers, so patients' views of themselves can be deeply affected by the way they feel the analyst relates to them. For this reason, I have come to think of those aspects of the psychoanalytic experience that have this effect upon patients as being related to self-experience. I therefore regard self-esteem and self-image as products of self-experience—*reflecting how others have related to the Self.* In analysis, therefore, we need to recognize the many ways in which analysts affect their patients' self-experience through their ways of interpreting and through the nature of their responses to the patients' communications.

Feelings Experienced as Manageable

A most important self-experience for many patients is when they discover that the analyst is able to accept the expression of difficult feelings as a communication. Feelings can then begin to lose the associations of a lifetime, either as feared or as something to be ashamed of. There are many occasions in analysis when patients discover, perhaps for the first time, that feelings—however intense—can be communicated and can be understood; they do not have to be repressed any more. There is much therapeutic gain for a patient when the analyst is seen to be surviving in the face of intense feelings that are being expressed by the patient, when previous figures in the patient's life had either collapsed or retaliated.

The value of the analyst's survival is most particularly impressive when he/she is working with projective identification as a communication from the patient. Feelings that could not previously be managed by the patient alone can then be found to have been communicated to the analyst, who is made to experience these feelings instead of the patient. Projective identification may unconsciously aim to get rid of unmanageable feelings but it also serves to get help with feelings. And, when that help is forthcoming in the analysis, a patient will have the experience of finding a response that had been looked for in the past but which had been significantly lacking from the key figures of childhood.

The Implications of Care

There are many other gains in self-experience for patients to be found in the analyst's attention and presence: of being a person who is taken seriously; who is listened to carefully; over whom the analyst takes trouble at many different levels of communication. Patients can sense when the analyst is in touch with what they are experiencing, and they can be deeply affected when they realize that they are with someone who is surviving what they are communicating, when they did not believe anyone could survive that, and much else. In all these respects patients have opportunities to discover fresh aspects of themselves, and a different self-image, reflected in the analyst's responses.

Through the experience of these parallels in the analytic relationship, a patient may also rediscover something of the experience of the mother's face as the first "mirror," in which the Self can be reflected as good, as lively and to be enjoyed.[5]

There is, however, a problem about change that is brought about through the patient's experience of the analytic relationship. Sometimes, an experience that may have seemed helpful to the patient turns out not to be lasting. The first of the following examples is intended to illustrate this problem.

CLINICAL EXAMPLES

It is Not Enough to be a "Better Parent"

Example 16.1
A female patient aged twenty-six (Miss J.), who had already been in therapy some years before, sought further help in analysis. She acknowledged that she had gained a lot from her former therapist—in fact, in that earlier therapy, Miss J. had been helped out of a prolonged depression and she had begun to find new purpose in life. For the most part, therefore, she had remained grateful to her therapist but she had since begun to feel that there was something important missing in that therapy.

It transpired that, some two years into the earlier therapy, Miss J. had continued to regard her life as meaningless. One day, her therapist had apparently said to her: "But there is a lot you could do with your life—you have a lot to give to others." Now, for someone who had felt starved of affirmation, such words had been like nectar and the patient had felt flattered; and Miss J. told me that she had been very moved by her therapist's affirmation of her. So, when her therapist later offered the further suggestion that she might feel more fulfilled if she had a job working with people, Miss J. felt strongly motivated to enquire into the possibility of a change in her career. She subsequently applied for social work training and, from then, her life had seemed to take on a new sense of direction. However, after that therapy had ended, this patient had found herself once again questioning the meaning of her life. Her depression had returned, which is why she had asked for analysis.

A significant dream
Early in her analysis with me Miss J. recounted a dream from her earlier therapy:

> "I had been projecting a photograph of grasses on to a screen. To my surprise and intense excitement this photograph appeared to be three-dimensional. I then fetched my mother to look at this but she could not see anything unusual about it. My sister, however, was able to see the real-life quality of the photograph; but she then rearranged the grasses and they began to fall to pieces. The picture which had been so remarkable became totally destroyed."

Miss J. further commented: "I awoke from that dream beside myself with anger."

The previous therapist had interpreted this dream as a projection of the hidden good in the patient, representing herself as having a value she had failed to own because it had not previously been adequately affirmed by others. The mother's not noticing and the sister's interference both seemed to be in character with Miss J.'s experience of them. The therapist's interpretation therefore had a great impact on the patient, and she had continued to regard this dream, and the work around it as a central gain in that therapy.

However, what of Miss J.'s later experience? She had finished the social work training and was beginning her new career, but she reported that she felt a fraud when seeing clients; she didn't know why. Even though her previous therapist had clearly helped her to feel more positively about herself, that benefit had not lasted. I therefore came to wonder whether it could have been that Miss J. had identified with a view of herself that seemed to have been accepted from an idealized therapist, which had however failed to become truly autonomous. If that were so, it might explain why the change in self-image had collapsed when Miss J. no longer had the continuing presence and influence of the person who had expressed a belief in her.[6]

Discussion. I think that this brief example raises some important issues. Providing a patient with an experience that was meant to be helpful often does not produce the therapeutic results that might be expected. Why does this attempt fail?

I think we get some clues here in the patient's much valued dream and the therapist's interpretation of it. What had previously been picked up from this had been the disowned (not recognized) good aspects of the patient that were seen in projection (the three-dimensional photograph), and that interpretation had its own validity. But what seems not to have been picked up then was the unconscious prompt to the therapist which can also be seen in that dream, for it represents the patient as having been interfered with. The thoughts of changing her career, which had been prompted by the therapist's interventions shortly before this dream, might unconsciously have been recognized as originating from just such an interference. In addition we find a reference to the now lifelike arrangement of grasses going to pieces. Perhaps this had been an unconscious metaphor for the false-self adjustment which was resulting from the patient fitting in with her therapist's suggestions. Later, when she was asking for analysis, Miss J. had consciously begun to recognize that something was going to pieces in herself.

The very fact that Miss J. felt a need to seek further analytic help grew out of her becoming aware of how precarious had been the adjustment in her self-esteem through the previous therapist's influence. It only later became clear that Miss J.'s earlier life had been dogged by many false-self adjustments, whereby she had offered changes in how she was, in an attempt to please (or placate) parents and significant others.

The previous therapist appeared to have offered herself as a "better parent." This could have seemed justified as a corrective emotional experience, using Alexander's "principle of contrast." But what was most important in the later analysis was found in the patient's discovery that she could eventually use me to represent precisely those ways in which she had been let down in the past, as with her parents and her sister. Feelings about those early relationships, which had continued to preoccupy her and which she had expected to remain unmanageable, could then be reexperienced and worked through in the transference relationship. In particular, Miss J. discovered that her explosive and previously repressed anger could be allowed expression in the analysis, and that this did not lead to either the collapse or the retaliation she had been accustomed to expect in her earlier relationships but led to a new vitality in herself and in her approach to life.

In the course of this analysis Miss J. also recovered a freedom to choose whether to continue with her new career or to do something different. She no longer had to please her therapist or her analyst.

A Different Use of Contrast

Example 16.2
Mrs. K., a woman in her early thirties, had come into analysis from a mental hospital. She had been briefly admitted there after the birth of her second child—a girl. Her first child was a boy.

I soon learned from Mrs. K. that she had been intensely jealous of her brother, born when she was two, and that her mother was then said to have become unable to cope with her. As a result, Mrs. K. had been lodged with her grandmother for a while, the family hoping that this would give her mother time to settle down with the new baby, her brother. When she returned home she had become very withdrawn, which was easier for her mother to manage. Inwardly she was feeling unwanted and very unhappy, but she no longer felt able to turn to her mother for help with that unhappiness.

It soon became evident that Mrs. K. had felt the birth of her second child to be a repetition of her own childhood experience. She had identified with the baby girl as representing herself just born. But, at another level, she also identified with her mother of that time—the mother who now had two children. (It transpired that her mother had suffered a post-puerperal depression after Mrs. K.'s birth.) So there was now a powerful spilling of the past into the present, and Mrs. K. felt as if she was about to lose her mother all over again. Her panic and withdrawal into hospital therefore had partly represented an "identification with aggressor," by means of which she was passing on to her new-born baby something of her own experience of desertion by *her* mother. Her baby, instead of herself, now became the one who lost a mother.

Mrs. K. began to feel some relief from gaining insight into this sequence around her daughter's birth, but the gains at first were limited because that insight continued to be split off from being experienced within the analytic relationship. However, when those conflicts did emerge in the transference, the patient's early experiences began to be reenacted most vividly within the analysis.

The Transference Neurosis

When we passed into the third year of her analysis, Mrs. K. became obsessively concerned with problems related to my waiting-room.

She felt shut out and excluded if she arrived early whilst I was seeing another patient. However, rather than protect herself from that distress by not coming so early she began to come earlier still. This also created a problem for me, as her presence in the waiting-room was felt by the patients before her to be intrusive. The end of sessions too became difficult, with Mrs. K. sometimes being extremely reluctant to leave.

It became clear that what was now emerging in the transference was her experience of me as the mother who was attending to another child. She became possessively jealous and very angry; she began to rage in her sessions that I should alter my schedule so that she could be protected from this distress; she should not have to be aware of other patients; and she complained that I was a bad analyst in not having more space between sessions, etc.

For several weeks it seemed as if I could not do anything right with Mrs. K. No interpretation from me seemed to make any difference. Whatever I said was dismissed, argued with or ignored; and if I did not speak—that was interpreted by the patient as rejection.

The crunch came soon after my summer holiday. Upon my return Mrs. K. was very withdrawn. When I wondered about this, she began to complain that she felt "shaky" and afraid that she might explode with what she was feeling inside. Then, in my second week back, Mrs. K. began to pour out her rage at me. "Be honest," she shouted, "you can't cope with me! No one can. Send me back to hospital. That's where I belong. All I'm good for is pills and electric shock treatment. Go on, ring up the hospital to come and fetch me. (*Pause.*) Why are you not saying anything?"

During this outburst I was aware of feeling intensely anxious. Was she right? Was it perhaps true that I could not manage her? But there were other clues. Her withdrawal after my absence reminded me of her return home after having been sent away to her grandmother. She had been two then and her brother had recently been born. She had been in analysis for two years and we had been working on this in relation to the waiting-room obsession. Nevertheless, to an almost delusional degree, *I had now become the mother of her as the two-year-old child.* And here she was bringing into the transference the feelings she'd had before, that her mother had not been able to manage, but this time she was able to give voice to them and to put them into words.

I eventually said to Mrs. K.: "You are reexperiencing feelings that belong to the time when your brother was born. You therefore expect me, as your mother, to prefer other patients to you. And you assume that I will not to be able to cope with what you are feeling. So, as with her, you expect me to send you away rather than to continue to be available to you for the needs that you are bringing to me."

Mrs. K. began to calm down, and she was able to leave at the end of the session without the difficulty that both she and I had anticipated.

Discussion: In this case we can see that it had not been enough for me merely to be the empathic analyst, or "better" parent, who could help the patient to understand her reactions around the birth of her new baby. Although that interpretive work had helped to relieve some of her immediate anxiety, through her beginning to understand this better, *she still had feelings within herself that no one had been able to manage*. Her mother had not been able to attend to her needs sufficiently after her brother was born, and eventually she had been sent to her grandmother. Also, when she had become so depressed after the birth of her second baby, her doctor had felt that she could not be managed at home. He too had sent her away, this time to hospital. Those same feelings had therefore continued to haunt her as if they might at any time explode and repeat the rejections of her childhood.

Mrs. K. could not be helped by any experience of simple contrast between her relationship to me, and the relationship she had had to her mother. Instead, she experienced me as the mother who had rejected her. She then felt justified in expressing towards me the repressed feelings that had so dominated her since that early time.

Far from providing this patient with an experience that was designed to *contrast* with what she had experienced in her childhood, Mrs. K. had found her own way to use me as if I were the *same* as her mother. Only then could she find a therapeutic difference in her experience with me that could help to bring about real and lasting change. The difference was that I could tolerate being treated as if I were the rejecting mother of her early life, and I could survive being subjected to those feelings that had first been associated with that early experience of rejection.

WHAT IS THERAPEUTIC IN ANALYSIS?[7]

The primary task of analysis is usually thought of as that of understanding unconscious conflict and unconscious phantasy. But, as I have already indicated, changes in self-image and self-esteem also reflect the quality of the analytic relationship. However, as Example 16.1 shows, what is therapeutic in analysis is not to be attained through any simple provision of better parenting. Patients often need to use the analyst for working through feelings about early experiences *as they had been* (see Examples 15.5 and 15.7). It is not enough simply to have experience in the analytic relationship that might seem to be "corrective."

Other therapeutic benefit, however, does often develop from a patient discovering within the analytic relationship a whole range of relating that allows for stages of development to be worked through afresh, and this often includes the meeting of needs that had been insufficiently met before. This relating ranges from merging to separation, from part-object relating to whole-object relating, from a preconcern use of the analyst to concerned relating, from hating to loving, etc. At times, the patient also needs the analyst to be capable of resonant empathy, whereby he or she can sense the patient's own most difficult or delicate feelings that are not always communicated solely in words. And when containment is needed, or confrontation, it is also important that the analyst can then respond with a firmness that can survive being tested.

An analyst is helped into these different ways of relating by the cues that emanate from a patient's unconscious search for what is necessary to meet unmet needs. By responding to these unconscious prompts, and not being afraid to follow them, an analyst can often get closer to what is appropriate for the patient at the different stages of an analysis. This can also lead to surprising results because what is most deeply needed by a patient, for recovery, is not always what the analyst might have expected.[8]

So, how does this fit in with the notion of "corrective emotional experience"? The main difference, in my opinion, is that *therapeutic experience in analysis is found by the patient—it is not provided.* Earlier bad experience may be repeated in the search for understanding, or for "mastery" of the anxieties related to it. But when better experience is also found in an analysis it is always important that this should have arisen spontaneously. It cannot become a matter of deliberate technique, for if it is in any way set up by the analyst it will be artificial and will eventually be experienced as false.

THE PAIN OF CONTRAST

Finally, I wish briefly to consider an issue related to any therapeutic experience that highlights a contrast between the present and the past—particularly when a patient's childhood has been significantly bad or depriving.

It is well known that patients can become resistant to receiving, or to holding on to, good experience in the analysis. This reaction is sometimes regarded as a "negative therapeutic reaction." Or it is interpreted in terms of envy, on the grounds that the analyst is assumed to have something that the patient lacks—the patient being thought of as preferring to attack this rather than to accept the benefit of it.

However, I believe that there is a further way of understanding this kind of reaction: I call it "the pain of contrast." A negative response to experience that might appear to be "good" seems to be an unconscious attempt by the patient to preserve childhood memories from comparison, particularly when there is a risk of exposing the depth of early deprivation or the true nature of damaging experience in childhood. Thus, when good experience is encountered, and is recognized as good, the shock to any defensively held view of childhood (as better than it was) can be very acute. Recognizing when a patient is reacting to the *pain of contrast* may help us to understand why experiences that might otherwise be thought of as good, and therefore as therapeutic for the patient, can lead some patients to be so resistant to them.

Example 16.3
A patient suddenly began crying bitterly during a session without any reason that I could identify. When eventually she was able to speak again she said: "It is your voice. You sounded kind." I still could not understand why this had so upset her, but a few minutes later she was able to add: "My most common childhood memory is of my parents being harsh with me, even cruel. I cannot ever remember them being kind."

It was with that patient I first recognized this type of reaction to good experience, and I have encountered many other examples of it since.

CONCLUSION

On the part of the analyst, the meeting of unmet needs in analysis is usually more incidental than deliberate. The analyst, by sticking to his/her analytic task, provides the patient with opportunities for finding what is needed—that is unconsciously looked for. The patient's experience of finding what is needed within the analytic relationship may then contribute deeply, but often silently and unseen, towards eventual therapeutic change. The part played by this kind of experience is often overlooked.

The meeting of needs *is not provided by the analyst*: it is in this fact that it is most singularly different from Alexander's own use of the corrective emotional experience. But the meeting of needs *can be found by the patient*. It then becomes possible for development and growth, which had been retarded through early environmental failure, to be resumed.

Whether or not Alexander's notion of the corrective emotional experience can be reclaimed from its history, the patient's unconscious search for necessary attention to unmet needs must be recognized as a valid process, and that search can become a powerful ally in the analytic endeavor.

AFTERTHOUGHT

Professional and Personal Needs in Analysis: Divergent Perspectives?

I have suggested in this chapter that a key therapeutic factor in analysis is to be found in the patient's experience of the analytic relationship itself. This raises some questions about training, and how students are taught to think about the analytic process, particularly if there is a notion that what had seemed right for the trainee will be right for all other patients too.

A significant difference between the treatment experience of students in analysis and that of other patients can result from the students being concurrently involved in learning how to become an analyst or therapist. I believe that this can have the effect of tilting the focus of the analytic experience too much towards the efficacy of words (being the most tangible tool of analysis), theoretical teaching adding a further emphasis upon words and upon traditional ways of thinking about the analytic encounter.

Of course, words do have a critical function in an analysis, in identifying unconscious conflict, tracing the evolution of false connections in the mind, clarifying what belongs to whom, and providing the relief of having put into words what could not be spoken about—helping to find sense where before there had been confusion and/or non-sense. So, words are indispensable in analysis, not least in helping patients to move beyond omnipotent ideas of communication towards something more realistic. Nevertheless, we need more than words.[9]

The traditional emphasis upon the work of interpretation can lead analysts to overlook an important aspect of a patient's emotional needs: it is not always enough to have needs described and explained analytically and "worked through" in the transference. But any idea of a fuller meeting of needs within the analytic relationship seems taboo in a training analysis, with the result that this level of experience is often withheld from patients.

Now, there is a natural tendency for students to be influenced by the standard thinking of their training body, on what counts as "real" analysis and what counts as "therapeutic." There is also likely to be an implicit reliance upon the authority of the analyst, students gradually coming to accept (as their own) much of the thinking and ways of working they have experienced in the analysis. And if the clinical style of the training analyst is accepted as therapeutic, even when it has been combative and sometimes even quite sadistic, it may be identified with and acted out against others as if this were a proper part of the analytic experience. (See also Chapter 20, Note 1.) There is much to be concerned about here.

What in particular may be overlooked by some students in analysis is that one of the most deeply therapeutic factors in an analysis is the extent to which a sensitive analyst parallels, in his/her way of working, the earliest relationship between a responsive mother and her infant: learning to follow the patient's cues, learning the patient's language, being open to correction by the patient when an essential communication is being missed, etc. Interpretations do not necessarily have their deepest effect because of their content: the principal function of interpretation for many patients is in indicating the degree to which the analyst has been following, is in touch with the patient, or (maybe) not really in touch.[10] *The experience of being understood is at least as important as the detail of any insight that is conveyed.* (Students are not, however, readily encouraged to feel that they can safely prompt the training analyst to think again when there has been some misunderstanding.)

I think that, at the extremes, there are two quite different models of analysis here—but most analysts are able to combine the merits of each in some kind of balance, including both a timely firmness and an appropriate responsiveness. One model seems to stress intellectual understanding: even though affect is acknowledged as strongly linked with the gaining of insight, a premium is often placed upon trying to get the patient to understand his/her unconscious communications "correctly." The other model more clearly acknowledges the value of a patient's emotional experience in the analysis, insight being *discovered with* the patient rather than being *given to* the patient.[11]

✤17✤

Unconscious Hope[1]

When behavior is recognized as communication this can often be seen to contain cues for the caregiving world, indicating unmet needs and an unconscious search for these to be more adequately attended to. This may be an important factor in the analytic process as well as in other walks of life.

INTRODUCTION

Having focused upon the meeting of needs in psychoanalysis in the previous chapter, I now wish to consider some of the ways in which these needs are indicated—in life as well as in analysis. I shall therefore be taking a fresh look at some familiar phenomena, developmental and clinical, in order to examine an aspect of these that seldom gets any attention. I shall be speaking of hope.[2] I am not thinking of hope that is conscious, nor of hope which is projected—when one person may "carry" hope on behalf of another (though I shall touch upon that); nor am I thinking of the unrealistic expectations sometimes attributed to the "transformational object" (Bollas 1987). I am suggesting that there may be an unconscious search (or hope) for what is needed to meet unmet needs; and that parents and analysts are given clues to what is needed in behavior, and even in some forms of defense or pathology.

I shall be focusing here upon hope that is essentially healthy, even if it may later be expressed through pathology. To that end I find it useful to make a distinction between different forms of unconscious communication. When communication is intentional even if unconscious, it has the active aim of reaching out to another person. By contrast, incidental communication (not knowingly intended) may also indicate unmet need, but more obliquely.

PRECURSORS OF HOPE

It is hard to tell at what point in development we can think of hope beginning to be established. I shall therefore begin with the meeting of basic needs, such as the infant's need for secure holding, for feeding, for being played with and enjoyed, and the over-all need that responses to the infant's cues should be in tune with these expressions of need.

When essential needs *are* met, and met with adequate consistency, an infant learns to expect that what is needed will continue to be provided by the mother or mother-substitute. It is this consistency which forms the basis for security, and for a developing expectation that good experience will be repeated and that bad experience will continue to be dealt with. It is on this basis that an infant begins to be hopeful, even if only preconsciously.

In this context I find it helpful to use the distinction described in Chapter 16, between needs and (libidinal) demands or wants. As development procceds we can see that the needs I shall be speaking of are not necessarily synonymous with libido. Here I am considering, in more detail, needs that are fundamental to growth which I think of as growth-needs.

To begin with, therefore, I am using unconscious hope to include any form of striving towards what is needed. When it is something as basic as food that is searched for we can speak of instinct. When an older child shows signs of needing fresh adaptation (in others) to changing needs, it is not so easy to explain the unconscious sureness with which this seems to be sought out or indicated. What is needed, at times of transition into a new phase of development, has not yet been experienced and yet it is indicated by means of unconscious cues to parents or to the caregiving world. We can also see much evidence of this in our clinical work.

Let me give an example to illustrate some of what I have been saying so far. Bion considers a hypothetical first feed, and suggests that the infant has a preconception of a breast before the breast is first encountered (Bion 1967b: 111–12). Winnicott, somewhat similarly, suggests that the infant (out of experienced need) "creates" an illusion of a breast (Winnicott 1958: 238-9; 1988: 100-5). When the mother places her actual breast within reach of the infant we notice the familiar rooting for the nipple, finding it, and eventually suckling. We can then postulate that the infant has found what it had been looking for, even though suckling at a breast had never been experienced before. Subsequently, because of that first feed, we can interpret the infant's repeated search for the breast (when hungry) as based increasingly upon experience.

Now, if we think of this sequence in terms of unconscious hope we could say the mother recognizes that her infant's first rooting for the nipple indicates an expectation of finding it. Later, based upon repeated experience, the infant may develop a sense of hope that what is needed can again be looked for and found: hope here lies in the infant's capacity to offer cues which is reinforced by another person's capacity to respond to them.

NEEDING AND WANTING

One could say that needing and wanting are synonymous during most of the first year of life. And yet there are signs of some distinction between them even in the newborn. For instance, when an infant is giving clear indications of hunger it does not always follow that the breast is immediately accepted when presented. The hunger (wanting food) is still evident; but sometimes there is also a recognizable need for something else. It may be, as Winnicott has suggested, that the infant needs "a period of hesitation" in which to rediscover the breast; or it may be that the breast has been invested by the infant with persecutory qualities, due to a prolonged delay in being available, or in being too quickly presented for feeding. The infant then needs the mother to understand this reluctance to feed, or to have an intuitive patience whilst her baby rediscovers a good breast, as it were "beyond" that which may have been experienced as bad and to be avoided. Through the mother's tolerance of this period of hesitation, the infant is better able to rediscover the breast subsequently as a good object, again able to nourish.

What makes the problem more difficult to resolve is when a mother is too anxious to see herself as a good object to her hungry infant. This can result in premature attempts at feeding. The offered breast may then be experienced as an impingement, fitting into a phantasy of the breast as an attacking object. The infant's need to be allowed time to rediscover the breast as a good object may be overlooked because the infant is also showing signs of wanting to be fed.

Sometimes there is a similar problem between the patient and analyst, often due to an experience which has led the patient to perceive the analyst as persecutory. This can dovetail with a need to use the analyst as a bad object, representing some past bad experience which has become dynamically present in the transference. There is then a need to work through unresolved feelings towards the earlier object-relationship that is now represented in this so-called "negative transference." (Incidentally, I question the unqualified description of this as "negative" because some very positive results are frequently achieved through working with this form of transference.)

The patient's unconscious hope here is, in my opinion, that the analyst will be better able to tolerate this use of him in the transference than the original object(s) had been. If this is the case, important steps can be achieved towards recovery from past traumatic experience. The patient may press the analyst to demonstrate his presence as a good object in order to ward off the bad experience that is being relived in the transference. But this is not in the patient's best interest. The wanting and the needing here are quite contrary (see Chapters 7 and 15).

UNCONSCIOUS HOPE EXPRESSED IN CHILD DEVELOPMENT

I find it interesting that at each stage of development we can see some evidence of what I am calling unconscious hope in a child's behavior which could alert the mother (or parents) that there is some fresh growth-need to be attended to. And it is then that we also see evidence of a growing distinction between needing and wanting. But, in each case, someone has to recognize behavior as a cue for what is needed. For instance:

1. The more mobile child begins to get into everything, wanting to explore and to gratify a widening curiosity about the world around. The fresh need then is for a greater alertness to the infant's safety. And, when this is lacking, behavior often follows that expresses the unmet need ever more clearly.

2. A child who is beginning to negotiate the difficult problem of facing even manageable degrees of frustration will often have tantrums. And when a child is in a tantrum it is all too apparent

that it is wanting something, desperately wanting it—even if it is only in order to have its own way. But what the child is also needing is something very different. The unconscious hope here, I would suggest, is for someone to provide a parental firmness that can help the child to cope with frustration that is age-appropriate. This firmness can only be effectively provided by a parent who has the confidence to bear the rage which may often follow when limits are set upon the child's demands (Casement 1969).

I believe that we could think of the sequence here as indicating an unconscious search for a framework that can provide a child with a much needed security. Without this the child develops a sense of an unstoppable rage within. This can only become tamed when it is experienced as manageable by another. If that containment by another person continues to be lacking, I do not think that the hope I am speaking of necessarily ceases to exist. The child continues to present parents (or others) with behavior that demonstrates the search for what is needed.

3. If a child finds one parent easy to get round, compared with the other who is trying to set limits, it is likely to take advantage of that split. But this is always a hollow triumph. Often, therefore, a child will press ever more noticeably for further gratification from the permissive parent, to a point where this may bring about more open discord between the parents over their different handling of the child. I think that we could see this as expressing an unconscious hope that such parents will eventually begin to see a need to get together on the issue of limit-setting. The child's need for containment may then begin to be attended to.

A brief example, taken from my work with Joy (Chapter 13), will illustrate what I am saying.

Example 17.1
Joy had been behaving in ways that clearly indicated *a need for firmness* handling her anger, which she had previously not been able to find. Her mother seemed to have indulged her when Joy was angry with her; her father had often been absent. Consequently, when Joy was with me, she would sometimes become almost uncontrollable—to the point where I had to be very firm in preventing her from scratching, kicking or biting, when she was angry with me for not letting her have her own way. Without my firmness she seemed to be quite unable to control herself.

I eventually had to hold Joy's wrists to control her, whilst she shouted: "Let go, let go!" (see Session 21). *I had to control her with my holding of her until she was ready to hold herself.*

Several times we went through a similar sequence, with the same kind of shift from destructive behavior to something positive. I believe that her difficult behavior had been expressing an unconscious hope that she might eventually find the holding that she needed, from someone able to survive her rages. Only thus was she able to experience herself as controllable, at first by someone else —then by herself.

In the analytic encounter, in different ways, we are presented with similar needs for firmness. We meet these differently, without having to provide a physical holding; but we still have to meet this challenge if the patient is going to feel securely held in the analytic relationship.

UNCONSCIOUS HOPE IN THE "ANTISOCIAL TENDENCY"

Unconscious hope is quite specifically expressed in predelinquent behavior, which Winnicott calls "the antisocial tendency." He says of this: "[It] *is not a diagnosis*. It does not compare directly with other diagnostic terms such as neurosis and psychosis. The antisocial tendency may be found in a normal individual, or in one that is neurotic or psychotic" (Winnicott 1958: 308). Later, he says: "The treatment of the antisocial tendency is not psychoanalysis but management, a going to meet and match the moment of hope" (Winnicott 1958: 309).

Older children, when their parents fail to respond to their prompting for them to be better parents, often extend the unconscious search for what is missing by behaving towards other parental figures in similar ways. Teachers, and sometimes the police, are then prompted to provide a firmness that has not yet been found within the family. But it is a caring firmness that is being looked for; and when that is still not forthcoming, the consequent antisocial behavior may become more truly delinquent. I believe that this shift into delinquency, when it occurs, is often motivated by a sense of let-down that follows from the unconscious hope for containment (or understanding) not having been met. Subsequently, the secondary gains from delinquency may eventually mask, even obliterate, the original search that had remained unfulfilled. But I do not think the hope then ceases to exist; instead it enters the repressed unconscious, and becomes evident through more oblique derivative communication.

When a child has been deprived of some necessary provision,

and has missed this for longer than can be managed by internal resources alone, the child may sometimes go in search of what is missing—symbolically—through stealing—*when hopeful* (Winnicott 1958: 310).

Example 17.2
When I was a probation officer, I came to see the parents of a ten-year-old girl (Mary) who had been picked up for shoplifting. I was told that this child had taken a number of objects from several different shops, before she was noticed. The police had been called and she was taken to her home, whereupon her father had been called in to be present whilst she was being questioned. Her father, I discovered, was a policeman.

Thinking about this now, we can readily imagine some of what Mary may have wanted. She may have felt that she wanted what she had stolen; she may have wanted to punish her father for spending time more readily with her two older brothers than with her; and she may have unconsciously wished him to be a policeman to her, an externalized superego. But *what Mary needed was a father who could also be a father to her.* It was therefore important to help this couple recognize her unmet need, particularly as the father's first response had been to lose his temper and to shout: "I never thought that we would have a thief in our own family."

It was, of course, necessary to work with this family for some time for Mary's need to be convincingly met. Fortunately, the father was later able to see that he had been showing preferential treatment to the boys, and he began to find time in which Mary could also be special to him. So, she found what she had been unconsciously looking for—and she did not need to steal again.

In this example, the unconscious hope (a search for a father for herself) was not disappointed. Sometimes, however, such predelinquent behavior is not recognized for what it is—an unconscious search for something missing—and the moment of hope is wasted (Winnicott 1958: 309).

OTHER MANIFESTATIONS OF UNCONSCIOUS HOPE

It can be a useful exercise to think of some examples of behavior difficulty, in child development or later, and to wonder about these in order to distinguish what the different elements of unconscious communication may have been in each. For instance:

1. In the familiar phenomenon of an older child's bed-wetting when a new baby is born, we can readily recognize a wish for mother's attention, and probably also a wish to be allowed to be the baby again. Equally we can imagine unconscious phantasies, wishing to attack the mother with urine and probably the baby too; or we may postulate a wish to create a substitute warmth in this experience of wetting, perhaps to replace the mother's warmth, and so on. But if we think more specifically of what is *needed* here by the older child we may be able to discern an element also of unconscious hope: a hope that the mother might understand and attend to her older child's jealousy and distress. If the mother is then able to respond sensitively to that need, it often happens that the bed-wetting (as a communication that has achieved its aim) may begin to be less frequent, until it stops.

2. If we think of the seductive behavior of an Oedipal child we can readily see a wish to get some special attention from the opposite-sex parent. We can also imagine various unconscious phantasies to do with getting rid of the rival parent and an unconscious wish to replace him/her. But it is also useful to consider what the unconscious hope may be. The growth-need is for the child's budding sexuality to be affirmed: not to be ignored, run away from, or exploited.

UNCONSCIOUS HOPE IN THE CLINICAL SETTING

When there has been some degree of failure in meeting the growth-needs, we are likely to find these re-presented in the clinical setting.

For instance, when there has been some failure in meeting the needs of Oedipal development, it is important that the unconscious hope should be recognized as it comes to be expressed in the analytic relationship. Typically, a patient may demonstrate a continuing need for sexuality to be affirmed—to be treated as a positive force in the patient, not as bad or overwhelmingly strong, nor as non-existent. It is therefore important that analysts can interpret a patient's sexuality, when this becomes evident within the analytic relationship, in ways that indicate an awareness of the unmet needs. It is not helpful to interpret evidence of a patient's sexuality in the session merely as being seductive—as if this were bad or as if the patient should not be expressing this sexuality towards the analyst. It is often more productive if such behavior can be understood in terms of a search for affirmation and containment. And, once again, it is essential that we do not confuse needing with wanting here. The patient might want to seduce the analyst; but the unconscious need and hope will be to find an analyst who is not afraid of this seductiveness, and who is able to contain it by understanding why this behavior is being presented in the analysis by the patient.

I now wish to give some brief references to the various ways in which I think that patients contribute hopefully towards finding the clinical setting that is needed. And I find it uncanny, sometimes, that patients who have had no experience of analysis or psychotherapy nevertheless seem to have a sense of what is necessary for them to progress therapeutically. I felt this most particularly during my work with Joy (Chapter 13).

For example, when a patient is using previous changes in arrangements as a basis for expecting further exceptions, this may also be a tacit prompt for more firmness in these arrangements: frequently, we will discover that a caring firmness had been absent in childhood. Similarly, any deviation by the analyst from the usual professional boundaries is often taken advantage of—the patient wanting more; but this too may be an unconscious cue that the analytic boundaries need to be more clearly established and maintained. Sometimes, I believe, we can see both a wish to exploit a weakness in the professional setting and a hope that the issues pointed to in this way will be better attended to. These unconscious prompts are, I think, essentially hopeful.

THE UNCONSCIOUS SEARCH FOR NEW SOLUTIONS

In Repetition Compulsion

A typical expression of unconscious hope may be found in repetition compulsion, when unresolved conflicts continue to generate attempts at solutions which do not really work. Once a genuine solution is found then the compulsion to repeat will usually diminish and eventually stop.

In Role-Responsiveness

When analysts allow themselves to be responsive to their patients' unconscious cues, they will be prompted into becoming different with each patient (Sandler 1976; 1983). What can follow from this responsiveness is sometimes strangely specific to the patient's life experience. Occasionally, the analyst may find himself being prodded into behaving in some way that is similar to a significant person who had let the patient down in earlier life. He will then be used to represent an element of parental failure from the past, becoming the object of whatever feelings had been associated with that earlier failure (see Chapters 15 and 16). It is thus within the immediacy of this experience in the transference relationship, that the patient has a further opportunity to work through feelings that had been unmanageable in the past and therefore repressed.

Example 17.3

I was once seeing a patient in twice-a-week psychotherapy. (I will call him David.) His sessions had originally been on Mondays and Thursdays, but the gap between these had become an obstacle to continuity in the therapy. As David was not able to come more frequently I had suggested that he might come on consecutive days, and this had resulted in a quite new shift in his therapy. He was able to use the first of each pair of sessions more freely because of there being a session on the following day; and the bigger gap in the week was less of a problem than might have been expected.

It so happened that David is a twin. He and his brother had been breastfed until they were about three months old. Then the mother had become suddenly ill and had to be admitted to hospital. The twins went too but had to be fed by a number of different nurses, the mother being unable to attend to them for about three days. Upon her recovery it was found that breast feeding could not be reestablished. The "older" twin would then not allow anyone else but the mother to attend to him. David, however, had become compliant—allowing himself to be fed by anyone available. This compliance was not recognized as a signal of his distress but had been mistaken for contentment.

About six months after the sessions had been established on consecutive days, I was having difficulty in finding a time for a new analytic patient. I am sure that it was no accident that I first thought of asking my most obliging patient (David) to change one session to another day, with one day between sessions, and he readily agreed. However, the next week (for the first time since I had started seeing him) David came to a session two minutes late. Before that he had always been either early or exactly on time.

When I thought about this quite unusual lateness, and the silence with which he began the session, I began to realize that this was a whispered protest against the change in days—probably representing a rage that David did not feel able to express more directly. Fortunately, I was able to recognize this protest and to attend to it. I was able to let him keep to his usual session-times instead of persisting with my request for this further change.

What followed then was David becoming able to be more force-ful, with a fresh belief that protest could be heard. And, as part of that new protesting, I was soon to be subjected to the feelings of rage that originally belonged to the mother, who (like me) had exploited this twin's readiness to fit in with what was expected of him.

In this experience with me, David was able to have attention given to his very early need. His mother had not recognized his distress beneath the defense of compliance; she was therefore not able to attend to that distress. But I believe there had remained an unconscious hope that, in some way, the unmet needs (which remained concealed beneath his compliance but were also indi-cated by it) could one day be recognized and be met. And that repeating pattern of compliance, so often exploited by others, had been an expression of that continued striving for attention to be given to the distress that had been overlooked before.

It is here too that an essential and therapeutic difference can be discovered by the patient, in that the analyst is able to recover from an element of his own failure in the analytic relationship. But that recovery cannot occur unless the analyst is willing to respond to the patient's corrective cues: it is this readiness to rethink, when things have gone wrong, that has often been missing in the patient's past relationships—particularly when parents had too often believed that they were in the right.

In this unconscious role-responsiveness we find something of what Winnicott had been referring to when he wrote of the patient "using the analyst's failures" (Winnicott 1958: Chapter 22; 1965: Chapter 23), and here he invokes a notion very close to that of unconscious hope. In another passage he writes of a defense against specific environmental failure by a *freezing of the failure situation*.

> Along with this [freezing] goes an unconscious assumption (which can become a conscious hope) that opportunity will occur at a later date for a renewed experience in which the failure situation will be able to be unfrozen and reexperienced, with the individual in a regressed state, in an environ-ment that is making adequate adaptation. (Winnicott 1958: 281)

The patient uses the analyst's failure in the here-and-now to repre-sent past failures in parental care. And when the analytic relation-ship feels secure enough, the patient rages against the analyst and so acts upon his feelings more fully than had been possible in relation to the original mother or mother-substitute, who had failed the patient in ways now being reenacted in the transference relationship. This is very different from any question of trying to be the better parent. If anything better *is* to be found in this, it grows out of the analyst's capacity to tolerate the feelings which come to be directed at him/her, when the analyst is used to represent the earlier *bad* experience. The original parent(s) had usually been unable to deal with those feelings even if only because they could not be spoken about. (Often, an important factor of early trauma had been that it could not be put into words.)

In Projective Identification

Another powerful way in which unconscious hope may be expressed clinically is through projective identification—when patients seek to get rid of, into the analyst, aspects of the self (or states of feeling) that cannot be managed alone. The unconscious hope here is that the analyst will be able to manage that which is being projected into him/her which patients cannot manage in themselves without help.

When projective identification is understood in this way it is clear why it is so important that analysts should be able to manage within themselves whatever is being "put into" them, and to do so with a sensitivity to the patient's need to seek help in this way.

THE PROJECTION OF HOPE AND DESPAIR

An important example of communication by means of projective identification is encountered when a patient presents in a state of despair. Superficially, it might look as if despair were the ultimate negation of hope. But I believe that we can see evidence of unconscious hope here in two forms.

More commonly recognized is the projection of a patient's hope into the analyst, the patient not being able to preserve that hope alongside the experience of despair. At such a moment we might say that the analyst has to carry the hope for the patient until such time as it can be accepted by the patient as his/her own. A common response, outside of analysis and psychotherapy, is to try reassuring the despairing person with sayings such as: "There will be light at the end of the tunnel." A more analytical response would be to say something like: "While you are feeling so much despair, I think you are needing me to hold on to the hope that you cannot feel in yourself just now."

Though that interpretation may be adequate (as far as it goes) it is likely to leave the patient still alone with the despair. If the other person can only feel the patient's projected hope, and not the despair, it could seem as if that despair cannot be tolerated. I have often noticed how important it is for a despairing patient to be able to communicate the despair directly—so that the analyst or therapist feels it too. What is then received by the analyst is the patient's own intolerable experience, and the patient is no longer so alone with it. This suggests that the analyst should be capable of a benign split within himself; being able to take in and experience the patient's despair, and yet being able still to see the possibility of not having to give up under the weight of it (see Example 15.7).

The nature of unconscious hope here is subtle and important. Obviously, the patient is not conscious of the hope that is projected into the analyst. Also, when hope gives way to despair it becomes repressed. I wish to suggest that it is this unconscious and repressed hope that now shows itself in the form of despair. The unmet need is then for someone else to be available to the patient, with the capacity to be truly in touch with what the patient is feeling until things feel better. Often, in the patient's past, there has been a traumatic absence of this emotional holding. It is then in the analytic relationship that it will again be searched for.

THREATS OF SUICIDE

I believe that, almost always, when a person talks of suicide there is a double message. One part of this is saying that life (as it is) has become unbearable; the other part is appealing for someone to be available to help change it. There may be an element of unconscious hope even in threats of suicide. It is therefore important that there is someone available to respond to such a plea, however deeply it may be hidden, in order to do whatever can be done towards changing what can be changed. One change could be that someone is prepared to be in touch with the unbearable state of suicidal desperation. It is therefore a most dangerous, even though popular, assumption that the person who speaks about suicide will not die of suicide. This view just encourages people to become unresponsive to the unconscious hope that may be in the suicide's plea for some form of help that has not yet been forthcoming. If no one responds to that remaining element of hope, then a successful attempt at suicide may follow—a final act of despair and retaliation against a world seen as uncaring.

THE COMMUNICATION OF HURT

I believe that we can sometimes see evidence of unconscious hope in hurtful behavior. A hurt child will often behave hurtfully to others, identifying with some past or recent aggressor and attempting to pass on to others the hurt received. The unconscious hope here may simply be to get rid of that hurt: sometimes, however, it may be to receive help with it. When the unconscious meaning of hurtful behavior is understood in this way, it becomes easier to attend to the child's experience of hurt, and the behavior does not have to be regarded simply as bad let alone as sadistic. However, when the needed attention to the hurt is not forthcoming, the earlier search for help may give way to the secondary gains of some pleasure discovered in hurting. This, I believe, is a contributory factor in the etiology of sadism that is often overlooked. When the unconscious hope in hurtful behavior is disappointed it may be repressed, and subsequently be in evidence only through the unconscious derivative of sadistic behavior. When this becomes sexualized, it is yet further removed from the unconscious hope that may initially have been expressed in such behavior. As with delinquency, when the needs that are indicated in hurtful behavior continue to be unmet, there is a tendency to retaliate against those who have failed to meet that need. The hurt child then punishes those who fail him/her and the attachment to the secondary gains in sadistic behavior may become addictive.

CONCLUSION

I would like to summarize the factors that I believe to indicate the presence of unconscious hope. There is usually some problematic behavior (or attitude) that attracts the attention of others; the behavior is usually non-satisfying in terms of what is really needed; it frequently becomes more noticeable, and often more difficult for others to manage, until what is needed is recognized and appropriately responded to. When this form of communication is interpreted in terms of that unconscious search, or as evidence of some unconscious hope of finding what is needed, patients often indicate a sense of having been understood—and what is unconsciously being looked for may begin to be found.

Finally, I wish to stress that at no time is unconscious hope more vital than when a patient is putting an analyst through the roughest of times. Even though treatment may intermittently look totally hopeless, and the analyst may be made to feel entirely hopeless too, it is most important not to lose sight of the fact that such problems in treatment are often (in themselves) an expression of the patient's unconscious search for some help—never previously found—with serious emotional difficulties. What the patient needs is to find someone who can bear being really in touch with the patient's extremes of personal difficulty without having to give up, someone who (without being unrealistic or trying to be omnipotent) can find some way to see the patient through. If an analyst begins to feel convinced that this will not be possible, I believe that it is then essential that he/she should seek whatever outside help may be necessary in order not to reject a patient: often the problem in the analytic relationship crucially represents precisely what is needing to be worked at in the analysis. Therefore, if an analysis is not to be prematurely terminated, becoming able to see the patient through may involve the analyst in seeking consultation (at the very least) or on-going supervision for a time (perhaps). Occasionally, a similar impasse with several patients may indicate a need for further personal analysis (for the analyst) if patients are not going to be subjected to a repetition, in the analytic treatment, of earlier failures by others. But when an analyst is able to find the capacity to see a patient through such extremely difficult times, ultimately the unconscious hope is met.[3]

❖18❖

Inner and Outer Realities[1]

Which realities do we find in the analytic encounter? There seems always to be an intermingling of the objective and the subjective realities of each participant—an intermingling of how each sees the other as well as how each may believe him/herself to be. Inevitably, therefore, the analyst's ways of being with the patient will affect what passes between them—as will the impact of the patient upon the analyst. These interactive pressures can disturb the analytic process or become part of it, depending upon whether they are recognized and how they are understood.

INTRODUCTION

It is common knowledge amongst the psychoanalytically minded, but not so well known to others, that in all relationships the other person is seen in terms of the internal world of the perceiver.

In this chapter, I wish to consider various ways in which the external and internal realities of analyst and patient affect each other, and how these in turn can either disturb the analytic process or become an integral part of it. I also wish to illustrate ways in which patients can use the objective realities of the analytic relationship to represent aspects of their own internal world, and those experiences that still need to be worked through.

THE ENVIRONMENT AND THE INNER WORLD

The present is often viewed so determinedly in terms of past experience that it takes a lot of careful work before the present can be seen for itself—as separate and different from the past. In the course of that work we frequently find evidence of early environmental failure etched into the patient's internal world, which in turn affects how subsequent experience is viewed and related to.

Example 18.1

Some time ago a man (Mr. L.) came to see me, saying that he needed help to change his life. Then, to explain this, he added: "You see, I suffered a severe environmental setback in my infancy." What he was trying to tell me was that his mother had died before he was two.

As well as telling me this detail of his early life, Mr. L. was demonstrating a number of other important facts about himself. His stilted way of talking reflected his experience of institutionalized life: he had spent most of his childhood in care. It also illustrated how far removed he had become from the emotional impact of his mother's death, which had remained beyond words— at least beyond those that had any warmth or emotional significance for him.

There was little or no warmth in his inner world. He had no conscious memory of his mother. So he had no available sense of an internal mother from whom to derive warmth or inner security. Instead, in this man's inner world there remained an absent mother; or, to be more precise, he had a repressed memory of a caring presence that had suddenly been replaced by an absence. An indelible link had thus come to be established in this man's mind between a warm presence and traumatic loss; as if death, or some other rejection, would inevitably follow any good experience with another person. As a result he had come to expect everybody to let him down in one way or another. Any possibility of warmth in a relationship had been shunned throughout his life, because he regarded this as a warning sign that he would again be hurt if he dared to expect it to continue.

So, we find here a common pattern: the nature of inner reality is largely based upon early experience and is little affected for the better by subsequent changes in the external world. Mr. L.'s early experience of loss had come to color his perception of all subsequent relationships. As a result, caring relationships, although desperately needed, had come to be feared and fiercely avoided.

I referred this patient to a female colleague, who later told me of his problems in that analysis. In particular, it had been difficult for her to find an appropriate balance in her technique. On the one hand, Mr. L. had experienced her more usual stance of clinical distance as confirming his view of the world as anonymous and uncaring; and yet, because it was familiar, that felt "safe" to him. On the other hand, when Mr. L. sensed a genuine caring in his analyst, he experienced that warmth as a danger-signal because of the link in his mind between warmth and loss. Much analytic work had therefore been necessary in order to build a bridge between the reality of the patient's inner world and a different reality in which caring did not necessarily have to lead to rejection or loss.

The Inner World Realized

I will now give some details from part of an analysis in which I had to find my own way of dealing with a similar conflict, between a patient's need to find security in a dependent relationship and her experience of dependence as dangerous.

Example 18.2

Miss M. was the only child of her unmarried mother. She came to me for analysis when she was twenty-two. Having been brought up in Europe she had come to this country to escape from what she had felt to be the grip of a possessive and cruel mother.

Miss M. described her mother as if she only felt hated by her. From an early age she had, apparently, been treated as her mother's slave. From about four years old she had been expected to wash up and clean, and from the age of ten she had to do much of the cooking after school whilst her mother was still at work. But whatever Miss M. did, her mother would invariably find fault: she seemed to be totally unpleasable.

Miss M.'s mother, I was told, used also to respond with sarcasm, denigration or abuse, to any emotional needs expressed by her daughter. There seemed to be one sacred rule—that she should never disturb her mother in any way. So, from very early on, if Miss M. ever expressed distress to her mother she was fobbed off with various tranquilizers. Any expectation that her mother should attend to her (except for giving pills) was immediately attacked as being "selfish."

Rather inevitably, Miss M. had learned not to turn to people but to substitutes. Initially she turned to food for comfort. Then, during her last year at school, she had become addicted to drugs. A few years later she nearly died after an unintended overdose, which so frightened her she developed a phobia against drugs and against almost any kind of medication. Subsequently, she turned to cigarettes and drink as alternative ways of trying to banish difficult feelings, and she was well on her way to becoming an alcoholic when she first came to me. Her reason for seeking analysis was that she felt she was in danger of going mad.

In the early stages of seeing Miss M., I was given many details of her life—but it was noticeable that she barely related to me as a person. I might sometimes be told of difficult situations, or of difficult feelings, but I was not expected to be of any help with either. Her inner reality cautioned her that, under no circumstances, was any person to be trusted or to be turned to because of need.

One defense used by Miss M. was that of creating splits in herself. She saw herself as having several distinct selves, one that was public and seemingly self-sufficient and another that was very needy but carefully hidden. Another version of this split was to be found in her illusion of never being alone: she always had a pretend companion—and sometimes she had voices. She felt that she kept herself "sane" by having conversations between her different selves. Between them they could safely criticize her mother, and could mock at people who needed people: her different selves had each other and therefore needed nobody. She eventually told me that one of her voices had been constantly deriding me, throughout the first years of her analysis, for thinking that she might eventually let me help her.

In the transference I was sometimes the person whom she needed to be a mother to her; but, at the same time, I represented her actual mother in relation to whom she had to demonstrate that she had no needs. So, when I tried to interpret her real need of me, and most particularly when I expressed the view that she needed me as a mother to her, she either scorned me for my stupidity or she became terrified that I was threatening to *become* her mother. "What is the matter with you?" she said. "Are you trying to drive me crazy?"

A major problem here, I had to realize, was that my use of the word "mother" had nothing but frightening associations for Miss M. In her experience, a mother had been someone who attacked her for being needy. The person whom she still needed to find was someone who could be different from her mother and who could really take care of her. She had no word for this, but that person was certainly not thought of as a mother. It was therefore a long time before Miss M. could discover that a mother could also be someone who attends to the needs of her child.

The patient's criticisms of me became increasingly fierce and sarcastic. Whatever I said was disagreed with. Every interpretation was challenged and mockingly treated as wrong. She began withdrawing into silence, often hiding under a blanket on the couch, or she would sullenly chain smoke throughout a session.[2] She didn't need me, and she had her conversations—so why should she speak to me? And yet she never failed to attend for her analysis.

Gradually it dawned upon me how the transference had shifted. The patient was "identifying with the aggressor"; and I was now being used to represent herself as the victim whom she attacked with her mother's derision. Like herself as a child, I was now regarded as failing to get anything right.

When I first tried to interpret this view of what was happening I failed to anticipate that Miss M. was more likely to respond to the form of my interpretation than to its content. I had said to her: "You are now treating me as your mother treated you." She reacted immediately to the implied criticism in my use of the word "now," as if I were adding yet another complaint to other complaints. She said, scornfully: "If you can't stand it then you shouldn't be pretending to me that you can help me."

Sometime later I tried a different approach. I said to her: "I believe that you are communicating to me something very important. I believe that you are unconsciously trying to get across to me *what it was like to be you in the presence of your mother*; so that I can now have a clear sense of the frustration and pain that you endured as a result of her always finding fault with you, and of her scorn and criticism. I think that this is why you have needed to treat me in ways similar to how your mother treated you." This time Miss M. was unusually reflective. She eventually replied: "I think that you are beginning to understand."

That session proved to be a turning point in this difficult, but eventually productive, analysis. The essential difference (this time) was that I had been more careful to create an atmosphere of understanding, in which the patient's behavior could be seen as a communication, and accepted, before trying once again to look at that behavior which the patient expected me to criticize.

I believe that Miss M. had needed to recreate a central feature of her mother's treatment of her within the relationship to me. Her inner reality thus came to be *actualized* within the analysis (Sandler 1976), whereby she made real to me that experience of her mother—at least as she had herself experienced it. (See also King 1978.)

Here, as with any patient, we have to face a further problem in deciding which reality we are dealing with. Miss M. could give me only her own account of *her experience with her mother,* and that would inevitably be deeply colored by her feelings and fantasies towards her. So, as well as the mother's real cruelty (which seemed to be verified independently by other people's views of her), I had to consider the possibility of the patient's own attacking that might have been projected on to the mother. But that too was complex, as I could sense a vicious circle in which any attacking that may have been projected by the patient would have been reinforced by the attacking behavior of her mother. It was therefore not possible to be sure, at any given moment, which was primary. But, on balance, I felt that the mother's inability to respond to her daughter's appeals to her, to be a mother, remained consistent and central to the clinical picture. In addition, it is quite likely that Miss M. used to project *into* her mother the unmanageable rage and distress that she could not cope with alone. The result then would probably have been that the patient's rage and distress were experienced as repeatedly "thrown back" at her, made worse by the fact that the mother was also unable to manage these things in herself—let alone take on what her daughter could not manage (Bion 1967b: 114–16).

In the patient's internal world, then, there was certainly a persecutory mother. There was also a split between the patient's needy self and her self-as-companion upon whom alone she felt that she could depend. This split had been developed very early through her discovery that the only attention she could expect to find for her needs was that which she provided for herself. And it is significant that Miss M.'s own word here was "companion" (someone friendly who stayed with her). It was a long time before she could tolerate any link between this and my notion of her need for a mother's care and holding.

What eventually began to shift this defensive self-sufficiency was the patient's discovery that I could understand and tolerate her use of me as the object of her attacks. From that discovery she was able to recognize that I could bear to remain in touch with her own most painful experiences, which was precisely what her mother could not bear being expected to help her with.

Then, from that earlier self-sufficiency and dependence upon substances rather than upon people, Miss M. began to allow herself to depend upon me in the analysis. These changes in the transference relationship reflected changes that had occurred within her internal world. She had now discovered a different reality, based upon her objective experience of me, in which it began to feel safe for her to relate to people and to risk becoming dependent—at first upon me and subsequently upon the man who later became her husband. The word "mother," too, ceased to be synonymous with cruelty; and, some years later, Miss M. was able to become a sensitive and imaginative mother to her own child.

THE ANALYST'S ENVIRONMENTAL PROVISION

Implicit in this second example was the need for the patient to discover that she was in the presence of someone whose underlying attitude to her sustained a wish to understand her behavior rather than to criticize it. But she could not believe *that* so long as my way of interpreting really did sound critical to her. It had then not been enough for me merely to suggest that Miss M. was experiencing me as her critical mother and therefore reading criticism into what I was saying. That interpretation had been dismissed by her as *my refusal to consider the truth of what she was saying.* But, by trial-identifying with the patient, I could more readily recognize an implied criticism in what I had said and I could see the need for me to find other ways of interpreting to her that were more clearly neutral.

It is, therefore, important to remember that some patients are acutely sensitive to the hidden meanings in what the analyst says. And I believe that it is harmful to the analytic process when analysts appear to ignore a patient's accurate perception, or interpret defensively in the face of it.

The Analyst's Style of Working

There are certain clinical states that are especially affected by the analyst's style of interpreting. I am thinking of compliant or false-self states, in patients who have adapted to a regime of parental impingements by taking over their parents' definition of what is real. I am also thinking of patients who have suffered narcissistic injury, having been made to feel bad about themselves in relation to their primary object(s).

With patients who are suffering from compliant or false-self states, much will depend upon whether the analyst behaves in an impinging way or allows adequate space for the patient to risk being more real. Too much interpretation, or interpretation that is given in a dogmatic way, is likely to invite further compliance. What is more helpful with such patients is a more tentative style of interpreting and an analytic presence that is less obtrusive (Balint 1968: Chapter 25).

In relation to narcissistic injury, much will rest upon whether the analyst remains sufficiently sensitive to the patient's underlying vulnerability, and avoids becoming too intent upon eliminating the symptomatic behavior. Pathology serves a communicative as well as a defensive function (see Chapter 17). This is sometimes overlooked when an analyst is confronted by narcissistic defenses: for, when these defenses are aimed at protecting the vulnerable self, they are frequently destructive of the capacity for object relating.

If narcissistic pathology is interpreted too insistently as due to an innate destructiveness in the patient, rather than understood as a defense against unbearable anxieties, an analyst can fall into an attitude towards a patient that is more critical than understanding. What then follows can amount to a battle between an attacking analyst and a patient whose defensive posture may largely be a response to the analyst. It is all too easy to fall into such an interaction, particularly if the analyst fails to recognize his/her own part in this, and it can further develop into a transference-counter-transference enactment that has its roots in the history of both combatants. The analyst will then urgently need to recover a more neutral stance from which to reflect upon such moments as these.

The wounding interpretations that narcissistically vulnerable patients sometimes attract, based on the analyst's desire to break through the narcissistic shell, can also become a reenactment of an original trauma. Such reenactments may therefore have diagnostic significance, pointing to a similar breakdown of early parental containment.

Another feature with narcissistically damaged patients is that, whilst conscious guilt may apparently be absent, the patient's unconscious guilt is often already extreme and unbearable.[3] This can lead to a form of interpretive work that, in itself, becomes persecutory, particularly if the compliant patient finds a superego role-responsiveness in the analyst. Unfortunately, patients may then show changes in symptomatology which are brought about by virtue of a strengthening of the already harsh superego, or an intensification of splitting. Furthermore, a sadomasochistic relationship can develop which is not always recognized as such by either patient or analyst.

Reality and Impasse in the Analysis

There are some occasions when an analysis begins to fail, or fails completely, because an impasse has developed between analyst and patient.[4] Often this has resulted from a loss of the analytic space, which can easily happen if the analyst has objective reality come too much like a key figure in the patient's internal world. When that happens the analysis cannot continue effectively until a sufficient difference has again been established between the analyst and the particular transference use of the analyst by the patient (see Chapter 15). If the analyst denies his or her contribution to this similarity, that adds a pathogenic dimension to the analytic relationship, which then makes it quite unanalyzable until the objective reality has been attended to by the analyst (see Example 17.3). Some analysts have a problem about admitting their mistakes which, they fear, might be personally revealing or might seem to involve some loss of face. My impression, however, is that patients ultimately feel more secure (not less) when they discover that the analyst can acknowledge and learn from mistakes.

THERAPEUTIC USE OF REENACTMENT

Reenactment by the analyst, if it is not understood and remedied, is always likely to disturb the analytic process. Sometimes, however, this reenactment seems to evolve from the analytic process itself. I am thinking of those occasions when an uncanny parallel to a key experience in the patient's life develops around some real event involving the analyst. This then takes on a double significance. At one level it becomes a trigger for transference; at another it involves the analyst in a way that enables the patient to feel justified in expressing towards the analyst, in the present, feelings that belonged originally to some earlier bad experience.

Finally, therefore, I wish to give a brief example to show how a patient's inner reality can sometimes be stumbled upon in this way.

Example 18.3
Mrs. P., as I shall call her, was in her early thirties when she came into analysis with me.

In her second year she came into a session in a state of great agitation. She demanded to know why I had allowed the patient before her to come back into the waiting-room whilst she was there. (He had, in fact, left a briefcase there and had gone back to fetch it.)

A few weeks later that man did the same thing again. Mrs. P. then became utterly enraged, and she expressed her views on this very forcefully: I should have been more watchful; I should have seen what he was up to; I should have made sure that he would never do that again; how could I have let it go on happening? And what kind of analyst did I think I was, allowing that to have happened at all let alone more than once? This incident became the focus for weeks of angry protesting and distrust. It was clear that the patient regarded me as careless, perhaps even as not caring. But the intensity of Mrs. P.'s distress suggested that there was something more in this that we did not yet understand.

A dream then helped to clarify what this sequence had come to represent. In this dream Mrs. P. was in her parents' home. She was quite small. The man from my waiting-room had come into where she was, in her bedroom. She had started screaming for her mother but nobody came. She had woken up in a state of terror.

Mrs. P. was very disturbed after dreaming this. It brought back vivid memories. It reminded her of the man who lived next door to her childhood home, whom she hated. There was something wrong about him and she could remember hiding from him whenever he visited her parents. But, strangely, even though she was so obviously frightened of this man, her mother continued to ask him to babysit. When, much later, Mrs. P. had asked her mother why she had continued to use that babysitter, of whom she was so clearly frightened, she was told that it didn't seem to matter as long as she was asleep when he came. (I gathered that her parents sometimes went down to the pub in the late evening, at which times this neighbor used to babysit for them.) But Mrs. P. then remembered, with great alarm, that she had token up to find herself alone with this man in her bedroom. She was quite small. She was also sure that this had happened on several occasions.

So, the man in my waiting-room had come to represent the man next door, this neighbor. And I, as the person who had not stopped him intruding upon the patient, had become the mother who was allowing something intolerable to continue happening. A few months later in the analysis it became clear that there had been actual sexual interference by this neighbor. Thus, through a chance real event in relation to the analysis, this patient had begun to get in touch with that traumatic experience, and eventually to remember.

The feelings about that repeated trauma could now be worked through in the transference. However, I had first to regain my position as an analyst who could be more alert and sensitive to what was happening to the patient. Only then could she feel safe enough to use me, and the events that had impinged upon her analysis, to represent those other realities of her inner world, and for the memories of her childhood trauma to be recovered from repression.

CONCLUSION

In the examples I have given there is always more than one reality operating. There is the reality of "environmental provision," in the analysis as well as childhood, and there is the reality of the inner world. But that inner reality is also partly based upon early environmental realities—in terms of which much subsequent experience may be perceived and interpreted. Thus, Mr. L. (Example 18.1) saw all relationships, particularly any that might be caring, as a potential threat; and Miss M. (Example 18.2) had come to regard anyone she experienced as a mother as someone who would be cruel to her.

There is also a distortion of how external reality is perceived, due to what is projected on to others, and I have indicated how this had to be allowed for in thinking about any account of childhood experiences—as with Miss M.. And yet, not all bad experience with others can be attributed to such projections. How the analyst works can also become a bad experience, especially if the effects of this are not acknowledged or remedied by the analyst, which can lead to impasse or breakdown in the analysis.

In addition, there is the overlapping of different realities that will inevitably occur as part of the analytic process. Here there are triggers for transference, with transference elaborations by the patient that result in aspects of his/her past being relived within the analytic relationship. But not all that is experienced in relation to the analyst is transference.

Unconscious reenactment by the analyst, if it is attended to, can sometimes have an important diagnostic function, as when the analyst's failure represents a key feature in the patient's past. It may thus represent what is needing to be dealt with in the analysis—and dealt with in a new way, which can help to relegate the past to the past, as with Mrs. P. (Example 18.3).

I have, in particular, wished to emphasize *the analyst's own part in the analytic process,* and the need for recognizing the effects upon the patient of the analyst's ways of working and interpreting. (I shall return to this in the next chapter.) Ignoring these effects can be as detrimental to the understanding of the patient as overlooking the real effects of early environmental failure. Not all of the analytic experience is to be understood in terms of inner reality or as projections by the patient. The analyst, as much as a parent, has a real impact upon the patient.

❖19❖

Trial Identification and Technique[1]

Once we accept the fact that the analytic process is affected by the impact of the analyst's way of working, it becomes important that the analyst can develop ways of monitoring the possible effects of this, from the patient's point of view. Examples are given, and technical "exercises" suggested for interest's sake, which can help to heighten an awareness of this dimension to the analytic relationship.

INTRODUCTION

A central issue in analysis is the freedom to work with the transference, to be able to interpret to the patient those ways in which the past is spilling into the present—affecting the patient's perceptions of the other and therefore his/her ways of relating. But for this interpretive work to be convincing to a patient, it is important that the objective realities in the analytic relationship do not mask or blur these manifestations of transference. It is therefore useful for analysts and therapists to monitor the ways in which they work with their patients so that they can recognize more readily the extent to which patients' responses are determined as much by these objective realities as by what is transferred to the analyst.

In the course of running clinical workshops, and in supervision, I have sometimes used clinical vignettes to create opportunities for practicing technique. When musicians are having difficulty in playing a particular passage, they often break the problem down into manageable "bits" in order to see where the difficulty lies. And, having identified this, they invent "technical exercises" in order to develop fluency in playing difficult passages. This use of exercises—for practice outside the consulting-room—is likewise useful in clinical practice. For it is when the analyst is *with* a patient, and under the pressures that are often an integral part of experiencing the patient's presence, that it is least possible to have this freedom to reflect and to explore the technical implications of how we might respond to the patient.

I have been referring to trial identification from time to time throughout this book, and I have already described in some detail the different uses of trial identification (see Chapter 14). I now wish to focus more extensively upon *trial identification with the patient in the session* order to get a better sense of how the patient may be experiencing the analyst, in what is being said or in the analyst's manner in the session, and how the patient may hear (or mishear) what the analyst has it in mind to say.

SOME EXAMPLES

I shall first mention some common technical issues illustrating the value, in relation to technique, of trial identification with the patient in the session.

The Timing of Transference Interpretations

One of the most frequent problems of technique is that of the timing of transference interpretations. If we consider the implications of such interpretations from the patient's point of view, it becomes easier to distinguish between those occasions when the patient needs a transference interpretation without delay and other times when it is important not to interpret too quickly.

For instance, if a patient is caught up in a transference to the analyst as someone felt to be hostile to the point where this is threatening the analytic work, then of course it is important to identify where this transference comes from (having first checked that it is not based upon some objective reality in how the analyst has been speaking to the patient). That interpreting of the transference can free the patient to continue with the analysis, which might otherwise have become blocked. Similarly, if a patient is beginning to get caught up in an erotized transference, it is important not to delay in interpreting this for what it signifies.

However, there are times when a patient gets into strong feelings (such as anger or hating) which key figures in the patient's past may not have been able to tolerate. At such times it could be a mistake to interpret straight away that these feelings really belong to someone other than the analyst. Instead, it can become a valuable experience if the analyst stays with these feelings long enough to demonstrate that they can be taken on the chin, as if they did belong solely to the analyst (see Example 18.3). Otherwise, he/she may be experienced by the patient as being too much like others before, also unable to bear being the object of such feelings. By waiting long enough before interpreting the transference here, a number of gains may follow: first, the details of the transference experience now being relived may become clearer, so that a more specific interpretation later becomes possible; also, the patient is able to have the experience of being with someone who is not backing off from a difficult experience. That can help to alter the quality of the patient's feelings here: they can be recognized as a form of communication; they do not have to be sheltered from or retaliated against. So it is often important to recognize when a transference interpretation (if given too immediately) could be perceived by the patient as the analyst being defensive, as if he/she were saying: "Don't give *that* to me—it doesn't belong to *me*."

A typical example of staying with a patient's anger (say) may be found in dealing with a patient's reactions to a cancelled session. The absence has been real; it may also have come at a particularly bad time for the patient. The reasons for the patient finding this so difficult may reflect feelings about a sudden absence in childhood. Nevertheless, staying with the anger—as if it were only to do with the analyst's absence—often results in the emergence of fresh details about earlier desertions or absences. I think that opportunities are lost when a patient's anger is too quickly interpreted "away" from the analyst, as if it were all to do with some specific earlier experience. That is usually already known about. But more important details (perhaps of other absences) may still need to be discovered, and these often surface when the analyst accepts the immediate focus for the patient's feeling, such as the untimeliness of a canceled session for that particular patient, as if it might not have been transference at all. Subsequent experience often demonstrates the value of having allowed that fuller transference experience to develop, particularly when the patient needs to find that this is after all manageable by the analyst. However, at other times a patient will need early interpretation in order to feel contained. The problem is to discern which timing is likely to be most fruitful under which circumstances.

The Therapist is Experienced as Critical

Example 19.1
Suppose a patient has told us what he is thinking, and we feel that there is something strange about this which needs to be explored further. If we were then to say "Why do you think that?," how might a patient hear this apparently quite simple question?

First of all, because it is a question, there is an implied pressure upon the patient to reply. But, in this context, the question could also be felt as criticism. The patient could hear the question as indicating that he should *not* thinking in the way he has just described. He might then feel a need to justify this by defensively offering an explanation.

So, rather than ask a question here, we could simply make a statement (not requiring an answer) such as: "I wonder why you think this." But truly, although it is partly disguised it is still a question, even if in a gentler form.

We might just say: "You have some reason for thinking this"; or, "I am not yet clear about this." The patient can then help us to become clearer (or not) as he wishes.

The Therapist is Experienced as Defensive

Example 19.2
A patient has been describing a number of recent experiences in which she felt criticized. The therapist (a man) recognized that these could be displaced references to the transference. But he puts this as a question: "Do you expect me to criticize you too?" The patient immediately replied: "Oh, no: I know that you wouldn't be critical."

If we look at the therapist's response from the patient's point of view, we can readily sense that the question here is *expecting* the answer "No." The patient might then see the therapist as unwilling to accept that she could, in fact, be expecting him to be critical. A statement here would more clearly allow the patient a freedom to enter into the transference without being quite so anxious about whether the therapist could tolerate this. For example, the therapist could have said: "You are telling me about your experiences of being criticized. I think you may be expecting me to be critical too." The patient could then feel able to say that she does expect this, and she might go on to give examples from recent sessions when she had already been experiencing the therapist as critical. And that, in turn, might prompt the therapist to reflect upon the possible basis for that sense of being criticized.

With the benefit of a patient's feedback, we may also find that some implicit criticism had been conveyed in the manner of recent interpretations. And, if that had been the case, it is then important that the therapist find some way of dealing with that reality without treating all of the patient's experience as transference. That does not mean, necessarily, that the therapist should always admit to what his/her feelings may have been. It is often sufficient, in such a situation, to say: "I can see how you could have heard what I said as critical." Acknowledging the reality is sometimes a better way of approaching the transference. To focus first, and only, on the transference will be seen by the patient as defensive—even as the therapist denying the elements of objective reality in the analytic relationship. It is always detrimental to the working alliance to give that impression to a patient.

The Therapist is Experienced as Intrusive

Example 19.3
PATIENT (a woman): I had a dream about some kind of sexual encounter. It was quite confusing. There were two sexual organs in some kind of contact. They seemed disembodied as if they did not belong to anybody. I think that one organ must have been mine but I do not know whose the other was. The situation seemed dangerous. I think that there was a risk of some infection, but I do not know whether it was the man who was infected or me.

THERAPIST (a man): Was there anything else in the dream?

We can use this brief interchange for practice. If we trial-identify with the patient and consider the implication of this response by the therapist—what is the impression that we get? First, the question is intrusive. It also suggests that the therapist wants more. Further, if we consider the quality of the question in this particular context we can see that it could be experienced by the patient as voyeuristic. How then are we to assess the patient's response?

To the question "Was there anything else in the dream?" the patient replied: "Not really. I don't think that there was any actual intercourse. But I think it may have taken place by an open window—somewhere you could look into."

We might therefore wonder whether it was just coincidence that the patient replied in this way: it sounds almost as if she is apologizing to the therapist for disappointing his voyeuristic expectations. But she adds that the sexual encounter took place "somewhere you could look into." This too speaks to the therapist as if he were unconsciously perceived as having a salacious interest in peering into the patient's sexual activities. I regard this as a clear illustration of "unconscious supervision by the patient."

Different Uses of the Countertransference

Example 19.4

A therapist working in a therapeutic community found himself feeling very impatient with a particular resident. This resident had been frequently absent from community meetings, sometimes absent for a day or several days at a time, so that it was not clear whether she had really left, or what was happening.

The therapist eventually confronted this girl very directly with her behavior: "I cannot put up with any more of this coming and going, and the effects that this is having on the community, as it leaves us not knowing what has happened to you."

The intention of the confrontation was to set a limit to this disturbing and quite destructive behavior. It may even have been the most effective way of dealing with that particular resident at the time. We can nevertheless use this example for some practice. For instance, if we listen to the form of the therapist's statement we can readily recognize the superego quality of it: the resident should not go on behaving in this way.

Now, under some circumstances, this kind of confrontation could be quite appropriate if a patient needs to be faced with the implications of difficult behavior, even if this means that the therapist intermittently becomes an auxiliary superego to the patient. This could arise if the patient's own superego control is either absent or so severe that it is defensively disowned (projected), which can have the effect of inducing in others a superego response that appears then to have come from "outside" the patient rather than from "inside."

When I learned that this particular resident had been abandoned by her natural parents, had been fostered but then placed in a series of children's homes, it was possible to see the countertransference response here in a different light. The therapist had been affected by the resident's repeated "comings" and "goings", and he was beginning to feel angry about these—confused and not knowing what was happening. It is possible then to see that the resident may unconsciously have been communicating something of her own distress and confusion about the comings and goings in *her* life. Perhaps, by means of her absences, she had been stirring up feelings in others that echoed her own unmanageable feelings about absences, which others (through projective identification) were picking up in her stead.

With this in mind it is possible to consider other ways in which the therapist might have responded. He might have been able to draw upon his own feelings in order to offer to the resident the thought that she might have been behaving towards the community as others had towards her. It would be possible then to consider how she probably had similar difficult feelings in response to other absences and other losses in her life. Her behavior could thus have been recognized as a form of communication rather than being treated as difficult behavior. And if she *had* been communicating unmanageable feelings, then we can see that the therapist's reaction to this could have been experienced by her as evidence that he too was unable to bear them.

Interpreting Behavior as Communication

One of the problems about interpreting behavior as communication is that a patient is often so sensitive to anything like criticism that almost any interpretation is likely to be experienced first as criticism. Of course it is possible to interpret that reaction by a patient as evidence of transference, which it almost certainly is, but when that happens too often it can deflect from what might have been a more fruitful exploration of the communication that the behavior had conveyed. There clearly are times when the more important communication is to be found in the behavior rather than in a possible transference from critical parents.

How Much to Put into an Interpretation

Not all interpretations need to be as long or as full as they sometimes are. When they are too full we can usefully wonder about the implications of this for the patient.

Example 19.5

A trainee therapist in analysis with me had been upset that his first training patient had already left therapy whereas he still needed to be in analysis. I knew that my patient had been quite seriously deprived by his own inattentive mother who had consistently disregarded his need for her attention. I therefore interpreted: "I think it is possible that you get something out of your patients still needing you, maybe because it gives you a way of being the attentive mother to your patient seen as a needy child—doing for someone else what your mother seems not to have done for you."

Now, if we look at my interpretation we can see that I have done more of the analytic work for the patient than is really necessary. I could have left the interpretation with just the first part: "I think it is possible that you get something out of your patients still needing you...." Leaving it there could have left the patient to do his own analytic work around this observation. As it was, the patient's response to this mostly echoed what I had said, which prompted me to realize that I had said too much.

A Balance Between Not-Knowing and Being Firm

When might it be most useful to make interpretations that leave the patient free to explore further and when is it more appropriate to make an interpretation that is more definite?

There are certainly times when it is better to make a statement that can be challenged, in particular in the area of character defenses (those things about the self that the patient least wants to acknowledge), because the resistance to facing painful truth about the self is unlikely to shift if the form of an interpretation is too mild, too tentative. Also, it is important for the analyst to offer understanding with a sufficient sureness to be able to contain a patient in crisis.

However, if the analyst's whole style of working appears to be based upon certainty, this will have far-reaching implications. A patient has then to do battle with the analyst's dogmatic attitude, with the risk of being beaten down by the analyst who can always have the last word—"the analyst (like some parents) always knows best," or the patient may give up and comply. A greater possibility for creative interchange is at times preserved when the patient is invited to respond to the analyst's shared not-knowing or to play with half-interpretations. Then the patient, as someone invited to take part in the working alliance, can work with the analyst towards fuller (and shared) understanding.

I shall not be giving examples of this here but analysts and therapists can readily find their own.

Interpretations that Reenact

Not infrequently the analyst or therapist gets drawn into a reenactment with the patient to a point where even the attempts at interpreting become a part of that reenactment. It is useful to scan for the potential reenactment that may be concealed within the form of interpretation that may first come to mind.

One of the more common ways in which interpretations can become a reenactment is in the realm of sexual abuse. It is well known that rape victims (and it must also be true of child-abuse victims) experience the subsequent police questioning as a repetition of the original trauma. Analysts have to be watchful that they do not do something similar when they interpret sexual matters to such a patient (see Example 12.6).

When there has been incest in a patient's childhood there is a strong unconscious push to repeat aspects of that trauma in the transference, as a way of communicating this to the analyst. Sometimes the trauma has been "forgotten" and only reemerges into consciousness through these partial repetitions, but there are many pitfalls on the way to recovering such memories.

Not infrequently an incest-victim has experienced a double trauma, not only suffering an abusing father but also a mother who remained blind to the abuse of her own child (see Example 18.3). The analyst is then faced with many problems of tact and timing. If the analyst interprets too swiftly, and too confidently, that the patient's free associations suggest something sexual—let alone assuming anything so specific as sexual interference by a parent—this attempt at interpreting may be experienced as forcing a sexual meaning upon the patient's more innocent-seeming associations.[2]

There is the counterpart problem—that of delaying too long before verbalizing the sexual implications of a patient's communications, and how these seem to point to something incestuous. Too long a delay in acknowledging what can no longer be overlooked can be experienced by the patient as the analyst being afraid to face facts: the analyst may then seem to have become a reenactment of the mother who turned a blind eye to what had been happening.

SOME TECHNICAL EXERCISES

The following "exercises" are offered for practice. They are not given as models for technique, but in the hope that they may inspire readers to make up their own exercises to heighten their awareness of the patient's point of view.

Identification with the Aggressor

A particular form of communication through behavior is evident when patients communicate something of their own experience through an identification with the aggressor. A patient may then behave towards the analyst in ways that represent some hurtful treatment the patient had previously experienced. By practicing with the different ways of trying to interpret this behavior we might find a way that does not too readily evoke the more likely response of feeling criticized.

> *Exercise A*
> A male patient has been putting the analyst down, attacking every inter-
> pretation to the point where the analyst is beginning to feel that whatever
> she says will be wrong. What are the options?

The analyst might feel like saying: "Whatever I say today seems to be wrong" and this could be justified in terms of confronting the patient. The intention here could be for the analyst to identify the transference, trying to understand this in terms of how someone has treated the patient in this kind of way. But if we put ourselves in the shoes of the patient, we can sense the quality of this response as critical, as complaining, and perhaps as retaliatory. How might a patient respond to that?

If the patient were then to say that he/she feels criticized, or attacked, by the analyst's confrontation we could not necessarily assume that this also points to some transference (see also Example 19.2). It could of course be that some unconscious role-responsive-ness was evoked in the analyst whereby she had become an embodi-ment of a complaining parent, and there is the possibility of some fruitful analysis along those lines. This would lead naturally to an interpretation of the patient's use of "identification with the aggressor" which may also be conveyed in this behavior and which it might be more important to understand.

It might however be more fruitful if we could find a way of approaching the patient's behavior that does not so predictably make the patient feel criticized. If that response is predictable I think we should wonder how much of it would necessarily be transference: some of it may be set up by the analyst's mode of intervention.

Another way of approaching this kind of problem is found through *creating an atmosphere of understanding* (as in Example 18.2) before attempting to confront the patient. The analyst could, for instance, start by saying something like: "I think that you may be communicating something to me in the only way that you can—by behaving towards me as your father (or mother) may have behaved towards you." The wish to understand the unconscious communication in this behavior is then clearly demonstrated as the priority, rather than any wish to criticize the patient for it, and the patient is likely to have a fuller sense of this and to respond accordingly.

Or the analyst could offer an interpretation first and then point to the basis for it in the patient's behavior. He could say: "I get the impression that you have had the experience of being often put in the wrong, and I think that that is why you have been putting me in a similar position in this session."

If, however, we practice further we might notice that this last interpretation (like so many) contains two statements rather than one. A further option could be to leave the patient with the first half only, to see what the patient does with it. One patient might take that up immediately with detail from the childhood, which could later be linked with the reenactment of this in the analytic relationship; another patient might first want to question where the analyst gets that impression from and, having been told, might then give detail from the childhood. Also, we might note, the fuller interpretation runs the risk of preempting a focus by the patient upon the analytic relationship (a common analytic preference) rather than leaving it open for the patient to respond to the first part of the interpretation in whichever way first occurs to the patient.

There is, of course, no particular "right way." In all these so-called exercises there is always a possibility of choice in how to interpret.

The Order of an Interpretation

An interesting point of technique which the exercise above can also illustrate is *the effect of order in an interpretation*. By choosing an order that is careful not to create a diversion (for instance through the patient's response to a sense of being criticized) it may be possible to explore something new in the analysis. If the patient still responds with feeling criticized then it would be clearer that this really is transference. Trial identification with the patient, before interpreting, can often help to highlight where a patient's sensitivities might lie and can help to point to different ways of interpreting and the possible implications of each (as in Chapter 14).

Reestablishing the Analytic Space

For analytic work to be possible there has to be sufficient analytic space within which the patient and analyst can together reflect upon what is happening in the session. There are times, however, when this gets lost and needs to be reestablished.

> *Exercise B*
> In supervision I encountered a stalemate in a session in which the female therapist and a female patient each felt that she was being double-bound by the other, and there seemed to be no way out of that without both parties getting into some kind of "You started it" interaction. How might one try to get out of that stalemate?

I thought it worth doing some practice with this vignette during that supervision. The analytic space had been temporarily lost, so we might think of some way in which this could be reestablished. Or, maybe, we could find a way of offering the patient some transitional space in which analytic reflection could be resumed. One might share an idea with the patient that could be played with, such as: "I am getting an image here of a parent and a child who are locked in a stalemate—with each blaming the other for what is happening between them." The patient might recognize enough validity in that to respond from her own experience. This might then lead to some clarification of which childhood experience(s) had been spilling into the present, trapping both parties in much the same way as had happened in the past. Enough analytic space might then be restored to explore the interaction between therapist and patient without continuing to prolong it through a process of mutual blame.

Internal supervision may make it possible to find a reflective viewpoint from which to explore the interaction rather than to remain caught up in it.

Linking the Past and the Present

Psychoanalytic interpretation is always at some level making links between the past and the present. It is, however, not always remembered that the *direction of an interpretation* has different implications for the patient. And again we are most likely to recognize the difference if we monitor from the patient's point of view what we might be about to say or what has just been said.

Exercise C
A patient comes to a session very angry, shouting at me for my absence of two weeks over the Easter holiday: "You were not here when I most needed you." I recognize the link with her past experience of abandon-ment, her mother having gone on holiday with her new baby leaving the older child (my patient) in the care of relatives. There are many ways in which I could make links here, so let us look at the contrasting implications for the patient in how the past and the present here might be interpreted as connected.

I could interpret: "You are angry with me now because I have been away and this has reminded you of the time when your mother left you shortly after your brother was born." The "direction" of this interpretation takes the focus away from myself (in the present) back into the patient's past. The patient might therefore feel that I could be deflecting her angry shouting away from me on to her mother, as if I were saying: "You are not really angry with me but with your mother." The patient could then see me as afraid of her feelings. She might then either become even more uncontained with her anger (if no one else can manage this then how can she?); or she might suppress her anger, or keep it deflected away from me, for fear that I might not be able to cope with such direct expressions of strong feelings. Clearly this is not the conscious intention of making an interpretation that has a direction towards the past. But it does often happen that interpretations are given in this mode, and I think the implications of that direction towards the past are not noticed often enough or monitored.

Another way of making the same interpretive link is to start with the past detail and to follow the direction of the transference—where the past is spilling into the present. We can then help the patient to see what it is that is happening in the session whilst at the same time being more clearly prepared to stay with those difficult feelings *in the present* until they come to be experienced by the patient as more contained. We could say: "At a time when you were most dependent upon your mother she went away with your brother. You were feeling particularly dependent upon me before the Easter break and then I went away, so you experience me now as the mother who left you when you most needed her." This way round offers some insight into the present distress whilst keeping the immediate focus still in the present where the patient's feelings are being expressed.

What I have said here, about linking past and present, applies equally to the use of material from a previous session. If there is something difficult in the present session, and the analyst makes a link between this and an earlier session, this linking can sometimes be seen by the patient as a defensive maneuver by the analyst—moving to the safer ground of clinical archaeology (the dead history of a past session) rather than staying with what is happening in the present. If it still seems useful, or necessary, to bring in something from an earlier session I think it is important to try to find a way of introducing it so that the focus remains quite clearly in the present. And if the patient's attention shifts from the present to the earlier session referred to, or in some other way remains focused outside the current interaction with the analyst, then it may be that the patient is giving the analyst an unconscious cue to recognize the deflective effects of a reference at that moment to something more safely in the past. It is always helpful if the analyst can recognize when the patient is reacting in this kind of way and to be alert to the possible reasons why.

It is well worth remembering that we do not need to go in search of the past: the unconscious brings the past to us—through the past becoming dynamically present in the session. The interpretive task is then to understand which elements of the patient's past are being reexperienced now, and why.

The Use of Strong Terms

Not infrequently we have patients use strong terms in describing themselves or others. I think that it is worth thinking about some of the problems that can develop around using a patient's language—when to use it too and when not to.

Exercise D
A patient has been describing her new boss who, she insists, is obstructive her work. The therapist refers to this description in his interpretation: "I see that you are having difficulties with this obstructive boss." What are the implications in this for the patient?

The patient could feel that the therapist accepts her own perception of the boss as obstructive—without question. This could temporarily limit the analytic space in which to analyze the patient's perception, and we do need to be able to wonder how valid that perception is. Whose obstructiveness is being referred to in the session? The boss's? The patient's in projection? And/or some transference on to the boss seen as obstructive? Or might this be a displacement from the therapist who may recently have been experienced in this way?

One way of keeping open the analytic space here would be for the therapist to play back the patient's description more clearly as the patient's perception: "You put great emphasis on how obstructive he seems to be." Or the therapist could make some comment such as: "A key theme in what you are saying is around someone being obstructive," thus opening up the question of whose obstructiveness is being alluded to. This does not presume that the focus is to be on the external world or upon the internal world of the patient. There is then plenty of room for the patient to take this observation further and for various other possible dimensions to be included in the analytic investigation.

We might also note, in passing, that for the therapist to accept too quickly that it is the boss who is being seen as obstructive could be an unconscious way of deflecting this criticism away from the therapist.

Exercise E
A patient has been talking to his therapist about himself and makes a reference to what he calls "my shitty feelings." The therapist adopts the patient's language here and makes an interpretation in which he speaks of "your shitty feelings" to the patient. How might the patient hear this?

It is possible that the patient could feel some relief that the therapist is accepting his own view of himself. Where else can that lead? Of course, without other detail we cannot know. But we can also sense that the patient might regard this use of his own self-description as confirming that his feelings really are "shitty." The therapist may have been invited into a judgmental attitude towards the patient which could be a reenactment from the past. But what about the analytic space? Has the patient the necessary freedom to examine this view of his feelings? If the therapist seems to see his feelings in the same way as the patient does, then what more is there to say about them? "They are shitty," so that would be that!

By contrast, we might consider how to address the patient's self-view without speaking as if it were being accepted as the only possible view. For instance the therapist could say: "You have come to regard your feelings as shitty . . .," which could lead to an exploration into how this has come about. Or, the therapist could say: "I think you expect me also to see your feelings as shitty . . .," which could lead to wondering about this invitation to have the therapist become the critical parent, or whoever. In either case there is more analytic space created here by the therapist addressing the same thing as the patient (the "shitty" feelings) without seeming to adopt the same perspective. The analytic work can evolve within that analytic space in a way that is less likely to happen if these feelings were just spoken of as shitty, as if that were the only way to speak of them, or as if there were no work to be done on how these feelings have come to be regarded in this way.

It is important, however, to be able to recognize when strong terms do need to be used, even if these are introduced by the analyst, and it is useful to notice examples when that is necessary. But how these strong terms are introduced will make a difference to how the patient is likely to experience them.

Exercise F

A patient has been complaining about other people putting him down and he has been feeling rather persecuted by this. He has also not been able to see why people have been treating him in this way.

His therapist has been aware of an arrogance in his patient and tries to point out that other people may be reacting to this. He says: "I think that people may have been reacting to your arrogance by putting you in your place."

There are a number of things we can notice about this, if we use it as an exercise, again bearing in mind that we do not have any background detail. For instance, we do not know if this is an old theme (that of arrogance), in which case this comment may be an entirely appropriate confrontation. Or, if the patient is someone who takes little notice of comments that are made with less impact than this, there may be a case for using a statement more likely to get through to him and for the therapist to deal with the consequences. On the other hand, if this is the first time that arrogance has been mentioned in the therapy it could feel to the patient as a further put-down, this time by the therapist.

With some patients the more important focus for analysis needs to be less upon the fact of arrogance than upon the reasons for this—in other words on the defensive function of arrogance. A less combative atmosphere is preserved, for shared work on such a defense, if some way can be found which also communicates an awareness of the insecurity that lies behind the arrogance. One way could be to say something like: "I think that a problem here is that when you are feeling threatened you try to appear big. Other people then see you as being arrogant without realizing that you are protecting yourself from feeling small." This is by no means the only way to tackle such an issue, but I give this alternative interpretation to illustrate the different quality in this compared to the potentially more hurtful confrontation used in the example.

Beware Assumptions

It is all too easy for analysts and therapists to fall into making assumptions which can deprive the patient of an important freedom to put things in his/her own way. Often these assumptions are left unchallenged by the patient.

Exercise G
I notice sometimes in supervision that a therapist evaluates an experience for the patient. For instance a therapist may say: "You must have found that very upsetting." What if the patient had not found it "very upsetting"?

I think that it is often better for the patient to be the one to add the word "very" rather than have to deal with the therapist's assumption that the patient's reaction will have been extreme. Of course, such a comment will not matter when the patient's experience was as assumed, but we may not discover when it is different if the form of an interpretation has been evaluative on behalf of the patient.

By contrast it leaves a patient more room to make his/her own evaluation of an experience if the therapist approaches this without assumptions. The therapist could ask: "How did you feel about that?" But that is a question and the patient is likely to feel it must be answered. Or, the therapist might make a statement such as: "I am not clear what you felt about this." As this is no more than an observation, and about the present limit of the therapist's understanding, the patient can feel invited to clarify what was felt, if anything.

However, if a patient has been in a situation that was almost certainly distressing, I think that it is necessary to find some way of acknowledging that feelings may have run high without assuming what kind of feelings these were. "You probably felt pretty strongly about this" can leave room for the patient to fill in with the detail of these feelings, which could range from feeling angry, frightened, guilty, excited—or whatever. If the therapist assumes that the patient would have felt anger, when it had been excitement that was felt, the patient is sometimes going to be inhibited from admitting to that. Also, if a therapist says: "You must have felt very guilty about this," it is likely that a patient will hear this as saying that this is what *should* have been felt. It does not always follow that this is how it was.

A patient whose younger sibling had died soon after birth could be assumed to have problems about guilt. But, in the early stages of getting to know such a patient, it is important not to assume that the patient is aware of this. "I wonder how you felt about this death" allows the patient to reflect upon it and perhaps to come out with a very different (and important) revelation, such as: "Well, actually, I remember feeling a great sense of relief.... I would not have to put up with a rival after all." If the therapist had assumed that the primary feelings would have been those of guilt it is unlikely that the patient will easily confess to these other feelings. There may then be induced guilt, or guilt at not having felt guilt, which is quite another matter.

Interpreting Unconscious Guilt

Exercise H
A patient had been raging against her hated husband. She could see no good in him at all. She would really like to get rid of him but she could not make him leave nor could she find anywhere to go if she left him. Then the husband had a heart attack and died. Following this, the patient clearly switched into a reaction formation against her former hatred, arranging an elaborate funeral and speaking nothing but praise for her dead husband. But she soon developed a crippling skin rash which she felt was threatening to drive her crazy. The therapist eventually made a link between the rash and her unconscious guilt. He said: "I think that you are unconsciously punishing yourself with this rash because you feel so bad about the hate that you used to feel for your husband before he died. Now, instead of attacking him, you are attacking yourself with the rash which is causing you so much distress." How might the patient experience this interpretation?

In the shoes of the patient we might expect her to feel criticized by this, even attacked by it, and that is almost certainly why she stopped coming to see her therapist. From that day she refused to see him again. (As a colleague once said of this kind of interpretation: "That is just adding insight to injury!")

We therefore need to anticipate a patient's likely reaction under similar circumstances so that we can interpret from a more neutral position. And we must remember that a patient's superego attacks at such times are often already so acute that it takes very little for an interpretation to be heard as from the superego in projection. To help deal with this it is necessary to be especially careful not to interpret in a way that is likely to amplify that process and to blur the distinction between external and internal realities.

When trying to interpret unconscious guilt I have found it helpful to use what I "know" analytically to find a way of approaching this through not (yet) knowing. For instance, if I were to have said to this patient: "You seem to be suffering a great deal from this rash" the patient might well have agreed, and she might have added other details of suffering. Eventually I might have been able to point out a more specific quality in these different forms of suffering: "It is almost as if you are experiencing this suffering as some kind of punishment." And, at some stage, I might even share the thought: "But, it is not clear what you are feeling guilty about." The patient might then feel free to explore this sense of guilt about something, perhaps still non-specific, or may begin talking about her mixed feelings for her husband about whom she used to be so nasty. At least the patient would not be so likely to feel that she was with someone who expected her to feel guilty, as if siding with the patient's superego, as the patient in the example probably felt.

The therapist could have taken more care not to side with the connection that the patient is making, between her having expressed some wish for the husband's death and his dying. When guilt is a reaction to this kind of false connection, based upon magical thinking, then we have to be careful that we do not appear to be assuming the same connection. If we speak as if we see the guilt and the connection all too clearly, from the patient's point of view that can be experienced as if we too believe that this is how the husband's death had been brought about, by her expressions of hate for him. Contrarily, "not knowing" the connection, but finding it in the patient's own communications, can help towards analyzing the unconscious guilt from a position that is not accepting any link between death and death-wishing as causal.

OTHER CLINICAL SITUATIONS

There are countless clinical events that we encounter in our daily work which can be used for practicing technique, creating "exercises" such as I have illustrated above, exploring each from the point of view of the patient. For instance:

- interpreting acting out (experienced as an attempt to contain through understanding or through superego control?)
- dealing with different kinds of silence (the risk of being intrusive or of being seen as retaliating with silence—the need to recognize the differences between silence as "being with," silence as resistance or as communication, etc.)
- dealing with a dilemma (recognizing that attention given to *this* could be seen by the patient as neglecting *that*, and vice versa)
- exploring the dynamics of reassurance (the patient's difficult feelings being seen as too much for the therapist)
- commenting on a patient's lateness (seen as attending to the communication in this or as rebuking the patient?)
- dealing with the therapist's lateness—offering make-up time (being fair or buying off the patient's anger?)
- offering an extra session at a time of acute distress (meeting a patient's need or communicating the therapist's view of the patient as not able to cope?)
- suggesting medication (seen as a necessary containment or as protecting the therapist from the patient's distress?)
- dealing with direct questions from the patient (seen as defensive in not answering or as seductive in doing so?).

The list could be endless.

CONCLUSION

Technical exercises such as those presented here may help us to see similar situations more readily when in the consulting-room. We may also be able to see more clearly why with a particular patient we might handle a difficult situation in one way and with another perhaps quite differently. This use of trial identification can therefore help us to work more specifically with the individual patient rather than fall into well-worn ways of thinking and interpreting. Herein lies the fascination in developing psychoanalytic technique and the reason why trying to find therapeutic ways of working within the analytic encounter remains for ever challenging.

❖ 20 ❖

The Analytic Space and Process

Some underlying themes of this book are highlighted here—two in particular: the nature of the mental and emotional space, which is provided by the analytic relationship, and the dynamics of the analytic process itself. It is suggested that, when the analytic space is kept sufficiently free from influences that could distort and disable it, the process that then unfolds can be trusted and followed.

> The frame marks off the different kind of reality
> that is within it from that which is outside it; but
> a temporal spatial frame also marks off the
> special kind of reality of a psycho-analytic
> session. And in psycho-analysis it is the existence
> of this frame that makes possible the full
> development of that creative illusion that
> analysts call transference.
>
> (MILNER 1952: 183)

INTRODUCTION

The mental and emotional space between people tends to be eroded by the claims that each person makes upon the other. The analytic space is unique in protecting the patient from such claims. The space within the analytic frame is kept separate from the world outside, allowing that particular kind of relating to develop in which the transference can freely emerge. Through the transference, the past experience of the patient represented in his/her internal world comes to be relived in the analytic relationship. It is this which so vividly brings into focus the ways whereby the patient's past still continues to spill into the present. In order to see these manifestations of transference most clearly, the world within this frame is protected as far as possible from influences other than those that emanate from the patient's past. If sufficient care is not given to this protection, the analyst can become a prime source of interfering influence. The analytic space will then be impaired and the analytic process deflected and/or distorted.

The analytic process is not created by the analyst. It has a dynamic of its own, a direction that expresses unconscious hope or the unconscious search of the patient, and often it seems to contain unconscious wisdom.

ANALYTIC SPACE

Rules and the Analytic Space

The analytic space needs to be protected from both external and internal influence. This protection is primarily provided by the arrangements for the analytic work.

The consulting-room space gives privacy and protection from intrusion by others; the set times, kept specifically for each patient, provide reliability and continuity; the professional ethic offers a guaranteed confidentiality and non-exploitation of the patient; and the relative anonymity of the analyst aims to keep to a minimum the impact upon the patient of knowing personal details about him/her. Normally, this framework can be taken for granted but many patients have to test it for themselves.

However, the analytic space is much more than this: it acknowledges the need for boundaries between people, and therefore respects a patient's need for boundaries, including those that are still needed to protect the ego from whatever it is not yet able to manage. When the need for such defenses has been sufficiently analyzed and understood, and when the patient is ready, they will be relinquished. They do not need to be removed by the analyst. The analytic space also offers a freedom from the intrusive pressures (influence, reassurance, advice, or moral judgment) that could arise from any personal or theoretical predisposition of the analyst. Pressure of any kind, in particular any sense of "ought" or "should" from the analyst, is antithetical to analysis, and so are preconceptions when these overrule the patient's experience and perception.

There are no rules for the patient. The only variation from this, which rarely has to be made explicit, is that communication can be in any form except through violence or physical contact. The only rules (in analysis) are those for the analyst, in particular those that protect the patient's space.

Freud never quite freed himself from some use of pressure: he still advocated the "fundamental rule" of free association. But his emphasis upon any departure from this (as a manifestation of resistance) could have the effect of bullying the patient, as if to say: "If you do not associate freely—we have ways of making you."[1] The concept and value of analytic space has therefore only gradually become apparent since Freud, and it was many years before Margaret Little said: "We no longer 'require' our patients to tell us everything that is in their minds. On the contrary, we give them permission to do so" (Little 1951: 39).

The Need for Space

The need, in analysis, for mental and emotional space is highlighted by the comparative absence of space in other relationships. To be healthy, every intimate relationship needs space and personal boundaries, and a corresponding respect by each person for the "otherness" of the other. Frequently, however, this space is either lacking or contaminated by intruding influences.

All parents, however well-intentioned, will impose pressures upon a child that come from needs and wishes of their own. With an infant, there will be such pressures as a wish for the baby to feed when expected, a wish for the baby to settle when convenient, and a need for the mother to be confirmed as a good mother by appreciative responses from her baby. The list could be endless. As we all know, such wishes and needs are not always met by the infant, nor should they be! But if a mother's expectations are too insistent, they can eventually result in compliant behavior and an impaired autonomy.[2]

With the older child, the wishes and needs of parents can be just as pressing but they are often more complex: a wish to see the child develop in a given way, a wish to influence choices, a need to be loved by the child: and so on. In all subsequent relationships, whether between friends, teacher and pupil, employer and employee, lovers or marital partners, etc., there will always be a pressure from each for some fitting into expectations, regardless of the needs of the other.

In these relationships there is less of the space that is typical of the analytic relationship. There may be physical space, leaving the other person alone, but that does not necessarily meet the emotional needs of the other. Spatial separation can amount to neglect; it can be experienced as rejection. Conversely, there may be insufficient separateness as in any relationship where one person controls or suffocates the other. The emotional needs of the person being possessed are often not recognized or attended to.

Frequently, therefore, it is an entirely new experience for a patient who comes into analysis (or into psychotherapy) to find that there can be space within an intimate relationship. And by "space," here, I am referring in particular to the freedom *to think* whatever, *to feel* whatever, *to express* whatever, and *to be* whatever belongs to the patient's spontaneity in the session and to his/her autonomous being.

Different Kinds of Playing

There are two particular realms of experience in which we can find precursors to what may later be found in the analytic space: I am thinking of *the capacity to be alone in the presence of another person* (Winnicott 1965: Chapter 2) and *playing*. These are closely related to each other, and I have tried to describe the interplay between them in my paper "Samuel Beckett's Relationship to His Mother-Tongue" (Casement 1982b).

> [Beckett] had intimately known this strangulation of his creativity from which there was no way on but back. He could not write whilst there was no room for creative play, and yet it was particularly in the ability to play with words, and with language, that his genius ultimately lay.
>
> Let us examine this area of creativity [at the point of its first appearance]. To be free to enter into imaginative and creative play a child needs there to be a space between himself and the mother, over which he has the autonomous rights of initiative. Given this space, which Winnicott (1965: Chapter 2) describes as "being alone in the presence of the mother," the child begins to explore the creative potential of this space. But this requires of the mother a sensitive reluctance to enter into this play area uninvited. If all goes well the playing child can put into this the products of his own imagination—being free to "include" her into, or out of, his play. He can use the mother's "absent" presence or her "present" absence as the warp and woof of his play. He can "create" or "uncreate" her at will, and thereby enjoy the magic of playing God and King over his own play-realm. The seeds of later creativity are sown and nurtured here. (Casement 1982b: 38)

Much else is nurtured here, not least of which is the capacity to offer to others a similar freedom to become and be themselves. Some people, however, can only discover this through the realization that this being "let be" had been missing for them in earlier life. Analysts in particular need to have, or need to develop, *a capacity to let the other person be.*

Unfortunately there are some parents who tend to take over their children's playing, which can result in a suppression of a child's natural spontaneity and capacity for imaginative play. Too many games, with rules invented by adults, can impair a child's development of autonomous playing. Of course there is a place for such adult-made games. But there is also a place for allowing a child to make up his/her own games without interference. For instance, a child left alone may use the counters for some board game—like Monopoly—to create an imaginary family, school, or farmyard, the different counters being used to represent whatever belongs to the invented game. It is a great loss if an adult intervenes by prematurely trying to impose the "rules" of the game, as if there were only one right way to play with a Monopoly set.

Creative play does not necessarily mean always playing alone; and this is the nature of an analysis when all is going well. In the first years this playing will often require the non-intrusive presence of a mother, or mother person, who is prepared to be included but equally prepared to be left out of her child's playing. The fact that she is not always included does not mean that her presence is not a necessary part of what is going on. It is often her background presence that provides the setting within which imaginative play can develop.

Example 20.1
A patient had been brought up by a mother who had frequently tried to control her play by providing whatever fitted in with the mother's idea of playing. When this patient herself became a mother she was careful not to impose a similar control upon her own child. Instead, she left toys and other objects around for her daughter to find, and to play with in her own way when she wished. Her baby soon developed a confidence in her own playing and she had very clear ideas about it.

When the grandmother was visiting, this baby (aged ten months) found her own imaginative play being interfered with: the grandmother tried to take it over, as she used to do with her own children and other grandchildren. This grandchild, however, had her own ways of dealing with her. Whenever the grandmother handed a toy to be played with, which did not fit into the child's own play, this toy would be tossed aside as something for which she had no use at the time. The child would continue with her own play, cuing the grandmother to keep out of it. She would not include her in this playing.

The mother had been more able to allow her daughter the freedom for creative play. She was often used as a background presence, providing security but not always being included, whilst at other times her child would actively draw her into taking part. There was no compliant playing here!

There are lessons in this for the analyst. Patients need to be allowed the freedom to use the analytic space in their own way, not to have imposed upon them the analyst's preconceptions. For some patients it is especially important that the analyst can remain in the background—not having to be the focus all the time of something called transference—to be included by the patient or to be used as a background presence whilst the patient continues with his/her own thoughts, feelings, associations.[3] The timing and nature of interventions by the analyst is a skill that is always having to be attuned to the individual patient.

Monitoring the Analytic Space

The analytic space represents a freedom to work with the patient at understanding whatever he or she brings. But this freedom depends upon there still being a "reflective viewpoint" within the analytic space, not entirely taken over by what is happening between analyst and patient, from which each can examine what has been going on between them.

The analyst needs to monitor regularly what is being put into the analytic space by him/herself, because whatever the analyst contributes to the interaction with the patient can either enhance the opportunities for analyzing what is happening in the analytic relationship, or it can deflect from this and confuse attempts at analytic understanding.[4] Within limits, an analyst can allow him/herself to be drawn into different kinds of relating to the patient (see below). But if the analyst begins to behave in ways that are too much like key figures in the patient's past, it will become difficult for the patient to recognize any transference element that may be attached to that behavior. The analytic space may then become lost—there being (at least temporarily) no "reflective viewpoint" possible from which to analyze anything as transference or projection. That loss of analytic space occurs whenever there is too little difference between what is now coming from the analyst and how others have previously behaved towards the patient. No analysis is then possible until a sufficient difference has been reestablished between the analyst's objective reality and whatever the patient may be putting on to the analyst (see Chapters 15 and 19).

THE ANALYTIC PROCESS

What happens within the analytic space, when all goes well, is the product of the analytic process. A primary element in this process is the unconscious expression of internal conflict and feeling-states that have previously been repressed for lack of any other way to "deal" with them. (This is a manifestation of unconscious hope; see Chapter 17.) However, contrary to the expectations of what common sense might suggest, the unconscious search here is not simply for better experience (see Chapters 15 and 16). It is for a sufficient security within which it may eventually come to feel safe enough for the patient to risk feeling again unsafe—in order to work through the feelings that had been associated with earlier difficult experiences. And whether that security can be found in the presence of the analyst will depend, to a large extent, on his/her ability to preserve the analytic space from the disturbances that can arise from the analyst's way of being with the patient.

When an analyst attempts to control the course of an analysis, the analytic space becomes constricted and the process is altered. What follows will then reflect the patient's responses to the analyst's influence. A lot may happen and changes ensue. However, changes that have been brought about under these conditions are not necessarily due to the analytic process: they may be more the product of an embattled relationship.

The analyst aims to be servant of the analytic process, not its master: firm when necessary, responsive to different kinds of need, but otherwise unobtrusive. The analyst's effectiveness is best demonstrated through learning to follow the analytic process, not in trying to control it. And when the analytic space is most clearly preserved for the patient, providing that unique opportunity for the patient to grow more fully into him/herself, the analytic process can be seen to have a life and direction of its own. Where it might lead cannot be anticipated, and what is then experienced by the patient goes far beyond the bounds of expectation.

The Analyst's Involvement with the Patient's Internal World

As we discover in the course of working analytically, all relating is mediated in some measure through the unconscious internal world of the patient by such processes as projection, projective identification, and transference. It is in order to identify most clearly the effects of these processes that the patient is given optimal freedom for these perceptual distortions to occur also within the analytic relationship.

It used to be suggested that the analyst should remain detached, an uninvolved observer and interpreter of the patient's transference as it unfolds. As I have already suggested (Chapter 18) it is now more widely recognized that the analyst, if he or she is not remaining defensively detached, will sooner or later become drawn into some interaction with the patient's internal drama, and this can be diagnostically useful. I believe that this level of response to the patient's unconscious is an essential part of the analytic process.

The technical point is that the analyst can allow him/herself, to a moderate degree, to become involved in the patient's psychic drama, as this emerges within the analytic relationship. I had provisionally called this "diagnostic response" or diagnostic countertransference (Casement 1973), and in 1976 Sandler said:

> Parallel to the "free-floating attention" of the analyst is what I should like to call his *free-floating responsiveness*. The analyst is, of course, not a machine in absolute self-control, only experiencing on the one hand, and delivering interpretations on the other, although much of the literature might seem to paint such a picture. Among many other things he talks, he greets the patient, he makes arrangements about practical matters, he may joke and, to some degree, allow his responses to depart from the classical psychoanalytic norm. My contention is that in the analyst's overt reactions to the patient as well as in his thoughts and feelings what can be called his "role-responsiveness" shows itself, not only in his feelings but also in his attitudes and behavior, as a crucial element in his "useful" countertransference. (Sandler 1976: 45)

When the analyst is drawn into some reenactment of the patient's internal drama different kinds of relating emerge. For instance, the analyst may become like one or other of the parents, or some other significant relationship, in ways that are typical of the patient's experience. It then becomes clearer what aspects of which object relationships are being relived. For this to be useful in the analysis, it is essential that the analyst also retain sufficient separateness from the interaction to be able to reflect upon it carefully before attempting to interpret (see Chapter 14). Otherwise there is a risk that the analyst may begin to "act-in," which will disturb the analytic process, making it more difficult to see what, in the current interaction, belongs to the patient and what to the analyst. It is then not easy to make use of such moments in a way that can be helpful to the patient. But when the reenactment is in response to the patient—and kept within careful limits—

the cues to what is needed are often being supplied (unconsciously) by the patient.

Example 20.2
A patient (Miss R.) had begun to talk more and more quietly in her sessions. I then had the problem of either continuing to point this out (at the risk of seeming to nag her, as I had already been asking her to speak up a bit) or trying to piece together as much as I could from what I was able to hear. Through listening in this way, I began to sense that there might be an important communication in the softness of her talking. As I could not hear her words, it was almost like having to listen to a preverbal child.

From the despairing tone of the patient's voice, I gradually formed the impression that she might be feeling hopeless because I was not understanding her. I then said to her: "I think that there is something important about the way in which you are talking to me—talking so that I can hardly hear. I could, again, have asked you to speak louder. Instead, I have realized that I will only pick up what you are trying to get across to me if I listen very carefully, as a mother might with her infant who does not have any words. And what I am sensing is that you are feeling that I am not in touch with you. I believe that this is what you need me to understand, that I am not at this moment understanding you."

The patient began to weep. When she was able to speak again she said: "But you understood that you did not understand. That is what makes the difference."

From this brief but important experience, Miss R. began to realize that her parents had seldom recognized when they had not been understanding her. They had too often assumed that they "knew." This realization was painful for her—the "pain of contrast." (This was all the more painful for Miss R. as she was still working through the loss of her earlier idealization of her parents, in particular that of her father.)

At different stages in an analysis the analyst is likely to be drawn into representing a wide range of "parental functions"—from that of the mother, who is drawn into a near-symbiotic closeness to her infant, to that of the father who needs to provide firmness and structure if the growing child is not to remain caught up in that earlier tie to the mother.

The analyst does not attempt *actively* to fulfill any of those parental functions. But, in my opinion, the analyst should not hold back from being used by the patient to represent them. And I would include here the mirroring function of the parent who is needed by the child for affirmation.

DIVERSE THEORIES: DIVERSE APPLICATIONS

The diversity of human experience defies definition, though the desire to demonstrate the notion that psychoanalysis is a science has tempted some analysts to offer definitive explanations of human interaction. There is an inescapable conflict in this. On the one hand, we need to be familiar with whatever can be established as common clinical experience: without a sufficient framework, we would be relying too much upon guesswork and intuition. On the other hand, we are constantly being challenged to discover what else may apply better to the individual patient. Because the diversity of human interaction goes so far beyond the strictures of any science, what we do as analysts will not always be manifestly consistent or without its contradictions.[5]

Different patients need different approaches. Most patients at some time need firmness, to provide containment for states that are chaotic or which threaten to get out of control. But also, many at some time need to feel that they are with an analyst who can offer an exploratory space within which the patient's own individuality and creativity can develop more fully. Analysts therefore need to acquire the capacity to work in different ways at different times.

I also think that it is salutary to remember that each school of psychoanalysis has been developed over years, from clinical experience viewed in different ways. Different schools have come into being (as with schismatic groups in religion) through a recognition that there had been some serious omission, or overemphasis, in the thinking of other schools. The part-truth newly highlighted by fresh thinking all too often comes to be elevated as being *the truth*, at which point this new position also begins to qualify for criticism and correction by others. In human affairs there cannot be any one view that excludes all others.[6]

The proponents of various analytic theories, and the different techniques that have evolved around them, often vie with each other as if one school of psychoanalysis were right and the others therefore wrong. What is overlooked in this rivalry is the degree to which individual analysts are drawn to theoretical and technical positions that *fit their own personalities*. Inevitably, analysts will themselves have been more helped by some theories than by others. It is natural that they will more readily see their patients in terms of those particular theories and the issues pertaining to them. Also, to some extent all analysts are influenced, in the way that they work, by the nature of their own personalities. Thus, the aggressive person may become a belligerent analyst, the insecure either dogmatic or passive, the indecisive exaggeratedly open-minded, the narcissistic too often insistent that they must be right, and so on. I believe that the personal contribution to styles of working is not recognized often enough for what it is and dealt with in the training analysis or, later, by means of self-analysis.

It is not just a matter of different styles that is needed: the analyst may also need to draw upon a range of different theories, to encompass the diversity of clinical phenomena that will be encountered. For example: the nature of many patients' problems still requires the analyst to draw especially upon Freud's theories of libido and theories of conflict. The problems of others, however, are so clearly related to early environmental failure that the analyst will be better helped by the theories of other writers such as Winnicott. With yet other patients, the analyst needs to be familiar with Kleinian contributions to our understanding of such phenomena as the dynamics of destructive narcissism. With others, again, the analyst will need to understand the search for ameliorative self-experience and may be better helped by ideas drawn from Kohut's self psychology.[7]

In my opinion, therefore, analysts cannot afford to be too monogamously wedded to one particular theory. They will be better helped in their clinical work if they are willing to learn even from analysts whose theories and technique are quite at variance with their own. The reluctance to do this is understandable. But without this inter-group learning there is a tendency for positions on theory and technique to become fossilized, with opportunities for creative interchange lost in the process of sterile rivalry.[8]

Important clinical opportunities are also missed if there is too fixed an adherence either to a technical position which stresses the malignancy of the patient's pathology, or to one that overstates the benign nature of the unconscious. Because of the diversity of the unconscious, in which contradictions can co-exist, we have to tolerate the discovery that logically opposite formulations can each, at different times, be true. Much discord between different theoretical positions may have grown out of an inability to face this clinical fact. Human truth cannot be unified. At times it requires paradox to contain it. And the patient will not necessarily be confused, as some people assume, in the face of different bodies of theory. When an analyst discovers insight *alongside* the patient, and does not impose it dogmatically, a process of synthesis takes place within the patient, from which a coherent understanding gradually emerges, based upon those insights that have most helped to make sense of the patient's experience.

DIFFERENT APPROACHES TO PSYCHIC DEPTH: THE PSYCHOTIC EXPERIENCE IN ANALYSIS

One crucial difference in technique distinguishes those who attempt to control the analytic process from those who attempt to follow it. These represent very different schools of thought about the "correct" approach to the deep unconscious.

One approach is to proceed from surface to depth—analyzing defense and resistance before content, ego before id. The rationale is that defenses have been necessary to the patient, so that "the analyst's interventions should aim at making the patient's reasonable ego better able to cope with the old danger situations" (Greenson 1967: 138).

The Kleinian approach, on the other hand, is to interpret the deepest anxiety immediately:

> My view, based on empiric observation, [is] that the analyst should not shy away from making a deep interpretation even at the start of the analysis, since the material belonging to a deeper layer of the mind will come back again later and be worked through. As I have said before, the function of deep going interpretation is simply to open the door to the unconscious, to diminish the anxiety that has been stirred up and thus to prepare the way for analytic work. (Klein 1932: 24)

For Kleinian analysts, therefore, the focus for an interpretation is aimed at the point of greatest urgency—the most immediate anxiety. But how that point of urgency is identified can be assessed in various ways by different analysts.

The Implications of Interpretive Activity

Different consequences follow from contrasting views of the analytic process and space, and these are demonstrated in the different levels of interpretive activity that reflect each view.

There are analysts who regard the dynamics of the patient's unconscious as potentially so destructive that they think they must always be in control of the analytic process. The result is often that the analyst is very active, and I think that the patient's responses to that activity often reflect the disturbing quality of these attempts to control everything that happens in the analytic space. It is debatable how much of the paranoid material that emerges in the course of such an analysis is necessarily a primary expression of the patient's internal world: *some* of it at least is likely to be in response to the analyst's manner of working.

> Once the analyst departs from sparing, provisional interpretations, he not only disturbs the listening situation but has made it difficult to reestablish it. He ought therefore to make up his mind beforehand what policy he is going to pursue. (Glover 1955: 96)

There is still a lot to be learned about how best to preserve the analytic space so that the analytic process can freely unfold. This is what I was intuitively trying to do in my work with Joy (Chapter 13) and more consciously ever since. It has been my experience that, though I do not actively search for the psychotic areas in a patient's personality, but address myself to whatever is emerging in the course of an analysis, patients eventually feel safe enough to bring their hidden psychotic states into the analysis. An important element in this development is the gradual building of trust during the analytic work that has gone before. This allows a patient to "abandon" that trust for a while and to enter into a state that may, intermittently, become deeply distrusting. However, the basic trust that had been built up before is not necessarily destroyed or completely lost. Instead, it seems to be relegated to a background position, to the working alliance. Sometimes, even that may seem to be in abeyance but, nevertheless, it is not altogether absent.

It is within this context, of allowing the analytic process to unfold in its own way, that a patient can feel safe enough to risk feeling psychotically unsafe within the analytic relationship. I therefore believe that, when sufficient time has been given (or has been possible) for establishing a background of trust, the timing of this emergence of psychotic states in the analysis reflects the patient's readiness for this and is a true expression of the analytic process.[9]

When a patient is manifestly psychotic it frequently requires extraordinary skill and mental agility to contain what has become uncontained. Therefore, when an analyst *goes* for the psychotic depth, I think that there may be some patients who feel stripped of the defenses that had been needed to keep psychotic areas contained. The result may then be that virulent psychotic states break out, as if to punish the analyst who has removed that defensive containment. Perhaps the patient is also challenging the analyst to take over total management of his/her unconscious, when the analyst has acted as if everything about the patient's thinking were within the analyst's competence to know and to control. Could it be, I have wondered, that some of the florid part-object material that seems typical of some analyses is the result of too much having been released from the unconscious too quickly? And may this kind of experience contribute to the view that some analysts seem to have of their patients—as if they were always dealing with such malignant forces in the unconscious that they do not feel able to recognize anything in the patient's deep unconscious that they can safely trust?

Every patient has some psychotic areas and these do usually come into an analysis sooner or later, if they are not deflected by the analyst. But I do not, personally, "go" for these depths. Instead, I try to make it possible for them to emerge more safely in the patient's own time, when sufficient ego strengths have been developed for the patient to be able to tolerate that experience. This may explain why I do not so often encounter fragmentation of the ego to quite the same degree as we find in some clinical accounts from analysts who work differently.

An issue of technique here is that, for mental and emotional space to exist between people, there have to be boundaries to the personality of each. When a patient's ego is unable to maintain these boundaries, the analytic space becomes at times invaded by "bizarre contents," resulting from the processes of splitting and projection taking place in the patient's mind. Analysts, therefore, have to be able to "field" these projections (or transferences) as best they can, to understand them and the dynamics behind them. But the degree of interpretive activity which may then seem to be necessary can also invade the analytic space. That is why I believe that it is preferable for analysts to meet whatever emerges from the patient's unconscious, with the firmness appropriate to contain it, rather than to get into the patient's mind in an anticipatory way. The attempt at analyzing what emerges from the patient's mind gets complicated if it arises largely in response to the analyst's ways of interpreting. And it is even more confusing for patients if they are then expected to own such responses as if they were originating, unprovoked, solely from within themselves.

PROFOUND EXPERIENCE

As indicated in Chapter 16, the gains in analysis are by no means limited to insight or to those changes that follow from interpreting the transference. There are times when significant change takes place around an experience that can be regarded as "profound" even if not specifically an experience of the transference. For instance, a patient can be profoundly affected by experiencing something quite new in the analysis, or by reexperiencing something that had been "forgotten" and lost. Unlike other profound experiences, which may be encountered in solitude, this always involves both participants in the analytic relationship.

Example 20.3
Mrs. S. (aged 44) was a patient who had remained hidden for most of her life behind a facade of false-self compliance. She did what was expected of her, fearing that if she did not she would be rejected.

One day Mrs. S. said to me: "You sometimes try too hard to understand me." This prompted me to realize that there was something else that she needed from me, but it was not yet clear what this was. A few weeks later she came very punctually to a session but she did not speak. For the whole session she remained silent. During this time I was wondering what to make of this. Was she resisting? (The atmosphere did not feel combative.) Was she needing me to reach out to her, to help her out of the silence? (She showed no signs of tension or anxiety.) Was she distressed, needing me to be aware of that? (There was a sense of calm and peacefulness in the session—no sense of distress.) I then felt that she needed me just to *let her be.*

Towards the end of the session I began to wonder how to deal with the ending. If I said nothing this could be unhelpfully ambiguous. It could be misunderstood as retaliatory. And, if the experience had been as I was now sensing, it would have been a pity to have spoiled that by leaving the patient with an uncertainty as to how I had understood it. I therefore said: "I have not felt that there was any need for me to speak in this session. But, before we end for today, it might help if I tell you where I have been in the silence. I have been remembering the time, a few weeks ago, when you told me that I had been trying too hard to understand." After a pause the patient got up to leave, and at the door she said: "Thank you."

The next day Mrs. S. lay in silence with the same atmosphere of calm. Throughout the session she said nothing and neither did I. There was no need now, I felt, to explain where I was in this further silence. At the end she got up to leave and, once again, she said: "Thank you." And the day following Mrs. S. said to me: "I want to thank you for not speaking. I felt more real in those last two sessions than I have ever felt before. *You allowed me to BE.*"

This experience, although profound, could not alone change this patient's life. But it could serve as a touchstone-experience, by which she began to recognize the difference between feeling real and being compliant. It could act as a pointer for the realness she still needed to find in herself.

Example 20.4

Since he had begun to go to school, Mr. T. (aged 29) had been crippled by the neurotic conversion of difficult feelings into a compelling need to go frequently to the toilet. There, in the form of faeces, he would symbolically get rid of his feelings, safely into the toilet.

Mr. T. had learned from his mother that she could not bear to be confronted by any distress of his. He had therefore developed ways in which he could keep his mother from breaking down, even keep her alive, by taking care that he never expressed to her any feelings that she might not be able to cope with. *He* mothered *her*. In particular Mr. T. could not express anger. I therefore began to feel sure that this patient had never been able to communicate through projective identification (getting his mother to feel what he could not manage on his own), and these feelings had come to be regarded by him as for ever unmanageable, even lethal.

In one session Mr. T. emphasized that it was largely to avoid humiliation that he had to go so frequently to the toilet. In association to this, he added that he felt sure that if he did ever express really what he felt he would be humiliated for that too. He was also afraid that I did not realize what I was asking of him when I spoke as if he might become able to show me more directly what he was feeling. He felt sure that I would retaliate if he did, like his parents. His mother could not bear to be confronted with what he was feeling, neither could his father.

I replied that he seemed to see me as a sadistic surgeon who, when lancing a boil, would blame the patient for the mess that emerged. I added that he seemed to have no sense that a surgeon who knows his business would also take care of the mess, as part of enabling the boil to discharge its poison. Mr. T. retorted that it was easy for me to say that: "But it's just words."

I reflected upon this response and realized that I had used this analogy before—with another patient some years ago. It was not new, so I could readily see how it might sound like "just words." Also, I had thought first of an analogy that was surgical and therefore distant. From this internal supervision a quite different image came into my mind.

I then said: "Another image has now come to me, and I am not going to bother whether it could be medically correct: I shall use it just as it comes to me. I see a mother holding her sick child on her lap. The child has an obstruction of the bowel from which the child will die if it cannot be relieved of this. But the mother senses that, if she can hold her child securely enough, he may be able to let this go and he will not die. I can then imagine the mother's tears of relief upon finding that her child's bowel has functioned again as it should. She will not give a thought to the mess this might have created in her lap, for the joy of knowing that her child will not die."

Mr. T. followed this description in silence, obviously moved. When I had finished speaking I noticed that he was silently crying. This was something quite new in his analysis.

After a period of quiet reflection Mr. T. said: "For the first time I can see the possibility that there can be some hope that I could become freed of my symptoms. Until now I have really just been going through the motions of analysis, not really believing that it could make any difference at all."

This was merely the beginning of a beginning. But, from that day, Mr. T. began to discover that he did not still have to protect me from his feelings by going to the toilet several times on most days before coming to his sessions. Instead, he began to bring his feelings to me more directly. At first he could usually tell me only about what he had been feeling before he came. Gradually, however, he began to express his feelings as he experienced them in the session: they did not have to be converted into symptoms and "got rid of" down toilets. Rather, a person could be available to him to receive whatever he was feeling and to help him with that. This was an entirely new discovery. It was a truly profound and transformative experience.

Mr. T. also began to discover that the analytic space was there specifically for him, and it was provided by a person. Into this space he now began to be able to express his own most dreaded feelings; and within this space he could find a *personal* containment which began to change his experience of them. They could become, once again, a communication of distress in search of a personal response—with a renewed hope of finding it.

When such changes occur in an analysis the implications can be far reaching, even to the point of changing a person's life. Some patients communicate and relate in new ways; their view of themselves and of others changes radically; the sense that feelings are dangerous gives way when they discover that another person has after all been containing and managing them so that the former view of these feelings (as unmanageable) does not have to dominate the rest of life. Without that beginning there can be no growth. But when the process of growth is renewed it can continue.

CONCLUSION

In this book and its predecessor (Part One) I have described some of my own clinical explorations and my wondering about the processes involved in the analytic encounter.

During this quest, I have had to recognize (like a climber) the limits of my own competence—to know when I must follow a guide or to stay on the "beaten track." And whilst I have been exploring away from the more usual routes, I have always sensed the need still to be held by the life-lines of classical theory and technique, to save me from falling or to help me find my way back when I have begun to get lost.

Inevitably, in the course of my journey I have made my share of mistakes, learning from which has always been important: but along the way I have also had many surprises. I have found much that has confirmed what I had previously accepted only provisionally (and reluctantly) upon the authority of others.

The analytic journey is often difficult and painful for analyst as well as patient, quite frequently bewildering, and at times awesome. Progress is slow and sometimes intermittent. Nevertheless, working with the analytic process can at the same time be extraordinarily enriching (to both participants) as true aliveness is rediscovered, as creativity is released from what had been blocking it, and as patients recover the capacity to be more fully themselves and to be playful.

The Question

Will you, sometime, who have sought so long and seek
Still in the slowly darkening hunting ground,
Catch sight some ordinary month or week
Of that strange quarry you scarcely thought you sought—
Yourself, the gatherer gathered, the finder found,
The buyer, who would buy all, in bounty bought—
And perch in pride on the princely hand, at home,
And there, the long hunt over, rest and roam?

(MUIR 1984: 122)

❖ APPENDIX I ❖

Knowing and Not-Knowing:
Winnicott and Bion

FROM WINNICOTT

"An infant is merged with the mother.... A change, however, comes with the end of merging.... The mother seems to know that the infant has a new capacity, that of giving a signal so that she can be guided towards meeting the infant's needs. It could be said that if now she knows too well what the infant needs, this is magic and forms no basis for an object relationship.... We find this subtlety appearing clearly in the transference in our analytic work. It is very important, except when the patient is regressed to earliest infancy and to a state of merging, that the analyst shall *not* know the answers except in so far as the patient gives the clues. The analyst gathers the clues and makes the interpretations, and it often happens that patients fail to give the clues, making certain thereby that the analyst can do nothing. This limitation of the analyst's power is important to the patient, just as the analyst's power is important, represented by the interpretation that is right and that is made at the right moment, and that is based on the clues and the unconscious cooperation of the patient who is supplying the material which builds up and justifies the interpretation. In this way the student analyst sometimes does better analysis than he will do in a few years' time when he knows more. When he has had several patients he begins to find it irksome to go as slowly as the patient is going, and he begins to make interpretations based not on material supplied on that particular day by the patient but on his own accumulated knowledge or his adherence for the time being to a particular group of ideas. This is of no use to the patient. The analyst may appear to be very clever, and the patient may express admiration, but in the end the correct interpretation is a trauma, which the patient has to reject, because it is not his. (Winnicott 1965b: 50-1)

"What I have to say... is extremely simple. Although it comes out of my psychoanalytical experience I would not say that it could have come out of my psychoanalytical experience of two decades ago, because I would not then have had the technique to make possible the transference movements that I wish to describe. For instance, it is only in recent years that I have become able to wait and wait for the natural evolution of the transference arising out of the patient's growing trust in the psychoanalytic technique and setting, and to avoid breaking up this natural process by making interpretations.... If only we can wait, the patient arrives at understanding creatively and with immense joy, and I now enjoy this joy more than I used to enjoy the sense of having been clever. I think I interpret mainly to let the patient know the limits of my understanding. The principle is that it is the patient and only the patient who has the answers." (Winnicott 1971: 86–7)

FROM BION

"Discard your memory; discard the future tense of your desire; forget them both, both what you knew and what you want, to leave space for a new idea. A thought, an idea unclaimed, may be floating around the room searching for a home. Amongst these may be one of your own which seems to turn up from your insides, or one from outside yourself, namely, from the patient." (Bion 1980: 11)

"Instead of trying to bring a brilliant, intelligent, knowledgeable light to bear on obscure problems, I suggest we bring to bear a diminution of the light—a penetrating beam of darkness; a reciprocal of the searchlight.... The darkness would be so absolute that it would achieve a luminous, absolute vacuum. So that, if any object existed, however faint, it would show up very clearly. Thus, a very faint light would become visible in maximum conditions of darkness." (Bion 1974: 37)

"Psycho-analysts must be able to tolerate the differences or the difficulties of the analysand long enough to recognize what they are. If psycho-analysts are to be able to interpret what the analysand says, they must have a great capacity for tolerating their analysands' statements without rushing to the conclusion that they know the interpretations. This is what I think Keats meant when he said that Shakespeare must have been able to tolerate negative capability." (Bion 1974: 72)

"...*Negative Capability*, that is, when a man is capable of being in uncertainties, mysteries, doubts, without any irritable reaching after fact and reason." (John Keats: Letter to George and Thomas Keats, 21 December 1817)

❖ APPENDIX II ❖

The Issues of Confidentiality and of Exposure by the Therapist

There are a number of important issues to be considered, around the question of confidentiality, before we can think of using clinical material for the purposes of shared learning about psychoanalysis and psychotherapy.

It is generally accepted that patients in analysis and therapy have an absolute right to expect total confidentiality. They must, therefore, always be protected from exposure in any clinical material that is used for teaching or publication. So, every analyst and therapist is faced with the ethical question "Whether or not to publish, or to use for teaching, clinical material that others might be able to learn from?"

There are various ways of dealing with this dilemma. We could try to ban any shared learning, in the name of preserving a total confidentiality; but it is doubtful that we could help our patients even as much as we sometimes do, if we were unable to learn from the work of others in the field. We could insist that we never publish, or use for teaching purposes, anything from a patient's treatment without permission from that patient. However, asking a patient about possible publication, during the course of therapy or analysis, introduces an intrusive factor into the analytic process. Some patients are unable to cope with this "rocking the boat" of the analytic experience, and it will always rock it. We cannot always assess correctly when it is right to ask for that permission from a patient. It may never be right.

We could, instead, confine ourselves to clinical material from patients who have finished their treatment, asking then for permission to publish. This too is not without its problems. When patients leave therapy it is their right to be left free from continuing contact with the therapist. One

359

would not want to interfere with the achieved separateness that is aimed for at the close of therapy or analysis. Moreover, such continuing contact can get in the way of a patient's freedom to return for further treatment.

One safeguard could be to wait a minimum period (some say ten years) after treatment is concluded before publishing any clinical material; but this slows down the process of shared learning. Another way to preserve patients' freedom, and their right to absolute confidentiality, is to use clinical material from other people's work with patients. This has many advantages; but it can shift the burden of the problem onto others. It can also be a way of therapists preserving themselves from the critical assessment by others which they may *need* in order to improve their understanding.

For this reason I have decided not to hide my work from examination by others; and I have been influenced in this by my impression that clinical presentations (spoken or published) too often show the presenter in a good light. Analysts and therapists do not so readily share their failures, but I think that more can be gained by all when some are prepared to do so.

I have also used disguised examples from clinical work that I have supervised. I trust that no student therapist will feel a sense of injury from this sharing of their struggles to become better therapists. Having decided to publish, I have dealt with the issues of confidentiality and permission for publication with careful consideration of the over-all situation for each patient concerned, and for those I have supervised.

I hope that the clinical vignettes in this book, and the longer clinical presentations, will provide useful learning material. There were certainly many lessons for me contained in these examples. If others can learn from the self-exposure involved I believe that this will have been worthwhile.

I cannot speak for the patients concerned or for the people I have supervised. Those who have given their permission for publication will, I trust, recognize the care with which I preserve their anonymity. I wish to believe that those others from whom (for whatever reason) I have preferred not to ask permission, will not recognize themselves. If any patient or student does, I trust that they can still preserve their own freedom not to have themselves identified by anyone else.

I hope that this book will not deter any patient from seeking analytic help. Rather, it is my wish that it may help to promote an analytic atmosphere in which patients can expect to be better listened to.

I am indebted to all those I have worked with, for what I have learned from them, without which this book could never have been written. If patients (or those I have supervised) have gained as much from the clinical encounter as I have, I hope they may be glad that I have considered it to be worth sharing some of this with others.

❖ ❖

Notes

Chapter 1

1. I first heard of Matte Blanco's use of these concepts, unconscious symmetry and sets, in a paper presented to the British Psycho-Analytical Society in 1980, by Eric Rayner. A version of that paper has now been published: "Infinite Experiences, Affects and the Characteristics of the Unconscious" (Rayner 1981).

2. Since writing this chapter, I have been pleased to find Sandler expressing similar thoughts in his paper "Reflections on some Relations between Psychoanalytic Concepts and Psychoanalytic Practice." In this he says:

   > The conviction that what is actually done in the analytic consulting room is not "kosher", that colleagues would criticize it if they knew about it, comes from the reality that any analyst worth his salt will adapt to specific patients on the basis of his interaction with those patients. He will modify his approach so that he can get as good as possible a working analytic situation developing. To achieve this he needs to feel relaxed and informal with his patient to an appropriate degree, and at times he might have to depart quite far from standard technique. (Sandler 1983: 38)

3. Sandler begins his paper (quoted above) by saying:

   > If one looks carefully one can find an implicit unconscious assumption in many psychoanalytic writings that our theory should aim to be a body of ideas that is essentially complete and organized, with each part being fully integrated with every other.

   He later continues:

   > There are advantages to emphasizing the developmental-historical dimension in psychoanalysis when we think of theoretical matters. It allows us to escape—it we want to—quarrels about which theory is right and which is wrong. Rather, it puts us in the position of asking Why

was this, that or the other formulation put forward? and What did its authors mean? (Sandler 1983: 35)

Chapter 2

1. In the paper referred to (originally presented to social workers) I suggest that, when there are two people working together with a family or marital couple, it is important to establish a "supervisory viewpoint" to which each worker can refer in thinking about what is happening in the interview or session. From this viewpoint, the social workers concerned can examine the interaction between them for ways in which this may be reflecting unconscious aspects of the family or marital interaction. The clinical value of this later prompted me to consider using a similar reference point, within the single worker or therapist, which I now call the "internal supervisor." (I outline this paper here as it is likely, by now, to be out of print.)

2. It may help the reader to know that all the extended clinical presentations in this book (Chapters 3, 5, 7, and 9) were written before my thinking in this present chapter had been formulated. In fact it was that work, with those earlier patients, which prompted me to examine more closely the processes upon which I have in particular focused in this chapter.

3. I outline what I mean by an interactional viewpoint in the next chapter.

Chapter 3

1. I am indebted to Langs for prompting me to look more closely into this dimension of the therapeutic relationship. He speaks of "the interactional-adaptational viewpoint," and sets out a detailed and systematic schema for listening (Langs 1978). I do not wish to describe that here. I wish only to outline an attitude to listening that includes an awareness of the patient's perception of the therapist's reality, and some responses to that reality.

2. The clinical account presented in this chapter is an extract from my paper "The Reflective Potential of the Patient as Mirror to the Therapist." In James O. Raney (ed.) (1984) *Listening and Interpreting: The Challenge of the Work of Robert Langs*, New York: Jason Aronson.

3. Marion Milner compares the function of the analytic frame to the part that is played by the frame of a picture in art:

> The frame marks off the different kind of reality that is within it from that which is outside it; but a temporal spatial frame also marks off the special kind of reality of a psycho-analytic session. And in psycho-analysis it is the existence of this frame that makes possible the full development of that creative illusion that analysts call transference. (Milner 1952: 183)

Chapter 4

1. Earlier in the same paper, Freud wishes to:

distinguish between using the words 'conscious' and 'unconscious' sometimes in a descriptive and sometimes in a systematic sense, in which latter they signify inclusion in particular systems and possession of certain characteristics (Freud 1915: 172).

He later goes on to say:

Perhaps we may look for some assistance from the proposal to employ, at any rate in writing, the abbreviation *Cs.* for consciousness and *Ucs.* for what is unconscious, when we are using the two words in the systematic sense. " (Freud 1915: 172)

2. A similar description of this process is give by Wangh (1962), in which he speaks of the "Evocation of a Proxy."

3. Projective identification as a concept is variously used to describe aspects of early psychic development in the infant (Klein 1952; Segal 1964), a primitive form of communication (Bion 1967b, for example), and for describing psychotic processes (Rosenfeld 1965; Bion 1967b). I am aware of the emphasis that Kleinians put upon splitting as involved in projective identification, but I am not including this in my present discussion of this concept. Projective identification is also used differently by Kleinians and other analysts, as discussed by (Grotstein (1981) and Ogden (1982).

4. Rosenfeld (1971) distinguishes between projective identification used for communication and projective identification used for ridding the self of unwanted parts. He adds a third use of this, where the psychotic patient aims at controlling the analyst's body and mind. He points out that this seems to be based on a very early infantile type of object relationship. He also emphasizes that these three types of projective identification exist simultaneously in the psychotic patient, and that it is important not to concentrate on one form of this process alone when dealing with psychotics. (I am confining myself here to considering the use of projective identification by non-psychotics.)

5. The notion of "double-bind" was first suggested by Bateson et al. 1956). It is used to describe a situation in which contradictory demands are being put upon a child (or patient, see Laing 1961) in such a way that there is no avenue of escape or challenge. (See also Rycroft 1968.)

6. Lucia Tower gives a similar example, in her paper "Countertransference," in which she forgot a patient's session. This prompted her to recognize that her repressed irritation with this patient had been maintained by a reaction formation of "infinite patience." She adds that a denied negative countertransference can at times result in "a negative countertransference structure, virtually a short-lived countertransference neurosis," unless something precipitates the necessary resolution of this which her own acting out against her patient helped to bring about (Tower 1956: 238).

7. See, for instance, Orr (1954), Kernberg (1965), Laplanche and Pon-

talis (1973), Sandler, Dare and Holder (1973), Epstein and Feiner (1979).

Chapter 5

1. The clinical sequence presented in this chapter is an extract from my paper, "The Reflective Potential of the Patient as Mirror to the Therapist." In James O. Raney (ed.) (1984) *Listening and Interpreting: The Challenge of the Work of Robert Langs.* New York: Jason Aronson.
2. I have noticed, with a number of patients, that the experience of *feeling better* is sometimes treated by the patient as a signal for further anxiety. Some analysts might treat this as a fear of losing the "secondary gains from illness." Others might regard it as "negative therapeutic reaction." However, I believe there are some occasions when a patient is indicating that an unconscious link has been formed between an earlier experience of trauma and the prior sense of safety, as if that "safety" had been a warning signal for the pending disaster. Perhaps an unconscious set is formed in which feeling safe and subsequent catastrophe are seen as forever linked.
3. Winnicott says: "That which has been dreamed and remembered and presented is within the capacity of the ego-strength and structure" (Winnicott 1965: 254).

Chapter 6

1. I am not confining myself to Bion's view of containment, but it may be useful to have a description of that. In his book *Splitting and Projective Identication,* Grotstein says of this:

   Bion's conception is of an elaborated primary process activity which acts like a *prism* to refract the intense hue of the infant's screams into the components of the color spectrum, so to speak, so as to sort them out and relegate them to a hierarchy of importance and of mental action. Thus, containment for Bion is a very active process which involves feeling, thinking, organizing, and acting. Silence would be the least part of it. (Grotstein 1981: 134)

Chapter 7

1. This chapter is a revised version of my paper "Some Pressures on the Analyst for Physical Contact during the Re-Living of an Early Trauma," which was presented at the 32nd International Psychoanalytical Congress, Helsinki, July 1981, and first published in the *International Review of Psycho-Analysis* (Casement 1982a).

Chapter 8

1. In speaking of an innate search for what is needed, I realize that this issue is more complex than I imply in the main text. I do not wish to overlook that an infant's perception of the "object" is distorted by his or her own feelings, by the aggressive or "death" instinct, by the splitting of good and bad, by the projection of bad feelings into the "feeding object," and by a multiplicity of other complicating factors.

"These get in the way of any easy finding of what is needed, or easy providing of it.

2. Winnicott speaks of "ego-needs" which are very similar to the growth-needs as described here (Winnicott 1965b: Chapter 4).
3. Since writing this, the paper by Fox, "The Concept of Abstinence Re-Considered" (1984) has been published. The author advocates a more discriminating application of the technical concept of abstinence. Part of his argument is based upon a discussion of the clinical sequence given above in Chapter 7, as previously published (Casement 1982a).
4. Analysts have been slow to drop the practice of giving the "basic rule" to patients, even though it has been realized that this can create resistance. Over thirty years ago, Margaret Little said: "We no longer "require" our patients to tell us everything that is in their minds. On the contrary, we give them permission to do so" (Little 1951: 39). In many training institutions the "basic rule" still seems to be given.

Chapter 9

1. Although this chapter follows on naturally from the preceding chapter, the work described was done before I had formulated my thoughts on the processes of internal supervision (described in Chapter 2). The reader will be able to recognize that I am here just beginning to find my way towards that.

Chapter 11

1. This chapter is a revised version of a paper that was originally entitled "Between the lines: *On Learning from the Patient*—Before and after," previously published in *The British Journal of Psychotherapy* 4: 86–93 (1987).
2. A description of projective identification, along with all the relevant references, may be found in *A Dictionary of Kleinian Thought* (Hinshelwood 1989: 179–208).
3. See Winnicott's "spatula game" (1958: Chapters 3 and 4; 1989: Chapter 40).
4. I am a member of the Independent Analysts' Group of the British Psycho-Analytical Society, as distinct from the Kleinians and what are now called the Contemporary Freudians.

Chapter 12

1. An earlier version of this chapter was presented as a paper at the British Association of Psychotherapists' Annual Conference, November 1985. It was also presented to numerous meetings of psychotherapists, and psychotherapy training associations, in and around London. It has been previously published in *Free Associations* 5:90–104 (1986); also in *The Bulletin of the British Association of Psychotherapists*: 3–16 (1986).
2. What I am describing as a "transferential attitude" to elements of

the clinical situation is not transference in the classical sense—nor is it truly countertransference. It does, however, have some similarity to the definition of countertransference as the analyst's transference towards the patient (Reich 1951; Gitelson 1952). Reich says of this: "In such cases the patient represents for the analyst an object of the past on to whom past feelings and wishes are projected" (1951: 26). What is transferred in the transferential attitude is, of course, not a past object relationship: it is the understanding of some other clinical experience which is attributed to present clinical phenomena. The sense of similarity triggers a transferential attitude, just as transference too is triggered by some element of similarity which is treated as sameness.

3. This example is described more fully elsewhere (see pp. 22–23).
4. I have discussed this case more fully elsewhere (see pp. 77–80 and 114–115).

Chapter 13
1. Dilys Daws, a child psychotherapist, said of this clinical sequence:

> The problem between Joy and her mother is not just that Joy is *not* a boy, but that she *is* a girl. As you point out, some of her exploration is to find her female genitals, as something positive, not just as lack of penis. However I think this is part of her problem, i.e. that she is the *same* as her mother with all the identification/rivalry issues that ensue.
>
> I cannot know, but would guess that her mother had a serious postnatal depression after Joy's birth, triggered by Joy being a girl. The lack of contact between them (which was not the case with the boys) may be the result of such a period, which makes it difficult for a mother to pick up cues from the baby and to respond to them. If there was such a period, and it was because Joy was a girl and not because of some other factor, then this might have been stirred up by the mother possibly having had a difficult relationship with her own mother, and the birth of a daughter facing her with having to deal with a mother-daughter relationship all over again. (Difficult births can also stir up the same sequence of postnatal trauma and a problem in making contact with the new baby.) Both mother and Joy may have felt that life would be much simpler if all these issues could be avoided by a preference for boys and penises! I think there are hints of all this from session 16 onwards. (Dilys Daws: personal correspondence)

I think that this hypothetical view offers a most plausible background for the relationship between Joy and her mother. My difficulty at the time was that I was not given proper referral information for psychotherapy with this child; and having been given the mixed brief that I was, to be a reading teacher "with an eye to the therapeutic need," I was hardly in a position to find out such personal details from the mother. And now, these many years later, I think it would be improper to ask. Further detail on the effects of postnatal depression upon the subsequent relationship between mother and infant can be found in *Through the Night* (Daws 1989: Chapter 13).

Chapter 14

1. This chapter is based upon a paper that was written by invitation, and published in *Contemporary Psychoanalysis 22*: 548–59 (1986). An earlier version was presented to the British Society of Analytical Psychology, London, December 1985; and subsequently to the British Psycho-Analytical Society, May 1986.
2. Bollas has given other cautions about the use of countertransference in interpretation; they are complementary to mine.

> As in any analytic intervention, it is exceedingly important to consider whether the patient can use an intervention, and this is why I place so much emphasis on the gradual presentation over time of the analyst's sense of the situation, as a prerequisite to any direct expression of the countertransference. Any disclosure on the analyst's part of how he feels must be experienced by the patient as a legitimate and natural part of the analytic process. If it comes as a shock, then the analyst has failed in his technique.... There are some patients to whom one could not ever usefully express one's experience as their object, and this must be accepted. (Bollas 1987: 210–11)

3. When I originally wrote the paper on which this chapter is based I was not familiar with the papers by Tansey and Burke (1985) and Burke and Tansey (1985), which are complementary to this chapter and offer interesting parallels. (See also Samuels 1985: 185–7; 1989: Chapter 9)

Chapter 15

1. The original version of this chapter was written, at the invitation of the editor of Free Association Books, as one of the papers to be published in memory of Dr. John Klauber, whose Freud Memorial Lectures (written just before his death) were the basis and inspiration of the book in which these papers were then published: *Illusion and Spontaneity*, ed. R. Young, London: Free Association Books (1987).
2. Klaus Fink has given us a most useful summary of Matte Blanco's theory in his paper "From symmetry to asymmetry" (Fink 1989), in which he summarizes the principles of "generalization" and "symmetry" that Matte Blanco has described, from which it follows that there is in the unconscious no distinction between past, present, and future; and the part is experienced as identical to the whole (see Matte Blanco 1975: 38–9 and 137–40).

Fink adds his own comments in relation to trauma:

> In the thought system of symmetry, time does not exist. An event that occurred yesterday can also occur today or tomorrow....This means that, for instance, traumatic events of the past are not only seen in the unconscious as ever present and permanently happening but also about to happen, hence the need or compulsion to repeat the defensive behaviour (Freud, 1914). (Fink 1989: 482–3)

And later he says:

> The whole object and its parts are equivalent and exchangeable

because any part of an object represents the whole object and the whole object may represent any of its parts. (Fink 1989: 483)

When we relate these thoughts to traumatic experience we can understand better why it is that a patient feels alerted by any similarity to part of that experience, and why something that has happened in the past can feel as if it is still about to happen.

3. I use this spelling to distinguish between unconscious phantasy, as in Isaacs (1948), and fantasy which can be a conscious imagining.

4. I focus in proper detail on the issue of corrective emotional experience in the next chapter.

Chapter 16

1. An earlier version of this chapter was written by invitation for a special issue devoted to the theme of "The corrective emotional experience re-visited" (*Psychoanalytic Inquiry 10*: 325–346, 1990).

2. Winnicott's handling of severe regression is illustrated in Margaret Little's accounts of her analysis with him (Little 1985; 1987).

3. It is also important not to make the opposite mistake, that of thinking of the patient as only an adult. Terrible misunderstandings can follow, as Jung demonstrated in his reaction to a patient who had dreamed of "an idiot child of about two years old. It was sitting on a chamber pot and had smeared itself with faeces." In his analysis of that dream, Jung says:

> In small children, such uncouth behaviour is somewhat unusual, but still possible. They may be intrigued by their faeces, which are coloured and have an odd smell.... But the dreamer, the doctor, was no child; he was a grown man. And therefore the dream image . . . is a sinister symbol. When he told me the dream, I realised that his normality was a compensation. I had caught him in the nick of time, for the latent psychosis was within a hair breadth of breaking out and becoming manifest. (Jung 1967: 157–8)

Jung concluded from this that he should stop treating this patient. This account is, of course, from a long time ago. But I am told that some psychotherapy students still quote this example as justifying a retreat from regressive material presented by a patient. When a patient begins to trust the analyst or therapist it will be just such disturbing aspects of the internal world that will be presented for understanding—not for a panic retreat by the therapist!

4. I realize that I am describing a view here that may be close to that of self psychology, but it has been arrived at independently.

5. See "Afterthought" at the end of this chapter for a consideration of what the consequences may be for the patient if the analyst has not had this kind of experience in his/her training analysis.

6. A major difference, in the experience of trainee patients, is that the ending of analysis/therapy is much more final for most patients than for those who go on to practise—joining a group of like-minded colleagues (which often includes the former training analyst). This continued (but often indirect) association with the former analyst/

therapist can mask a continuing dependence and the sustaining of change by means of that association. The irony is that few analysts or therapists are faced so starkly with an ending as most other patients are. This raises important questions about their sensitivity to the issues involved in ending and their competence to deal with these fully enough with those patients who will not be going on to train.

7. Other therapeutic factors not mentioned here are stressed by a number of other authors, quite apart from mutative transference interpretations as described by Strachey (1934). In particular I wish to draw attention to Blum's paper "The Position and Value of Extratransference Interpretation" (1983), Symington's paper "The Analyst's Act of Freedom as Agent of Therapeutic Change" (1983) and that of Stewart "Interpretation and Other Agents for Psychic Change" (1990).

8. In Chapter 7, I give details of a case that is also discussed in Example 15.5. I describe there how a patient unconsciously prompted me to let her use me in the transference to represent her mother who had fainted at a most crucial moment in her early childhood. The patient could then work through, in relation to me, the terror and rage that had belonged to that experience.

9. My comments here about the use of words need to be read alongside Freud's *Appendix* "Words and Things" (Freud 1915: 209–15) and other statements on this subject such as the papers by Olinick (1982), O'Shaughnessy (1983), and Tuckett (1983), for example.

10. Rycroft has some important observations to make on the subject of interpretation in his papers "The Nature and Function of the Analyst's Communication to the Patient" and "An Enquiry into the Function of Words in the Psychoanalytical Situation" (Rycroft 1968: Chapters 5 and 6).

11. There are a number of authors that I have not quoted here who also address the issues raised in this chapter. I am thinking in particular of Balint (1952, 1968), Kohut (1984), and Bowlby (1988) to name but a few. I also wish to highlight one other (J. Klein 1988) who gives us a valuable exploration of the literature along with her own contributions on this subject.

   What I have given here are my own observations, drawn from clinical experience, which I offer in parallel to the findings of others. It is my hope that some validation of what other practitioners have observed may arise from a comparison of these parallels.

Chapter 17

1. An earlier version of this chapter was presented to a meeting of the Independent Analysts' Group of the British Psycho-Analytical Society, October 1987; and subsequently at the Annual Training and Development Conference "Connections and Boundaries: Interfacing Traditional and Humanistic Psychotherapy" organized by the Association of Humanistic Psychology Practitioners, at Hawkwood College, Stroud, November 1987. It was also given (at the invitation of

the Swedish Mental Health Association) as "The Scandinavian Lecture" in Stockholm, March 1988; and in Athens, May 1989, as a public lecture organized by the Hellenic Society of Psychoanalytic Psychotherapy. Published (in Greek) in *Psychologika Themata 2*: 100–111 (1989), Athens.

2. The only reference to "Hope" that I could initially find in the psychoanalytic journals familiar to me was the paper "On hope: its nature and psychotherapy" (Boris 1976). That author had also noticed its absence in the literature:

> If one searches the standard psychoanalytic literature (I have in mind, for instance, Freud, A. Freud, Fenichel, Fairbairn, H. Segal) one is apt to find little in the index between "homosexuality" and "hysteria," save "hunger." "Hope" itself is nowhere to be seen (Boris 1976: 139).

Since then the following paper has appeared, "Hope and hopelessness: a technical problem?" (Mehler and Argentieri 1989).

3. If during an ongoing analysis or therapy it seems to be in the patient's best interests for him/her to be referred elsewhere, no action on this should be instigated except after the most careful examination of what a patient may be presenting for attention at such times of crisis and whether this could yet be managed without terminating treatment with that patient. It should also be clearly understood that, when treatment is prematurely ended, this is a treatment failure—not necessarily a fault of the patient. Nevertheless, every patient who is passed on will take this rejection as the latest of many, and (often) as evidence of some dreadful truth about themselves that is assumed to be hidden behind whatever reasons are given for that treatment decision.

Chapter 18

1. An earlier version of this chapter was presented at a Conference on "The Inter-relation of Inner World and the Environment: Problems of Interpretation in Clinical Work" held at University College, London, September 1988.

2. I did not then (in the 1970s) forbid patients to smoke in sessions. Instead I would occasionally invite a patient to explore the reasons for wanting to smoke *just then*. At this stage in Miss M.'s analysis I felt it would have been counter-productive had I tried to control her smoking, even if "only" by interpretation. She later gave up smoking quite spontaneously when she discovered that she no longer needed to turn to substitutes. That change, when it came, was truly autonomous; it was not compliant.

3. This is similar to the severity of superego found in the psychopath (Symington 1980).

4. Rosenfeld has given some important examples of impasse in analysis which clearly illustrate the analyst's contributions to this (Rosenfeld 1987).

Chapter 19

1. A somewhat different paper, but with the same title as that of this chapter, was presented to the British Society of Analytical Psychology, London, December 1985. The clinical substance of that earlier paper is now presented in Chapter 14.

2. In Chapter 12, I have already given an example of a patient who experienced her psychiatrist as behaving sexually towards her because of his frequent interpretation of Oedipal themes which she had also found exciting.

Chapter 20

1. Unfortunately, there are other forms of *bullying the patient* to be found in some descriptions of analysis. Most common (perhaps) is that of the attacking style of interpreting, usually rationalized as being aimed at "getting through defenses" or "dealing with resistance." This is particularly evident in some of the accounts of clinical work with narcissistic patients. The problem then is that this style of interpreting can too closely parallel the pathogenic behavior of primary figures in the patient's formative life, against which behavior the narcissistic defenses had been formed in the first place. This parallel, in the analyst's manner of working with such patients, can often result in an impasse or breakdown in the analysis; or it may lead to an idealization of the "strong" analyst and an identification with the aggressor. When this style of analyzing is encountered in the course of a training analysis, some victims of that identification will be found amongst the next generation of patients. I believe that there may be a divergent "strain" of analytic experience that is passed on in this way.

2. I am not advocating any notion of unlimited freedom for a child to have its own way. A child who is not given appropriate limits goes in search of them (see Chapter 13). It is in growing into a confident sense of Self that a child most needs to be "let be." Libidinal demands are another matter altogether (see Chapter 16).

3. I think of this as similar to the two uses of the spatula: (a) to be shoved down patients' throats—as in repeated transference interpretations; and (b) to be found and to be played with—as in Winnicott's child consultations (see Chapter 11).

4. The point of the exercises in the last chapter was largely in order to highlight these interferences in the analytic space and process. Trial-identifying with the patient can always provide some help in preserving the analytic space, or in restoring it when it has become impaired.

5. In my opinion, psychoanalysis is not a science. But, as far as can be compatible with the individuality of each patient, it is quite proper that analysts should try to be "scientific" in trying to establish the comparability between similar clinical situations. But, when the scientific attitude is taken too far—to establish the "repeatability"

that is a keystone to any science—the result can be interpretive work that becomes repetitive. It is then more likely to shape the process between patient and analyst rather than to follow it. I do not regard that as working in a truly psychoanalytic way.

6. I find it encouraging that Sandler suggests a similar openness to theories that relate more clearly to the clinical work in hand, rather than remaining chronically attached to a particular theoretical position. In his paper "Reflections on Some Relations Between Psychoanalytic Concepts and Psychoanalytic Practice" he says:

> If we abandon our search for the pot of theoretical gold at the end of the rainbow, then we may perhaps allow ourselves a greater degree of tolerance of concepts which are unclear and ill-defined, particularly those which have been created by people who have a different psychoanalytic background....
>
> To try to satisfy all "explanatory intents" with one comprehensive theory is clearly impossible, and I would urge the view that we have *a body of ideas*, rather than a consistent whole, that constitutes psychoanalytic theory. What is critical is not what psychoanalytic theory *should*, but what should be *emphasized* within the whole compass of psychoanalytic thinking. *And what should be emphasized is that which relates to the work we have to do.* This means that for most of us the theory needs to be a clinically, psychopathologically and technically oriented one, which also includes a central preoccupation, not only with the abnormal, but with the normal as well. (Sandler 1983: 37)

7. Valuable over-views of these various theories can be found in Greenberg and Mitchell (1983) and in J. Klein (1988). Bollas has also expressed some interesting views on these issues (Bollas 1989: Chapter 5).

8. The opportunity that is missed, for a creative interchange of ideas about clinical practice, is often illustrated when analysts of different persuasions respond to the presentation of a clinical paper. There are two particular trends noticeable in the discussion that follows. One approach to a paper, from a colleague who works differently, may be characterized by such a question as "What can I learn from this other view?" A creative dialogue may then follow. Often, however, the question seems to be: "What can I find, in the view expressed in this paper, that I can use to justify *not learning anything from it?*" The aim then seems to be to prove that the speaker had been wrong, leaving the respondent with his/her own practice undisturbed.

9. I have described some of my work with one such patient elsewhere (see pp. 123–127).

❖ ❖

References

Alexander, F. (1954). Some quantitative aspects of psychoanalytic technique. *Journal of the American Psychoanalytic Association 2*: 685–701.

Alexander, F., French, T.M. et al. (1946). *Psychoanalytic Therapy: Principles and Application*. New York: Ronald Press.

Balint, M. (1952). *Primary Love and Psycho-Analytic Technique*. London: Tavistock Publications.

Balint, M. (1968). *The Basic Fault: Therapeutic Aspects of Regression*. London: Tavistock Publications.

Bateson, G. et al. (1956). Toward a theory of schizophrenia. *Behavioral Science 1*: 251–264.

Bion, W.R. (1962). Learning from Experience. In *Seven Servants*. New York: Aronson, 1977.

Bion, W.R. (1967a). Notes on memory and desire. *Psychoanalytic Forum 2*: 271–80.

Bion, W.R. (1967b). *Second Thoughts*. New York: Aronson.

Bion, W.R. (1970). Attention and Interpretation. In *Seven Servants*. New York: Aronson, 1977.

Bion, W.R. (1974). *Brazilian Lectures 1*. Rio de Janeiro: Imago Editora.

Bion, W.R. (1975). *Brazilian Lectures 2*. Rio de Janeiro: Imago Editora.

Bion, W.R. (1980). *Bion in New York and Sao Paulo*. Ed. F. Bion. Perthshire: Clunie Press .

Blum, H.P. (1983). The position and value of extratransference interpretation. *Journal of the American Psychoanalytic Association 31*: 587–617.

Bollas, C. (1987). *The Shadow of the Object: Psychoanalysis of the Unthought Known*. London: Free Association Books.

Bollas, C. (1989). *Forces of Destiny: Psychoanalysis and Human Idiom*, London: Free Association Books.

Boris, H.N. (1976). On hope: its nature and psychotherapy. *International Review of Psycho-Analysis 3*: 139–50.

Bowlby, J. (1988). *A Secure Base*. London: Routledge.

Burke, W.F., and Tansey, M.J. (1985). Projective identification and countertransference turmoil, *Contemporary Psychoanalysis 21*: 372–402.

Casement, P.J. (1963). The paradox of unity. *Prism 69*: 8–11.

Casement, P.J. (1964). False security? *Prism 88*: 28–30.

Casement, P.J. (1969). The setting of limits: a belief in growth. *Case Conference 16*: 267–71.

Casement, P.J. (1973). The supervisory viewpoint. In W.F. Finn (ed.), *Family Therapy in Social Work: Conference Papers*. London: Family Welfare Association.

Casement, P.J . (1982a). Some pressures on the analyst for physical contact during the re-living of an early trauma. *International Review of Psycho-Analysis 9:* 279–86.

Casement, P.J. (1982b). Samuel Beckett's relationship to his mother-tongue. *International Review of Psycho-Analysis 9:* 35–44.

Casement, P.J . (1984). The reflective potential of the patient as mirror to the therapist. In J.O. Raney (ed.), *Listening and Interpreting: the Challenge of the Work of Robert Langs*. New York: Aronson.

Chesterson, G.K. (1908). *Orthodoxy*. Reprinted (1961). London: Fontana Books.

Daws, D. (1989). *Through the Night*. London: Free Association Books.

Doucet, P., and Laurin, C. (eds.) (1971). *Problems of Psychosis*. Amsterdam: Excerpta Medica.

Eissler, K.R. (1953). The effect of the structure of the ego on psychoanalytic technique. *Journal of the American Psychoanalytic Association 1*: 104–43.

Eliot, T.S. (1935). "Little Gidding." In *Four Quartets*. London: Faber & Faber, 1949.

Epstein, L., and Feiner, A.H. (eds.) (1979). *Countertransference*. New York: Aronson.

Fink, K. (1989). From symmetry to asymmetry. *International Journal of Psycho-Analysis 70*: 481–9.

Finn, W.R. (ed.) (1973). *Family Therapy in Social Work: Conference Papers*. London: Family Welfare Association.

Fleiss, R. (1942). The metapsychology of the analyst. *Psychoanalytic Quarterly 11*: 211–27.

Fox, R.P. (1984). The principle of abstinence reconsidered. *International Review of Psycho-Analysis 11*: 227–36.

Freud, A. (1937). *The Ego and Mechanisms of Defence*. London: Hogarth Press.

Freud, S. (1900). The Interpretation of Dreams. *Standard Edition 5*. (Standard Edition of the Complete Psychological Works of Sigmund Freud, London: Hogarth Press, 1950–1974.)

Freud, S. (1909). Notes upon a case of obsessional neurosis. *Standard Edition 10*: 153–320.

Freud, S. (1910). The future prospects of psychotherapy. *Standard Edition 11*: 141–151.

Freud, S. (1914). Remembering, repeating and working-through. *Standard Edition 12*: 145–156.

Freud, S. (1914/1915). Observations of transference-love. *Standard Edition 12*: 157–171.

Freud, S. (1915). The unconscious. *Standard Edition 14*: 159–215.

Freud, S. (1927). The future of an illusion. *Standard Edition 21*: 3–56.

Freud, S. (1933/1934). New introductory lectures. *Standard Edition 22*: 3–182.

Gill, M.M. (1982). *Analysis of the Transference, Vol. 1.* New York: International Universities Press.

Giovacchini, P.L. (ed.) (1975). *Tactics and Techniques in Psychoanalytic Therapy, Vol 11.* New York: Aronson.

Gitelson, M. (1952). The emotional position of the analyst in the psychoanalytic situation. *International Journal of Psycho-Analysis 33*: 1–10.

Glover, E. (1955). *The Technique of Psycho-Analysis.* New York: International Universities Press, 1968.

Greenberg, J.R., and Mitchell, S.A. (1983). *Object Relations in Psychoanalytic Theory.* Cambridge, MA: Harvard University Press.

Greenson, R.R. (1967). *The Technique and Practice of Psycho-Analysis.* London: Hogarth Press.

Grotstein, J.S. (1981). *Splitting and Projective Identification.* New York: Aronson.

Heimann, P. (1950). On counter-transference. *International Journal of Psycho-Analysis 31*: 81–4.

Hinshelwood, R.D. (1989). *Dictionary of Kleinian Thought.* London: Free Association Books.

Hoffer, W. (1952). The mutual influences in the development of ego and id: earliest stages. *Psychoanalytic Study of the Child 7:* 31–41.

Isaacs, S. (1948). The nature and function of phantasy. *International Journal of Psycho-Analysis 29*: 73–97.

James, M. (1960). Premature ego development: some observations on disturbances in the first three months of life. *International Journal of Psycho-Analysis 41*: 288–94.

Jung, C.G. (1967). *Memories, Dreams, Reflections,* London: Collins.

Kernberg, O. (1965). Notes on countertransference. *Journal of the American Psychoanalytic Association 13*: 38–56.

Khan, M.M. (1974). *The Privacy of the Self.* London: Hogarth Press.

King, P. (1978). Affective response of the analyst to the patient's communications. *International Journal of Psycho-Analysis 59*: 9–34.

Klauber, J. et al. (1987). *Illusion and Spontaneity.* London: Free Association Books.

Klein, J. (1988). *Our Need for Others and Its Roots in Infancy.* London: Tavistock.

Klein, M. (1932). The psycho-analysis of children. In *The Writings of Melanie Klein, Volume 2*. London: Hogarth Press, 1975.

Klein, M. (1946). Notes on some schizoid mechanisms. In J. Riviere (ed.), *Developments in Psycho-Analysis*. London: Hogarth Press, 1952.

Klein, M. (1952). Some theoretical conclusions regarding the emotional life of the infant. In J. Riviere (ed.), *Developments in Psycho-Analysis*. London: Hogarth Press (1952).

Klein, M. (1961). Narrative of a child analysis. In *The Writings of Melanie Klein, Volume 4*. London: Hogarth Press, 1975.

Kohut, H. (1984). In A. Goldberg (ed.), *How Does Analysis Cure?* Chicago: University of Chicago Press.

Kris, E. (1950). On preconscious mental processes. *Psychoanalytic Quarterly 19*: 540–60.

Laing, R.D. (1961). *The Self and Others*. London: Tavistock.

Langs, R.J. (1978). *The Listening Process*. New York: Aronson.

Laplanche, J., and Pontonalis, J-B. (1973). *The Language of Psychoanalysis*. London: Hogarth Press.

Leites, N. (1977). Transference interpretations only? *International Journal of Psycho-Analysis 58*: 275–87.

Little, M. (1951). Counter-transference and the patient's response to it. *International Journal of Psycho-Analysis 32*: 32–40.

Little, M. (1985). Winnicott working in areas where psychotic anxieties predominate: a personal record. *Free Associations 3*: 9–42.

Little, M. (1987). On the value of regression to dependence. *Free Associations 10*: 7–22.

Matte Blanco, I. (1975). *The Unconscious as Infinite Sets*. London: Duckworth.

Mehler, J.A., and Argentieri, S. (1989). Hope and hopelessness: a technical problem? *International Journal of Psycho-Analysis 70*: 295–304.

Milner, M. (1952). Aspects of symbolism in comprehension of the not-self. *International Journal of Psycho-Analysis 33*: 181–95.

Moberly, E.R. (1985). *The Psychology of Self and Other*. London: Tavistock.

Money-Kyrle, R. (1956). Normal counter-transference and some of its deviations. *International Journal of Psycho-Analysis 37*: 360–66.

Muir, E. (1960). *Collected Poems*. London: Faber, 1984.

Ogden, T. (1982). *Projective Identification and Psychotherapeutic Technique*. New York: Aronson.

Olinick, S.L. (1982). Meanings beyond words: psychoanalytic perceptions of silence and communication, happiness, sexual love and death. *International Review of Psychoanalysis 9*: 461–72.

Orr, D.W. (1954). Transference and countertransference: a historical survey. *Journal of the American Psychoanalytic Association 2*: 621–70.

O'Shaughnessy, E. (1983). Words and working through. *International Journal of Psycho-Analysis 64*: 281–9; also in *Melanie Klein Today*, Vol. 2. London: Routledge, 1988.

Priestley, J.B. (1972). *Over the Long High Wall*. London: Heinemann.

Racker, H. (1968). *Transference and Counter-Tranference*. London: Hogarth Press.

Raney, J.O. (ed.) (1984). *Listening and Interpreting: The Challenge of the Work of Robert Langs*. New York: Aronson.

Rayner, E. (1981). Infinite experiences, affects and characteristics of the unconscious. *International Journal of Psycho-Analysis 62*: 403–12.

Reich, A. (1951). On counter-transference, *International Journal of Psycho-Analysis 32*: 25–31.

Reik, T. (1937). *Surprise and the Psychoanalyst*. New York: E.P. Dutton.

Riviere, J. (ed.) (1952). *Developments in Psycho-Analysis*. London: Hogarth Press.

Rosenfeld, H. (1965). *Psychotic States*. London: Hogarth Press.

Rosenfeld, H. (1971). Contribution to the psychopathology of psychotic states. In P. Doucet and C. Laurin (eds.), *Problems of Psychosis*. Amsterdam: Excerpta Medica.

Rosenfeld, H. (1987). *Impasse and Interpretation*. London: Tavistock.

Rycroft, C. (1968). *Imagination and Reality*. New York: International Universities Press.

Rycroft, C. (1972). *Critical Dictionary of Psychoanalysis*. London: Penguin.

Samuels, A. (1985). *Jung and the Post-Jungians*. London: Routledge.

Samuels, A. (1989). *The Plural Psyche*. London: Routledge.

Sandler, J. (1976). Countertransference and role-responsiveness. *International Review of Psycho-Analysis 3*: 43–7.

Sandler, J. (1983). Reflections on some relations between psychoanalytic concepts and psychoanalytic practice. *Journal of Psycho-Analysis 64:* 35–45.

Sandler, J., Dare, C., and Holder, A. (1973). *The Patient and the Analyst: The Basis of the Psychoanalytic Process*. London: George Allen & Unwin.

Searles, H. (1975). The patient as therapist to his analyst. In P.L. Giovacchini (ed.), *Tactics and Techniques in Psychoanalytic Therapy*, Vol 11. New York: Aronson.

Segal, H. (1964). *Introduction to the Work of Melanie Klein*. London: Heinemann .

Sterba, R. (1934). The fate of the ego in analytic therapy. *International Journal of Psycho-Analysis 15*: 117–26.

Stewart, H. (1990). Interpretation and other agents for psychic change, *International Review of Psycho-Analysis, 17*: 61–70.

Strachey, J. (1934). The nature of the therapeutic interaction of psychoanalysis, *International Journal of Psycho-Analysis 15*: 127–59.

Symington, N. (1980). The response aroused by the psychopath. *International Review of Psycho-Analysis 7*: 291–8.

Symington, N. (1983). The analyst's act of freedom as agent of therapeutic change. *International Review of Psycho-Analysis 10*: 283–91.

Tansey, M.H., and Burke, W.F. (1985). Projective identification and the empathic process. *Contemporary Psychoanalysis 21:* 42–69.

Tower, L.E. (1956). Countertransference. *Journal of the American Psychoanalytic Association 4:* 224–55.

Tuckett, D. (1983). Words and the psychoanalytic interaction. *International Review of Psycho-Analysis 10*: 407–13.

Wangh, M. (1962). The "evocation of a proxy": A psychological maneuver, its use as a defense, its purpose and genesis. *The Psychoanalytic Study of the Child 17:* 451–69.

Winnicott, D.W. (1958). *Collected Papers: Through Pediatrics to Psycho-Analysis.* London: Tavistock.

Winnicott, D.W. (1965a). *The Family and Individual Development.* London: Tavistock.

Winnicott, D.W. (1965b). *Maturational Processes and the Facilitating Environment.* London: Hogarth Press.

Winnicott, D.W. (1970). Fear of breakdown. *International Review of Psycho-Analysis [1974] 1:* 103–07.

Winnicott, D.W. (1971). *Playing and Reality.* London: Tavistock.

Winnicott, D.W. (1988). *Human Nature.* London: Free Association Books.

Winnicott, D.W. (1989). In C. Winnicott, R. Shepherd, M. Davis (eds.), *Psycho-Analytic Explorations.* London: Karnac.

Index